NATURAL TOXINS

Characterization, Pharmacology and Therapeutics

Titles of Related Interest

DORNER and DREWS
Pharmacology of Bacterial Toxins

HARTMAN
Neuropsychological Toxicology

MASIHI and LANGE
Immunomodulators and Non-Specific Host Defence Mechanisms Against Microbial Infections

SAID EL SHAMI and MERRETT
Allergy and Molecular Biology

WEBBE
Toxicology of Molluscicides

Journals of Related Interest (sample copies gladly sent on request)

Current Advances in Pharmacology and Toxicology

Food and Chemical Toxicology

Reproductive Toxicology

Toxicology in Vitro

Toxicon

NATURAL TOXINS

Characterization, Pharmacology and Therapeutics

Proceedings of the 9th World Congress on Animal, Plant and Microbial Toxins, Stillwater, Oklahoma, August 1988

Edited by

CHARLOTTE L. OWNBY

Department of Physiological Sciences,
College of Veterinary Medicine,
Oklahoma State University,
Stillwater, Oklahoma,
USA

and

GEORGE V. ODELL

Department of Biochemistry,
Oklahoma State University,
Stillwater, Oklahoma,
USA

PERGAMON PRESS

OXFORD · NEW YORK · BEIJING · FRANKFURT
SÃO PAULO · SYDNEY · TOKYO · TORONTO

U.K.	Pergamon Press plc, Headington Hill Hall, Oxford OX3 0BW, England
U.S.A.	Pergamon Press, Inc., Maxwell House, Fairview Park, Elmsford, New York 10523, U.S.A.
PEOPLE'S REPUBLIC OF CHINA	Pergamon Press, Room 4037, Qianmen Hotel, Beijing, People's Republic of China
FEDERAL REPUBLIC OF GERMANY	Pergamon Press GmbH, Hammerweg 6, D-6242 Kronberg, Federal Republic of Germany
BRAZIL	Pergamon Editora Ltda, Rua Eça de Queiros, 346, CEP 04011, Paraiso, São Paulo, Brazil
AUSTRALIA	Pergamon Press Australia Pty Ltd., P.O. Box 544, Potts Point, N.S.W. 2011, Australia
JAPAN	Pergamon Press, 5th Floor, Matsuoka Central Building, 1-7-1 Nishishinjuku, Shinjuku-ku, Tokyo 160, Japan
CANADA	Pergamon Press Canada Ltd., Suite No. 271, 253 College Street, Toronto, Ontario, Canada M5T 1R5

First edition 1989

Library of Congress Cataloging in Publication Data

World Congress on Animal, Plant, and Microbial Toxins
(9th: 1988: Stillwater, Okla.)
Natural toxins: proceedings of the 9th World Congress on Animal, Plant, and Microbial Toxins, Stillwater, Oklahoma, August 1988 edited by Charlotte L. Ownby and George V. Odell.
p. cm.
Sponsored by the International Society on Toxinology.
Includes indexes.
1. Toxins—Congresses. I. Ownby, Charlotte L.
II. Odell, George V. III. International Society on Toxinology. IV. Title.
[DNLM: 1. Toxins—congresses. QW 630 W927n 1988]
QP631.W67 1988 615.9'5—dc19 89–3848

British Library Cataloguing in Publication Data

World Congress on Animal, Plant and Microbial Toxins
(9th: 1988: Stillwater, Oklahoma)
Natural toxins.
1. Toxins
I. Title II. Ownby, Charlotte L. III. Odell, George V.
615.9'5

ISBN 0–08–036139–0

Printed in Great Britain by BPCC Wheaton Ltd, Exeter

PREFACE

The International Society on Toxinology celebrated its 25th Anniversary during 1987 and at its 9th World Congress in Stillwater, Oklahoma, USA during 1988. The Society was organized to promote research on animal, plant and microbial toxins. With the establishment of the scientific journal, Toxicon, the Society began to promote the dissemination of knowledge about these toxins and further promote such research. Every three years the Society sponsors a World Congress during which toxinologists from all over the world assemble to exchange the newest information about these toxins. This book is the formal record of the plenary lectures presented at the 9th World Congress held during July 31- August 5, 1988.

The plenary lecture topics were selected to present a broad view of the science of toxinology as it stands in 1988. As can be seen by the great diversity of topics included in this volume, the science of toxinology covers a very broad and diverse area of interest. It is hoped that this volume will not only provide the reader with new and interesting information, but also with an idea of the diversity of this field as well as the status of the field of toxinology on the 25th Anniversary of the Society. The editors thank the many contributors for their hard work and diligence in preparing the manuscripts.

The editors would like to thank the other members of the Organizing Committee of the 9th World Congress, Dr. George Burrows and Mr. Terry R. Colberg. For financial support of the Congress we would like to acknowledge The International Society on Toxinology, The College of Veterinary Medicine, Oklahoma State University, Latoxan, Pentapharm Ltd., The Miami Serpentarium, The U.S. Army Medical Research and Development Command, and The Office of Naval Research. We would like to thank Ms. Sue Ann Hudiburg for proof-reading and Pergamon Press, Inc. for their assistance.

Stillwater, Oklahoma
1988

Charlotte L. Ownby
George V. Odell

CONTRIBUTORS

Pierre E. Bougis
Toxinology Department, Pathology Division, USAMRIID Fort Detrick, Frederick, MD 21701, USA

J-C. Boulain
Service de Biochimie, Departement de Biologie, CEN Saclay, 91191 Gif-sur-Yvette, France

George B. Brown
The Neuropsychiatry Research Program and the Department of Psychiatry, University of Alabama at Birmingham, Birmingham, AL 35294, USA

Joseph W. Burnett
Division of Dermatology, Department of Medicine, University of Maryland School of Medicine, Baltimore, MD 21201, USA

J.A. Campos
Departamento de Pediatria, Faculdade de Medicina da UFMG and Hospital Joao XXIII, Belo Horizonte, Brasil

Wayne W. Carmichael
Department of Biological Sciences, Wright State University, Dayton, Ohio 45435, USA

Richard D. Crosland
Pathology Division, U.S. Army Medical Research Institute of Infectious Diseases, Frederick, MD 21701-5011, USA

Lourdes J. Cruz
Department of Biochemistry and Molecular Biology, College of Medicine, University of the Philippines, P.O. Box 593, Manila, Philippines and Department of Biology, University of Utah, Salt Lake City, UT 84112, USA

J.C. Fontecilla-Camps
Laboratoire de Cristallographie et de Cristallisation de Macromolecules Biologiques-CNRS, Faculte de Medecine, Secteur Nord, Bd. Pierre Dramard, 13326 Marseille, Cedex 15, France

L. Freire-Maia
Departamento de Farmacologia, Instituto de Ciencias Biologicas, Universidade Federal de Minas Gerais, Belo Horizonte, Brasil

J.C. Genovesio-Taverne
Laboratoire de Cristallographie et de Cristallisation de Macromolecules Biologiques-CNRS, Faculte de Medecine, Secteur Nord, Bd. Pierre Dramard, 13326 Marseille, Cedex 15, France

D.S. Griffin
Environmental Protection Agency, Washington, D.C., USA

G. Guignery-Frelat
Service de Biochimie, Departement de Biologie, CEN Saclay, 91191 Gif-sur-Yvette, France

E. Habermann
Rudolf-Buchheim-Institute of Pharmacology, University of Giessen, 6300 Giessen

C. Habersetzer-Rochat
CRMC[2]-CNRS, Campus Luminy, Case 913, 13288 Marseille, Cedex 9, France

Bruce B. Jarvis
Department of Chemistry and Biochemistry, University of Maryland, College Park, MD 20742, USA

M.W. Lame
Department of Veterinary Pharmacology and Toxicology, University of California, Davis, CA 95616, USA

K.L. Martin
Chemical Defence Establishment, Porton Down, Salisbury, Wiltshire, United Kingdom

Andre Menez
Service de Biochimie, Departement de Biologie, CEN Saclay, 91191 Gif-sur-Yvette, France

D.M. Morin
Department of Veterinary Pharmacology and Toxicology, University of California, Davis, California 95616, USA

Jon Robertus
Department of Chemistry, University of Texas, Austin, TX 78712, USA

Herve Rochat
Universite d'Aix-Marseille II, Faculte de Medecine Secteur Nord, Biochimie, UDC: CNRS UA 1179- INSERM U 172, Bd P. Dramard, 13326 Marseille Cedex 15, France

T. Rubidge
Chemical Defence Establishment, Porton Down, Salisbury, Wiltshire, United Kingdom

H.J. Segall
Department of Veterinary Pathology, University of California, Davis, CA 95616, USA

Leonard A. Smith
Toxinology Department, Pathology Division, USAMRIID, Fort Detrick, Frederick, MD 21701, USA

G.R. Strichartz
Anesthesia Research Laboratories, Brigham and Women's Hospital and Department of Biological Chemistry and Molecular Pharmacology, Harvard Medical School, Boston, MA 02115, USA

T. Tamiya
Faculty of Science and Technology, Sophia University, Tokyo, Japan

R.W. Titball
Chemical Defence Establishment, Porton Down, Salisbury, Wiltshire, United Kingdom

D.W. Wilson
Department of Veterinary Pathology, University of California, Davis, California 95616, USA

C.K. Winter
Department of Entomology, University of California, Riverside, California 96521, USA

CONTENTS

I. Overview of Toxins

II. Interaction of Toxins with Ion Channels

III. Use of Cloning Techniques in the Study of Toxins

I. Overview of Toxins

Freshwater Cyanobacteria (blue-green algae) Toxins

Wayne W. Carmichael, Ph.D.

Department of Biological Sciences
Wright State University
Dayton, Ohio 45435, U.S.A.

ABSTRACT

Worldwide in natural or man induced eutrophic water bodies certain fresh/brackish water cyanobacteria (blue-green algae) species and strains in the genera *Anabaena*, *Aphanizomenon*, *Microcystis*, *Nodularia* and *Oscillatoria* are known to produce potent biotoxins. Two chemical groups of toxins are recognized, the first is a related family of hepatotoxic cyclic hepta- and pentapeptides, termed microcystin and nodularin. These peptide toxins produce similar gross and ultrastructural effects on hepatocytes resulting in hemorrhagic necrosis and death by hemorrhogic shock. Research suggests that the toxins are taken up via the bile acid transport systems and that the toxins exert an effect on the cytoskeletal system of the cell. The second group contains at least three types of neurotoxic alkaloids produced by strains of the species *Anabaena* (anatoxins) and *Aphanizomenon* (aphantoxins). Anatoxin-a (a bicyclic secondary amine) is a potent nicotinic agonist acting as a depolarizing neuro-muscular blocking agent. Anatoxin-a(s) (a cyclic organo-phosphate) has been shown to act as a potent irreversible acetylcholinesterase inhibitor. The mechanism of inhibition is similar to known irreversible organophosphorus anti-cholinesterases such as diisopropylfluorophosphate (DFP). Aphantoxins have been shown to be the same as saxitoxin and neosaxitoxin, the potent sodium channel blockers, produced by species of marine dinoflagellates such as *Protogonyaulax*. The range of toxicity for these peptide and alkaloid toxins is between 10 and 500 μg/kg body weight (based on intraperitoneal mouse assay).

KEYWORDS

Cyanobacteria, blue-green algae, toxins, freshwater algae

INTRODUCTION

Reports of toxic algae in the freshwater environment are almost exclusively caused by strains of species that are members of the division Cyanophyta, commonly called blue-green algae or cyanobacteria. Although cyanobacteria are found in almost any environment ranging from hot springs to Antarctic soils, known toxic members are mostly planktonic. Published accounts of field poisonings by cyanobacteria are known since the late 19th century (Francis, 1878). These reports describe sickness and death of livestock, pets, and wildlife following ingestion of water containing toxic algae cells or the toxin released by the aging cells. Recent reviews of these poisonings and the toxins of freshwater cyanobacteria are given by Carmichael (1981, 1986, 1988), Codd and Bell (1985) and Gorham and Carmichael (1988).

While about 12 genera have been implicated in cyanobacteria poisonings only toxins from *Anabaena*, *Aphanizomenon*, *Microcystis*, *Nodularia* and *Oscillatoria* have been isolated, at least partially chemically defined and the toxins studied for their mode of action. In addition to the acute lethal toxins, some cyanobacteria produce potent cytotoxins. These secondary chemicals are not considered in this chapter but The reader is referred to papers by Barchi *et* al. (1983, 1984); Carmichael (1988); Moore et al. (1984, 1986); Mason et al. (1982) and Gleason and Paulson (1984) for further discussion on these compounds. These cytotoxins are also listed in Table 2.

Economic losses related to freshwater cyanobacterial toxins are the result of contact with or consumption of water containing toxin and/or toxic cells. These toxins are water-soluble and temperature-stable. They are either released by the cyanobacterial cell or loosely bound so that changes in cell permeability or age allow their release into the environment. Lethal and sublethal amounts of these toxins become available to animals during periods of heavy cell growth, termed "waterblooms," especially when the waterbloom accumulates on the surface, inshore, where animals are watering. Waterblooms can occur wherever proper conditions for growth, including irradiance, temperature, neutral or alkaline conditions, and nutrients are found. The increasing eutrophication of water supplies from urban and agricultural sources, which raises mineral nutrient levels, has increased the occurrence and intensity of these annual blooms. It should be noted that although there are several bloom-forming genera of cyanobacteria those that occur most often are also those that can produce toxins. Known occurrences of toxic cyanobacteria in water supplies (Table 1), include Canada (four provinces), Europe (12 countries, United States (20 states), USSR (Ukraine), Australia, India, Bangladesh, South Africa, Israel, Japan, New Zealand, Argentina, Chile and the Peoples Republic of China (Skulberg, et al., 1984; Carmichael et al., 1985, Gorham and Carmichael, 1988). Not all blooms of a toxigenic species produce toxins, however, and it is not possible to tell by microscopic examination of the cells whether they are toxic. Environmental conditions that favor bloom formation include (1) moderate to high levels of nutrients, especially phosphorus and nitrate or ammonia, (2) water temperatures between 15 and 30°C, and (3) a pH between 6 and 9 or higher (Skulberg et al., 1984). The economic impact from toxic freshwater cyanobacteria include the costs incurred from deaths of domestic animals; allergic and gastrointestinal problems after human contact with waterblooms (including lost income from recreational areas); and increased expense for the detection and removal of taste, odor, and toxins (although no approved method yet exists for removal of toxins, activated carbon has been tried in certain areas). This chapter summarizes the neurotoxins and hepatotoxins of fresh and brackish cyanobacteria. A summary of these compounds is given in Table 2.

NEUROTOXINS

Anatoxins

Neurotoxins produced by filamentous *Anabaena flos-aquae* are called anatoxins (ANTX) (Carmichael and Gorham, 1978). Two anatoxins [ANTX-A and A(S)] are available for structure and function studies. ANTX-A from strain NRC-44-1 is the first toxin from a freshwater cyanobacteria to be chemically defined. It is the secondary amine, 2-acetyl-9-azabicyclo (4-2-1) non-2-ene (Huber, 1972; Devlin et al., 1977), molecular weight 166 daltons (Fig. 1a). It has been synthesized through a ring expansion of cocaine (Campbell et al., 1977, 1979), from iminium salts (Bates and Rapoport, 1979; Peterson et al., 1984; Koskinen and Rapoport, 1985), from nitrone (Tufariello et al., 1984, 1985), from 4-cycloheptenone or tetrabromotricyclooctane (Danheiser et al., 1985) by construction of the azabicyclo ring from 9-methyl-9-azabicyclo [3.3.1] nonan-1-ol (Wiseman and Lee, 1986) and by starting with 9-methyl-9-aza[4.2.1] nonan-2-one (Lindgren et al., 1987).

ANTX-A is a potent, postsynaptic, depolarizing, neuromuscular blocking agent that affects both nicotinic and muscarinic acetylcholine (ACH) receptors at the ACH channel (Carmichael et al., 1979; Spivak et al., 1980, 1983; Aronstam and Witkop, 1981). Signs of poisoning in field reports for wild and domestic animals include staggering, muscle fasciculations, gasping, convulsions, and opisthotonos (birds). Death by respiratory arrest occurs within minutes to a few hours depending on species, dosage, and prior food consumption. The LD_{50} intraperitoneal (IP) mouse for purified toxin is about 200μg/kg body weight, with survival time of 4-7 min. This means that animals need to ingest only a few milliliters to a few liters of the toxic surface bloom to receive a lethal bolus (Carmichael and Gorham, 1977; Carmichael et al., 1977; Carmichael and Biggs, 1978).

Anatoxin-A(S) [ANTX-A(S)], produced by *A. flos-aquae* NRC-525-17, is different from ANTX-A. It produces opisthotonos in chicks, as does ANTX-A, but also causes viscous salivation [which gives the terminology its (S) label] and lachrymation in mice, chromodacryorrhea in rats, urinary incontinence, and defecation prior to death by respiratory arrest. Also observed is a dose-dependent fasciculation of limbs for 1-2 min after death. ANTX-A(S) has been purified by column chromatography and high-performance liquid chromatography (HPLC) (Carmichael and

Mahmood, 1984), but its structure is still being worked on. ANTX-A(S) is acid stable, unstable in basic conditions, has very low ultraviolet (uv) absorbance, gives a positive alkaloid test, and has a molecular weight estimated by gel exclusion chromatography and mass spectrometry of about 250 daltons.

Table 1. Known Occurrences of Toxic Cyanobacteria in Fresh or Marine Water (updated from Gorham and Carmichael, 1988)

ARGENTINA	EUROPE (continued)	U.S.A. (continued)
AUSTRALIA	Portugal	Minnesota
BANGLADESH	Sweden	Montana
BERMUDA	West Germany	Nevada
BRAZIL		New Hampshire
CANADA	INDIA	New Mexico
Alberta	ISRAEL	New York
Manitoba	JAPAN	North Dakota
Ontario	NEW ZEALAND	Oregon
Saskatchewan	OKINAWA (MARINE)	Pennsylvania
	PEOPLES REPUBLIC OF CHINA	South Dakota
EUROPE	SOUTH AFRICA	Texas
Czechoslovakia		Washington
Denmark	U.S.A.	Wisconsin
East Germany	California	
Finland	Colorado	U.S.S.R.
Great Britain	Hawaii (marine)	
Hungary	Idaho	Ukraine
Netherlands	Illinois	
Norway	Iowa	
Poland	Michigan	

World map showing areas (darkened) where toxic freshwater cyanobacteria have been found.

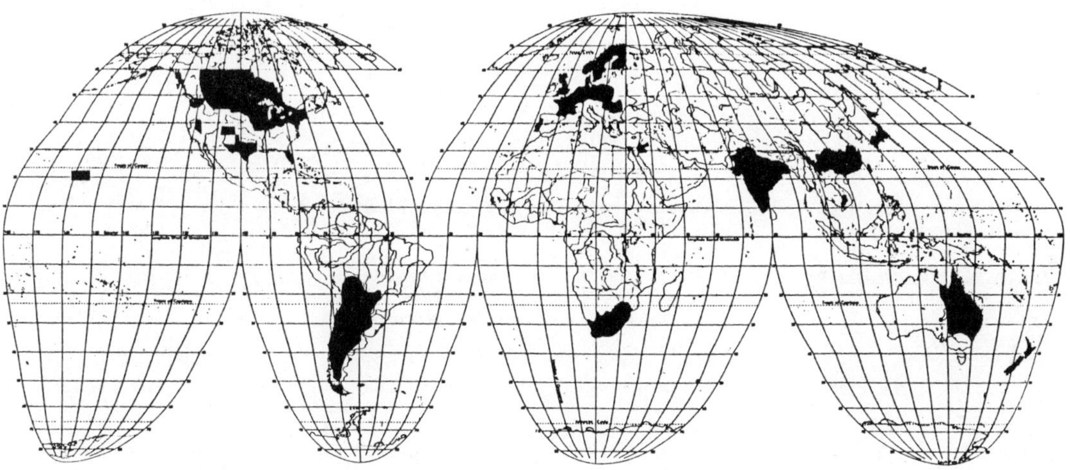

The LD_{50} IP mouse for ANTX-A(S) is about 30 μg/kg, six times more toxic than ANTX-A. At the LD_{50} the survival time for mice is 10-30 min. Mahmood and Carmichael (1986a) conclude that the toxicological and pharmacological signs of poisoning indicate excessive, cholinergic

Table 2. Toxins of Freshwater Cyanobacteria

Species, strain, and source	Toxin term	Structure	LD_{50} $\mu g/kg$ IP, mouse
Neurotoxins			
Anabaena flos-aquae	Anatoxin-A	Secondary amine alkaloid,MW 165	200
Strain NRC-44-1 (Canada, Saskatchewan)			
Strain NRC-525-17 (Canada, Saskatchewan)	Anatoxin-A(S)	Unknown	50
Aphanizomenon flos-aquae	Aphantoxin (neosaxitoxin)	Purine alkaloid MW 315 (neoSTX) MW 299 (STX)	10
Strain NH-1 & NH-5 (U.S., New Hampshire)	Aphantoxin II (saxitoxin)		
Hepatotoxins			
Anabaena flos-aquae	Microcystins[a]	Heptapeptides MW 994	50
Strain S-23-g-1 (Canada, Saskatchewan)			
Microcystis aeruginosa	Cyanoginosins[a]	Heptapeptides MW 909-1044	50
Strain WR-70 (=UV-010) (South Africa, Transvaal)			
(Waterbloom, Australia, New South Wales)	Cyanoginosin	Heptapeptide MW 1035	50
(Waterbloom, U.S., Wisconsin	Microcystin	Heptapeptide MW 994	50
Strain NRC-1(SS-17) (Canada, Ontario)	Microcystin	Heptapeptide MW 994	50
Strain 7820 (Scotland, Loch Balgaves)	Microcystin	Heptapeptide MW 994	50
(Waterbloom, Norway, Lake Akersvatn)	Microcystin	Heptapeptide MW 994	50
Microcystis aeruginosa	Microcystin	Heptapeptide MW 994 MW 1044	50
Strain M-228 (Japan, Tokyo)			
Microcystis aeruginosa	Cyanogenosin[a]	Heptapeptide MW 1039	not reported
Microcystis viridis	Cyanoviridin[a]	Heptapeptide MW 1039	not reported
Nodularia spumigena	Nodularin	Pentapeptide MW 824	30-50
Oscillatoria agardhii var. isothrix	Microcystins	Heptapeptides MW 1009	300-500
(Waterbloom, Norway, Lake Froylandsvatn)			

Oscillatoria agardhii var. (Waterbloom, Norway, Lake Kolbotnvatn)	Microcystins	Heptapeptides MW 1023	500-1000
Cytotoxins			
Scytonema pseudohofmanni Strain BC-1-2 (U.S., Hawaii)	Scytophycin A & B	Methylformamide A=MW 821; B=MW 819	650 (scytophycin B)
Scytonema hofmanni Strain UTEX-1581 (U.S., Texas)	Cyanobacterin	Chlorinated diaryllactone	not reported
Hapalosiphon fontinalis Strain V-3-1 (Marshall Islands)	Hapalindole A	Substituted indole alkaloid	not reported
Tolypothrix byssoidea Strain H-6-2 (U.S., Hawaii)	Tubercidin	Pyrrolopyrimidine	not reported
Oscillatoria acutissima Strain B-1 (U.S., Hawaii)	Acutiphycin	Macrolide	not reported

[a]See text for explanation of terminology.

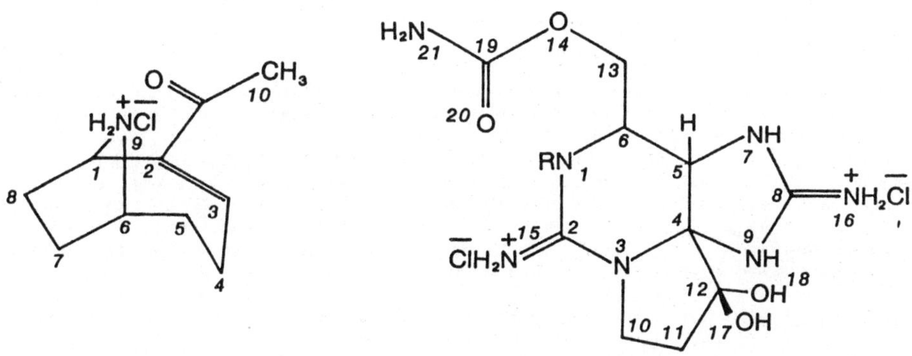

anatoxin - a hydrochloride

R=H; saxitoxin dihydrochloride
R=OH; neosaxitoxin dihydrochloride

Fig. 1.a. (left) Anatoxin-a (ANTX-A) hydrochloride. Produced by the freshwater filamentous cyanobacterium Anabaena flos-aquae NRC-44-1.

b. (right) Aphantoxin-I (neosaxitoxin) and Aphantoxin-II (saxitoxin) produced by certain strains of the filamentous cyanobacterium Aphanizomenon flos-aquae.

Mahmood and co-workers (1988) have identified ANTX-A(S) as the probable cause of death for five dogs, eight pups and two calves that ingested quantities of *A. flos-aquae* in Richmond Lake, South Dakota, in late summer 1985. At present all neurotoxic *A. flos-aquae* strains studied in the laboratory have come from North America. There are, however, some recent reports of neurotoxic *Anabaena* in Australia (Runnegar *et al.*, 1988a), Japan and Scandinavia (M. Watanabe, O.M. Skulberg, and K. Sivonen personal communication). It seems likely that once they are looked for, neurotoxic *Anabaena* will be found in all the same geographic areas as other toxic cyanobacteria.

Aphantoxins

Occurrence of neurotoxins (aphantoxins) in the freshwater filamentous cyanobacterium *Aphanizomenon flos-aquae* was first demonstrated by Sawyer and co-workers (1968). All aphantoxins (APHTXS) studied to date have come from waterblooms and laboratory strains of nonfasciculate (non-flake-forming) *Aph. flos-aquae* that occurred in lakes and ponds of New Hampshire from 1966 through 1980. Toxic cells and extracts of *Aph. flos-aquae* were shown to be toxic to mice, fish, and waterfleas (*Daphnia catawba*) by Jakim and Gentile (1968). Chromatographic and pharmacological evidence established that APHTXS consist mainly of two neurotoxic alkaloids that strongly resembled saxitoxin (STX) and neosaxitoxin (neoSTX), the two primary toxins of red tide paralytic shellfish poisoning (PSP) (Sasner *et al.*, 1984). The bloom material and toxic strain used in studies before 1980 came from collections made between 1960 and 1970. The more recent work on APHTXS has used two strains (NH-1 and NH-5) isolated by Carmichael in 1980 from a small pond near Durham, New Hampshire (Carmichael, 1982; Ikawa *et al.*, 1982). These APHTXS, as well as neoSTX and STX, are fast-acting neurotoxins that inhibit nerve conduction by blocking sodium channels without affecting permeability to potassium, the transmembrane resting potential, or membrane resistance (Adelman *et al.*, 1982). Mahmood and Carmichael (1986b), using the NH-5 strain showed that batch-cultured cells have a mouse IP LD_{50} of about 5 mg/kg. Each gram of lyophilized cells yields about 1.3 mg aphantoxin I (neosaxitoxin) and 0.1 mg aphantoxin II (saxitoxin) (Fig. 1b). Also detected were three unstable neurotoxins that were not similar to any of the known paralytic shellfish poisons.

Shimizu and co-workers (1984) studied the biosynthesis of the STX analog neoSTX using *Aph. flos-aquae* NH-1. They were able to confirm its presence in strain NH-1 and to explain the biosynthetic pathway for this important group of secondary chemicals.

HEPATOTOXINS

Low-molecular-weight peptide toxins that affect the liver have been the predominant toxins involved in cases of animal poisonings due to cyanobacterial toxins (Schwimmer and Schwimmer, 1968; Carmichael, 1986; and Gorham and Carmichael, 1988). After almost 25 years of structure analysis on toxic peptides of the colonial bloom-forming cyanobacterium *Microcystis aeruginosa*, Botes and co-workers (1982a,b, 1986) and Santikarn and colleagues (1983) provided structure details on one of four toxins (designated toxin BE-4) produced by the South African *M. aeruginosa* strain WR70 (= UV-010). They concluded that it was monocyclic and contained three D-amino acids--alanine, erythro-ß-methylaspartic acid, and glutamic acid, two L-amino acids--leucine and alanine--plus two unusual amino acids. These were *N*-methyldehydroalanine (Medha) and a nonpolar side chain of 20 carbon atoms that turned out to be a novel ß-amino acid; 3-amino-9-methoxy-2,6,8-trimethyl-10-phenyldeca-4,6-dienoic acid (ADDA). Based on fast atom bombardment mass spectrometry (FABMS) and nuclear magnetic resonance (NMR) studies, BE-4 toxin is now known to be a cyclic heptapeptide having a molecular weight of 909 daltons. Botes and co-workers (1985) also showed that the other three toxins of strain WR-70 all had the same D-amino acids and the two novel amino acids (Medha and ADDA). They differed in that the L-amino acids were leucine-arginine; tyrosine-arginine and tyrosine-alanine instead of leucine-alanine as in toxin BE-4. They were also able to show that the hepatotoxin isolated by Elleman and colleagues (1978) from waterbloom material collected in Malpas Dam, New South Wales, Australia, contained the five characteristic amino acids plus the L-amino acid variants tyrosine-methionine.

Instead of calling the BE-4 toxin microcystin, as previous *Microcystis* toxins were called (Konst et al., 1965; Murthy and Capindale, 1970; Rabin and Darbre, 1975) and using alphabetical or numerical suffixes to indicate chromatographic elution order or structural differences, Botes (1986) proposed the generically derived designation cyanoginosin (CYGSN). This name, which indicates the cyanobacterial species (*i.e.* aerginosa) origin, is followed by a two-letter suffix that indicates the identity and sequence of the two L-amino acids relative to the N-Me-dehydroalanyl-D-alanine bond. Thus toxin BE-4 was renamed cyanoginosin-LA since leucine and alanine are the L-amino acids. Microcystin (MCYST) is the term given to the fast death factor (FDF) produced by M. aeruginosa strain NRC-1 and its daughter strain NRC-1 (SS-17) (Bishop et al., 1959; Konst et al., 1965). A definitive structure for the toxin of strain NRC-1 (SS-17) is not yet available but is known to be a peptide (MW 994) containing the variant L-amino acids leucine and arginine (Carmichael, unpublished). Krishnamurthy and co-workers (1986a,b) have shown that the toxin isolated from a waterbloom of M. aeruginosa collected in Lake Akersvatn, Norway (Berg et al., 1987), has a structure similar to that of MYCST from NRC-1 (SS-17) and CYGSN-LR. This toxin has also been found to be the main toxin produced by the Scottish strain of M. aeruginosa PCC-7820 and a Canadian A. flos-aquae strain S-23-g-1 (Krishnamurthy et al., 1986 a,b). The identification of a peptide toxin from A. flos-aquae S-23-g-1 provides the first evidence that these hepatotoxins are produced by filamentous as well as coccoid cyanobacteria. A. flos-aquae S-23-g-1 and toxic M. aeruginosa from a waterbloom in Wisconsin also produced a second cyclic heptapeptide hepatotoxin, which has been found to have six of the same amino acids, that is, leucine-arginine, but has aspartic acid instead of ß-methylaspartic acid (Krishnamurthy et al., 1986a).

The filamentous genus Oscillatoria has also been shown to produce a hepatotoxin (Ostensvik et al., 1981; Eriksson et al., 1987a). From water blooms of O. agardhii var and O. agardhii var. isothrix, two similar cyclic heptapeptides have been isolated. Both toxins have the variant L-amino acids arginine-arginine and aspartic acid instead of ß-methylaspartic acid. The toxin from O. agardhii var. isothrix also has dehydroalanine instead of methyldehydroalanine (Krishnamurthy et al., 1986b). More recently M. viridis (Kusumi et al., 1987) and M. aeruginosa (Painuly et al., 1988; Harada et al., 1988) have been shown to produce the cyclic heptapeptide with an arginine-arginine "L" amino acid variant.

Nodularia spumigena has also been shown to produce a peptide with hepatotoxic activity. The more recent reports come from Australia (Main et al., 1977), the German Democratic Republic (Kalbe and Tiess, 1964), Denmark (Lindstrom, 1976), Sweden (Edler et al., 1985) and Finland (Eriksson et al., 1988; Persson et al., 1984). Recently structure information on Nodularia toxin has been presented by Rinehart (Royal Soc. Chem., Ann. Chem. Congress, Swansea, U.K., April 13-16, 1987, Paper A-12) for waterbloom material collected in Lake Forsythe, New Zealand in 1984; by Carmichael and co-workers (1988) for a clonal isolate from Lake Ellesmere, New Zealand; by Eriksson and co-workers (1988) from waterbloom material collected in the Baltic Sea in 1986 and Runnegar and colleagues (1988b) for a field isolate from the Peel Inlet, Perth, Australia. Structure work by these groups all indicate that the peptide is smaller than the heptapeptide toxins. Rinehart and co-workers (1988) showed that the toxin is a pentapeptide with a similar structure to the heptapeptides and containing ß-methylaspartic acid, glutamic acid, arginine, N-methyl-dehydrobutyrine and ADDA (M.W. 824) (Fig.2).

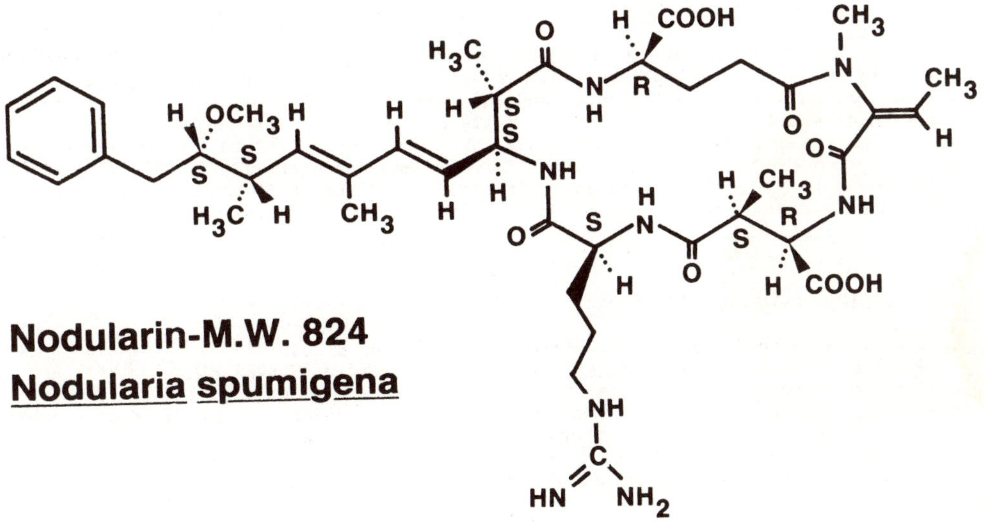

Fig. 2 Structure of nodularin (NODLN) produced by Nodularia spumigena waterbloom from Lake Forsythe, New Zealand and clonal isolate L575 from Lake Ellesmere, New Zealand (Rinehart et al., 1988).

Mode of Action for Microcystins

The liver has always been reported as the organ that showed the greatest degree of histopathological change when animals are poisoned by these cyclic peptides. The molecular basis of action for these cyclic peptides is not yet understood but the cause of death from toxin and toxic cells administered to laboratory mice and rats is at least partially known and is concluded to be hypovolemic shock caused by interstitial hemorrhage into the liver (Theiss et al., 1988). This work with small animal models is currently being extended to larger animals in order to study the uptake, distribution, and metabolism of the toxins (Beasley et al., unpublished data). There is evidence to show from studies using ^{125}I-labeled CYGSN-YM (MCYST-YM) that the liver is the organ for both accumulation and excretion (Falconer et al., 1986; Runnegar et al., 1986a). Brooks and Codd (1987), using C^{14} labeled MCYST-LR, showed that seventy percent of the labeled toxin was localized in the mouse liver after 1 min following intraperitoneal injection of the toxin.

Studies at both the light and electron microscopic (EM) level of time-course histopathological changes in mouse liver show rapid and extensive centrilobular necrosis of the liver with loss of characteristic architecture of the hepatic cords.

Sinusoid endothelial cells and then hepatocytes show extensive fragmentation and vesiculation of cell membranes (Runnegar and Falconer, 1981; Foxall and Sasner, 1981). Using microcystin-LR from M. aeruginosa strain PCC-7820, Dabholkar and Carmichael (1987) found that at both lethal and sublethal toxin levels hepatocytes show progressive intracellular changes beginning at about 10 min postinjection. The most common response to lethal and sublethal injections is vesiculation of rough endoplasmic reticulum (RER), swollen mitochondria, and degranulation (partial or total loss of ribosomes from vesicles). The vesicles appear to form from dilated parts of RER by fragmentation or separation. Affected hepatocytes remain intact and do not lyse. Use of the isolated perfused rat liver to study the pathology of these toxins shows similar results to the in vivo work. Berg and co-workers (1988) used three structurally different cyclic heptapeptide hepatotoxins (MCYST-LR; desmethyl MCYST-RR and didesmethyl MCYST-RR). All three toxins had a similar effect on the perfused liver system although both "RR" toxins required higher concentrations (5-7x) to produce their effect. This was consistent with the lower toxicity of the "RR" toxins, which was about 500 and 1000μg/kg i.p. mouse compared to 50 μg/kg for MCYST-LR.

In vitro studies on isolated cells including hepatocytes, erythrocytes, fibroblasts and alveolar cells continue to demonstrate the specificity of action that these toxins have for liver cells (Eriksson et al., 1987a; Runnegar et al., 1987 and Falconer and Runnegar, 1987). This has led Aune and Berg (1987) to use isolated rat hepatocytes as a screen for detecting hepatotoxic waterblooms of cyanobacteria.

The cellular/molecular mechanism of action for these cyclic peptide toxins is now an area of active research in several laboratories. These peptides cause striking ultrastructural changes in isolated hepatocytes (Runnegar and Falconer, 1986b) including a decrease in the polymerization of actin. This effect on the cells cytoskeletal system continues to be investigated and recent work supports the idea that these toxins interact with the cells cytoskeletal system (Eriksson et al., 1987b; Falconer and Runnegar, 1987). The apparent specificity of these toxins for liver cells is not clear although it has been suggested that the bile uptake system may be at least partly responsible for penetration of the toxin into the cell (Berg, et al., 1988).

Naming the Cyclic Peptide Hepatotoxins

The hepatotoxins have been called Fast-Death Factor (Bishop et al., 1959), Microcystin (Konst et al., 1965), Cyanoginosin (Botes et al., 1986), Cyanoviridin (Kusumi et al., 1987) and Cyanogenosin (apparently a misspelling of cyanoginosin) (Painuly et al., 1988). Continued use of this multiple naming system will create confusion and misunderstanding as more is published on these cyclic peptides. A number of investigators doing research on these toxins have therefore proposed a system of nomenclature based on the original term microcystin (MCYST) (Carmichael et al., 1988). Using this system the structures of known microcystins are given in Fig. 3.

Fig. 3 Structure of known microcystins (refer also to Table 2).

a. Structure of six microcystins varying only in L-amino acids and three microcystins with desmethyl portions of amino acids 3 and 7.

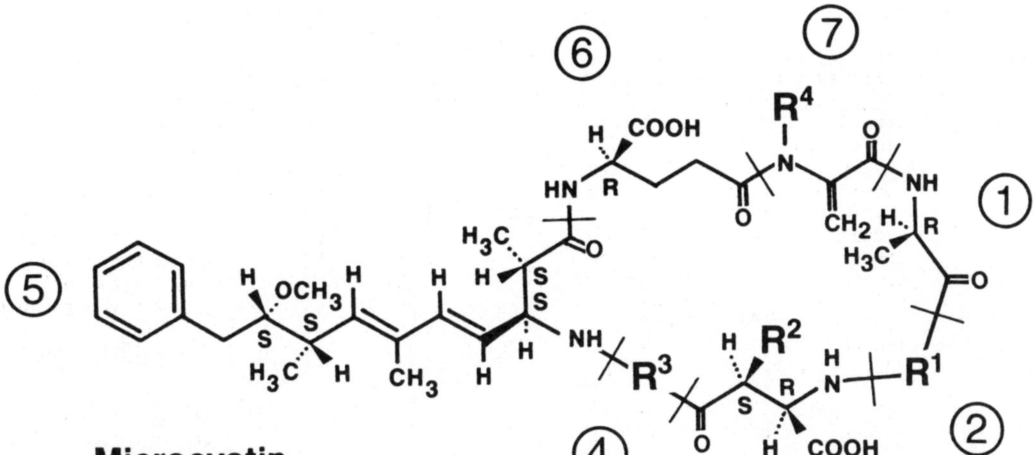

Microcystin (MCYST)

		M.W.
	MCYST-LA: R^1 = Leu; R^2 = CH_3; R^3 = Ala; R^4 = CH_3	909
	MCYST-YA: R^1 = Tyr; R^2 = CH_3; R^3 = Ala; R^4 = CH_3	959
	MCYST-LR: R^1 = Leu; R^2 = CH_3; R^3 = Arg; R^4 = CH_3	994
desmethyl 3-	MCYST-LR: R^1 = Leu; R^2 = H; R^3 = Arg; R^4 = CH_3	980
	MCYST-YM: R^1 = Tyr; R^2 = CH_3; R^3 = Met; R^4 = CH_3	1035
	MCYST-RR: R^1 = Arg; R^2 = CH_3; R^3 = Arg; R^4 = CH_3	1037
desmethyl 3-	MCYST-RR: R^1 = Arg; R^2 = H; R^3 = Arg; R^4 = CH_3	1023
desmethyl 3,7-	MCYST-RR: R^1 = Arg; R^2 = H; R^3 = Arg; R^4 = H	1009
	MCYST-YR: R^1 = Tyr; R^2 = CH_3; R^3 = Arg; R^4 = CH_3	1044

b. Structure of Microcystin-LR, the most commonly found toxin in this group.

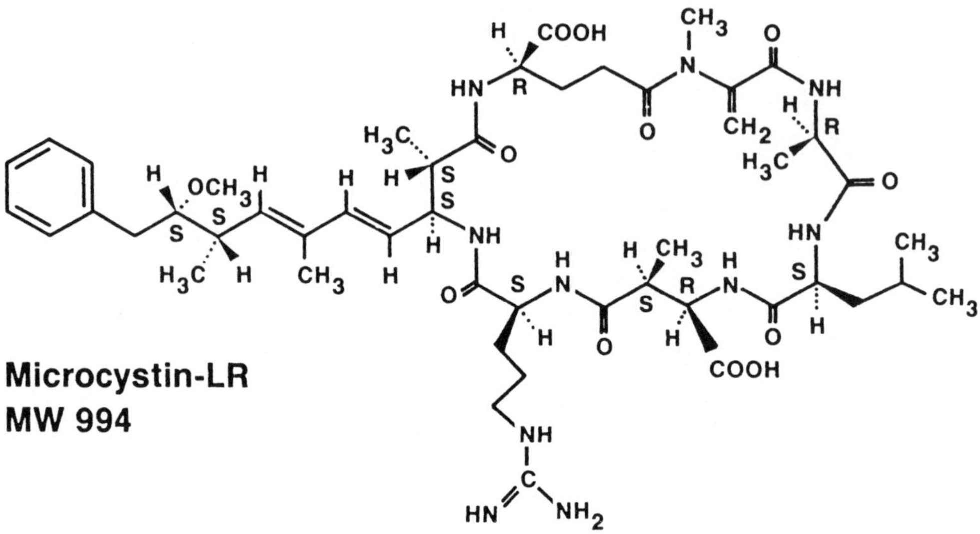

Microcystin-LR
MW 994

Other Water-Based Diseases of Toxic Cyanobacteria

Acute poisoning of humans by freshwater cyanobacteria as occurs with paralytic shellfish poisoning, while reported, has never been confirmed. Humans are probably just as susceptible as pets, livestock or wildlife but people naturally avoid contact with heavy waterblooms of cyanobacteria. In addition, there are no known vectors, like shellfish, to concentrate toxins from cyanobacteria into the human food chain. Susceptibility of humans to cyanobacteria toxins is supported mostly by indirect evidence. In many of these cases, however, if a more thorough epidemiological study had been possible these cases probably would have shown direct evidence for toxicity. Dillenberg and Dehnel (1960) described cases of human poisoning from accidental ingestion of blooms from lakes in Saskatchewan, Canada. Sargunar and Sargunar (1979) published an abstract which described a study in India involving human intoxication by *Microcystis aeruginosa*. Symptoms included nausea, vomiting, giddiness, stomachache, diarrhea, cramps, vague body paints and weakness. Aziz (1974) reported a diarrheic factor from waterblooms and laboratory cultures of *M. aeruginosa* collected from a city pond in Dacca, Bangladesh. The toxin caused a cholera type response but was not a protein-like cholera toxin.

In 1979, an outbreak of hepatoenteritis occurred among an aboriginal population on Palm Island, Queensland, Australia. It involved 148 people, mostly children, many of whom required hospitalization. The illnesses began shortly after copper sulfate was used to control a cyanobacteria bloom in Solomon Dam, the reservoir for the domestic water supply. The investigation that followed discovered a new hepatotoxic toxic genus and species identified as *Cylindrospermopsis raciborskii* (Wolosz) Seenaya and Subba Raju (Hawkins *et al.*, 1985).

Episodes of dermatitis and/or irritation from contact with freshwater cyanobacteria are occurring with increasing frequency as more eutrophic waters have been used for recreational purposes. Investigations in the U.S.A. (Billings, 1981); Canada (Carmichael *et al.*, 1985); Scotland (Codd and Bell, 1985); and Norway (Skulberg *et al.*, 1984) have shown that dermatotoxic blooms may be dominated by *Anabaena*, *Aphanizomenon*, *Gloeotrichia* and *Oscillatoria*, respectively.

In summary, it can be reported that toxic cyanobacteria can produce neurotoxic, hepatotoxic and dermatotoxic compounds that are a direct threat to animal and human water supplies. This threat increases as water bodies become more eutrophic, thus supporting higher production of toxic and nontoxic cyanobacteria. Presence of these potent natural product toxins pose an increasing threat to the maintenance of quality water supplies for agriculture, municipal and recreational use. However they also show promise for use as pharmacological tools in the study of basic cellular processes including certain neuromuscular diseases.

ACKNOWLEDGMENTS

Work with European toxic cyanobacteria was partially supported by a NATO collaborative research grant between W.W. Carmichael and G.A. Codd, University of Dundee, Scotland, and O.M. Skulberg, Norwegian Water Research Institute, Oslo, Norway. Toxin structure and function work is supported in part by U.S. AMRDC contract DAMD17-87-C-7019 to W.W. Carmichael.

REFERENCES

Adelman, W.J., Jr., J.F. Fohlmeister, J.J. Sasner, Jr. and M. Ikawa (1982). Sodium channels blocked by aphantoxin obtained from the blue-green alga, Aphanizomenon flos-aquae. Toxicon, 20, 513-516.

Aronstam, R.S. and B. Witkop (1981). Anatoxin-a interactions with cholinergic synaptic molecules. Proc. Natl. Acad. Sci. USA 78, 4639-4643.

Aune, T. and K. Berg (1986). Use of freshly prepared rat hepatocytes to study toxicity of blooms of the blue-green algae Microcystis aeruginosa and Oscillatoria agardhii. J. Toxicol. Environ. Health, 19, 325-336.

Aziz, K.M.S. (1974). Diarrhea toxin obtained from a waterbloom producing species, Microcystis aeruginosa Kutz. Science, 183, 1206-1207.

Barchi, J.J., Jr., R.E. Moore and G.M.L. Patterson (1984). Acutiphycin and 20,21-Didehydroacutiphycin, new antineo-plastic agents from the cyanophyte Oscillatoria acutissima. J. Am. Chem. Soc., 106, 8193-8197.

Barchi, J.J., Jr., T.R. Norton, E. Fursuawa, G.M.L. Patterson and R.E. Moore (1983). Identification of a cytotoxin from Tolypothrix byssoidea as tubercidin. Phytochemistry, 22, 2851-2852.

Bates, H.A. and H. Rapoport (1979). Synthesis of anatoxin a via intra-molecular cyclization of iminium salts. J. Am. Chem. Soc., 101, 1259-1265.

Berg, K., W.W. Carmichael, O.M. Skulberg, C. Benestad and B. Underdal (1987). Investigation of a toxic waterbloom of Microcystis aeruginosa (cyanophyceae) in Lake Akersvatn, Norway. Hydrobiologia, 144, 97-103.

Berg, K., J. Wyman, W.W. Carmichael and A.S. Dabholkar (1988). Isolated rat liver perfusion studies with cyclic heptapeptide toxins of Microcystis and Oscillatoria (freshwater cyanobacteria). Toxicon (In press).

Billings, W.H. (1981). Water-associated human illness in northeast Pennsylvania and its suspected association with blue-green algae blooms. In W.W. Carmichael (Ed.), The Water Environment: Algal Toxins and Health. Plenum Press, New York. pp. 243-255.

Bishop, C.T., E.F.L.J. Anet and P.R. Gorham (1959). Isolation and identification of the fast-death factor in Microcystis aeruginosa NRC-1. Can. J. Biochem. Physiol., 37, 453-471.

Botes, D.P. (1986). Cyanoginosins-isolation and structure. In P.S. Steyn and R. Vleggaar (eds.), Mycotoxins and Phycotoxins, Bioactive Molecules, Vol. 1. Elsevier, Amsterdam. pp. 161-167.

Botes, D.P., H. Wessels, H. Kruger, M.T.C. Runnegar, S. Santikarn, R.J. Smith, J.C.J. Barna and D.H. Williams (1985). Structural studies on cyanoginosins-LR, -YR, -YA, and -YM, peptide toxins from Microcystis aeruginosa. J. Chem. Soc. Perkin. Trans., 1, 2747-2748.

Botes, D.P., H. Kruger and C.C. Viljoen (1982a). Isolation and characterization of four toxins from the blue-green alga, Microcystis aeruginosa. Toxicon, 20, 945-954.

Botes, D.P., C.C. Viljoen, H. Kruger, P.L. Wessels and D.H. Williams (1982b). Configuration assignments of the amino acid residues and the present of N-methyldehydroalanine in toxins from the blue-green alga Microcystis aeruginosa. J. Chem. Soc. Perkin. Trans., 1, 2747-2748.

Brooks, W.P. and G.A. Codd (1987). Distribution of Microcystis aeruginosa peptide toxin and interactions with hepatic microsomes in mice. Pharm. Tox., 60, 187-191.

Campbell, H.F., O.E. Edwards, J.W. Elder and R.J. Kolt (1979). Total synthesis of DL-anatoxin-a and DL-isoanatoxin-a. Pol. J. Chem., 53, 27-37.

Campbell, H.F., O.E. Edwards and R. Kolt (1977). Synthesis of noranatoxin-A and anatoxin-A. Can. J. Chem., 55, 1372-1379.

Carmichael, W.W., V. Beasley, M-J. Yu, D.L. Bunner, T. Krishnamurthy, J.N. Eloff, R.E. Moore, I. Falconer, K. Rinehart, P.R. Gorham, M. Runnegar, K-I. Harada, O.M. Skulberg and M. Watanabe (1988). Naming of cyclic heptapeptide toxins of cyanobacteria (blue-green algae). Toxicon (in press).

Carmichael, W.W., J.T. Eschedor, G.M.L. Patterson and R.E. Moore (1988). Toxicity and partial structure for a hepatotoxic peptide produced by Nodularia spumigena Mertens emend. strain L575 (cyanobacteria) from New Zealand. App. Envir. Micro. (in press).

Carmichael, W.W. (1988). Toxins of Freshwater Algae. In A.T. Tu (Ed.), Handbook of Natural Toxins, Vol. 3, Marine Toxins and Venoms. Marcel Dekkar, New York. pp. 121-147.

Carmichael, W.W. (1986). Algal Toxins. In E. A. Callow (Ed.), Advances in Botanical Research, Vol. 12. Academic Press, London. pp. 47-101.
Carmichael, W.W., C.L.A. Jones, N.A. Mahmood and W.W. Theiss (1985). Algal toxins and water-based diseases. In C.P. Straub (Ed.), Critical Reviews in Environmental Control, Vol. 15(3). CRC Press, Boca Raton, Florida. pp. 275-313.
Carmichael, W.W. (1982). Chemical and toxicological studies of the toxic freshwater cyanobacteria Microcystis aeruginosa, Anabaena flos-aquae and Aphanizomenon flos-aquae. S. Afr. J. Sci., 78, 367-372.
Carmichael, W.W. (1981). The Water Environment: Algal Toxins and Health. Environ. Sci. Res., Volume 20. Plenum Press, New York. p. 491.
Carmichael, W.W., D.F. Biggs and M.A. Peterson (1979). Pharmacology of anatoxin-a, produced by the freshwater cyanophyte Anabaena flos-aquae NRC-44-1. Toxicon, 17, 229-236.
Carmichael, W.W. and D.F. Biggs (1978). Muscle sensitivity differences in two avian species to anatoxin-a produced by the freshwater cyanophyte Anabaena flos-aquae NRC-44-1. Can. J. Zool., 56, 510-512.
Carmichael, W.W. and P.R. Gorham (1977). Factors influencing the toxicity and animal susceptibility of Anabaena flos-aquae (cyanophyta) blooms. J. Phycol., 13, 97-101.
Carmichael, W.W., P.R. Gorham and D.F. Biggs (1977). Two laboratory case studies on the oral toxicity to calves of the freshwater cyanophyte (blue-green alga) Anabaena flos-aquae, NRC-44-1. Can. Vet. J., 18, 71-75.
Codd, G.A. and S.G. Bell (1985). Eutrophication and toxic cyanobacteria in freshwater. Water Pollution Control, 84, 225-232.
Dabholkar, A.S. and W.W. Carmichael (1987). Ultrastructural changes in the mouse liver induced by hepatotoxin from the freshwater cyanobacterium Microcystis aeruginosa strain 7820. Toxicon, 25, 285-292.
Danheiser, R.L., J.M. Morin, Jr. and E.J. Salaski (1985). Efficient total synthesis of (±)-anatoxin a. J. Am. Chem. Soc., 107, 8066-8073.
Devlin, J.P., O.E. Edwards, P.R. Gorham, N.R. Hunter, P.K. Pike and B. Stavric (1977). Anatoxin-a, a toxic alkaloid from Anabaena flos-aquae NRC-44h. Can. J. Chem., 55, 1367-1371.
Dillenberg, H.O. and M.K. Dehnel (1960). Toxic waterbloom in Saskatchewan, 1959. Can. Med. Assoc. J., 83, 1151-1154.
Edler, L., S. Ferno, M.G. Lind, R. Lundberg and P.O. Nilsson (1985). Mortality of dogs associated with a bloom of the cyanobacterium Nodularia spumigena in the Baltic Sea. Ophelia, 24, 103-109.
Ellman, T.C., I.R. Falconer, A.R.B. Jackson and M.T. Runnegar (1978). Isolation, characterization and pathology of the toxin from a Microcystis aeruginosa (= Anacystis cyanea bloom). Aust. J. Biol. Sci., 31, 209-218.
Eriksson, J.E., J.A.O. Meriluoto, H.P. Kujari, K. Osterlund, K. Fagerlund and L. Hallbom (1988). Preliminary characterization of a toxin isolated from the cyanobacterium Nodularia spumigena. Toxicon, 26, 161-166.
Eriksson, J.E., J.A.O. Meriluoto, H.P. Kujari and O.M. Skulberg (1987a). A comparison of toxins isolated from the cyanobacteria Oscillatoria agardhii and Microcystis aeruginosa. Comp. Biochem. Physiol., 89C, 207-210.
Eriksson, J., H. Hagerstr and B. Isomaa (1987b). Cell selective cytotoxicity of a peptide toxin from cyanobacterium. Biochem. Biophysc. Acta, 930, 304-310.
Falconer, I.R. and M.T.C. Runnegar (1987). Effects of the peptide toxin from Microcystis aeruginosa on intracellular calcium, pH and membrane integrity in mammalian cells. Chem. Biol. Interactions, 63, 215-225.
Falconer, I.R., T. Buckley and M.T.C. Runnegar (1986). Biological half-life, organ distribution and excretion of ^{125}I-labeled toxic peptide from the blue-green alga Microcystis aeruginosa. Aust. J. Biol. Sci., 39, 17-21.
Foxall, T.L. and J.J. Sasner, Jr. (1981). Effects of a hepatic toxin from the cyanophyte Microcystis aeruginosa. In W.W. Carmichael (Ed.), The Water Environment: Algal Toxins and Health. Plenum Press, New York. pp. 365-387.
Francis, G. (1878). Poisonous Australian lake. Nature (Lond.) 18, 11-12.
Gleason, F.K. and J.L. Paulson (1984). Site of action of the natural algicide, cyanobacterin, in the blue-green alga, Synechococcus sp. Arch. Microbiol., 138, 273-277.
Gorham, P.R. and W.W. Carmichael (1988). Hazards of freshwater blue-greens (cyanobacteria). In C.A. Lembi and J.R. Waaland (eds.), Algae and Human Affairs, Ch. 16. Cambridge University Press. pp. 403-431.
Harada, K.I., K. Matsuura, M. Suzuki, H. Oka, M.F. Watanabe, S. Oishi, A. Dahlem, V.R. Beasley and W.W. Carmichael (1988). Analysis and purification of toxic peptides from cyanobacteria by reverse phase HPLC. J. Chromat. (in press).
Hawkins, P.R., M.T.C. Runnegar, A.R.B. Jackson and I.R. Falconer (1985). Severe hepatotoxicity caused by the tropical cyanobacterium (blue-green alga) Cylindrospermopsis

raciborskii (Woloszynska) Seenaya and Subba Raju isolated from a domestic water supply reservoir. Appl. Environ. Microbiol., 50, 1292-1295.

Huber, C.S. (1972). The crystal structure and absolute configuration of 2,9-diacetyl-9-azabicyclo(4,2,1)non-2,3-ene. Acta Crystallograph., B78, 2577-2582.

Ikawa, M. K. Wegener, T.L. Foxall, and J.J. Sasner, Jr. (1982). Comparison of the toxins of the blue-green alga Aphanizomenon flos-aquae with the Gonyaulax toxins. Toxicon, 20, 747-752.

Jakim, E. and J.H. Gentile (1968). Toxins of blue-green alga: Similarity to saxitoxin. Science, 162, 915-916.

Kalbe, L. and D. Tiess (1964). Entenmass ensterben durch Nodularia - wasserblute am kleinen jasmunder bodden auf rugen. Arch. Exp. Vet. Med., 18, 535-539.

Konst, H., P.D. McKercher, P.R. Gorham, A. Robertson and J. Howell (1965). Symptoms and pathology produced by toxic Microcystis aeruginosa NRC-1 in laboratory and domestic animals. Can. J. Comp. Med. Vet. Sci., 29, 221-228.

Koskinen, M.P. and H. Rapoport (1985). Synthetic and conformatimal studies on anatoxin-a: A potent acetylcholine agonist. J. Med. Chem., 28, 1301-1309.

Krishnamurthy, T., W.W. Carmichael and E.W. Sarver (1986a). Investigations of freshwater cyanobacteria (blue-green algae) toxic peptides. I. Isolation, purification and characterization of peptides from Microcystis aeruginosa and Anabaena flos-aquae. Toxicon, 24, 865-873.

Krishnamurthy, T., L. Szafraniec, E.W. Sarver, D.F. Hunt, J. Shabanowitz, W.W. Carmichael, S. Missler, O. Skulberg and G. Codd (1986b). Amino acid sequences of freshwater blue-green algal toxic peptides by fast atom bombardment tandem mass spectrometric technique, P. 93. Proc. Am. Soc. Mass Spectrometry (ASMS) - 34th Annual Meeting, Cincinnati, Ohio, June 9, 1986.

Kusumi, T., T. Ooi, M.M. Watanabe, H. Takahagh and H. Kakisawa (1987). Cyanoviridin-RR, a toxin from the cyanobacterium (blue-green alga) Microcystis viridis. Tetrahed. Letters, 28, 4695-4698.

Lindgren, B., P. Stjernlof and L. Trozen (1987). Synthesis of anatoxin-a. A constituent of blue-green freshwater algae. Acta Chemica Scand., B41, 180-183.

Lindstrom, E. (1976). Et Udbrud af algeforgiftning blandt hunde. Dansk Vet. Tidsskr., 59, 637-641.

Mahmood, N.A., W.W. Carmichael and D. Pfahler (1988). Anticholinsterase poisonings in dogs from a cyanobacteria (blue-green algae) bloom dominated by Anabaena flos-aquae. Am. J. Vet. Res., 49, 500-503.

Mahmood, N.A. and W.W. Carmichael (1987). Anatoxin-a(s) an anticholinesterase from the cyanobacterium Anabaena flos-aquae NRC-525-17. Toxicon, 25, 1221-1227.

Mahmood, N.A. and W.W. Carmichael (1986a). The pharmacology of anatoxin-a(s), a neurotoxin produced by the freshwater cyanobacterium Anabaena flos-aquae NRC 525-17. Toxicon, 24, 425-434.

Mahmood, N.A. and W.W. Carmichael (1986b). Paralytic shellfish poisons produced by the freshwater cyanobacterium Aphanizomenon flos-aquae NH-5. Toxicon, 24, 175-186.

Main, D.C., P.H. Berry, R.L. Peet and J.P. Robertson (1977). Sheep mortalities associated with the blue-green algae Nodularia spumigena. Aust. Vet. J., 53, 578-581.

Mason, C.P., K.R. Edwards, R.E. Carlson, J. Pignatello, F.R. Gleason and J.M. Wood (1982). Isolation of chlorine-containing antibiotic from the freshwater cyanobacterium Scytonema hofmanni. Science, 215, 400-402.

Moore, R.E., G.M.L. Patterson, J.L. Mynderse and J. Barchi, Jr. (1986). Toxins from cyanophytes belonging to the scytonemataceae. Pure Appl. Chem., 58, 263-271.

Moore, R.E. (1984). Public health and toxins from marine blue-green algae. In E.P. Ragelis (Ed.), Seafood Toxins. American Chemical Society Symposium Series 262, Washington, D.C. pp. 369-376.

Murthy, J.R. and J.B. Capindale (1970). A new isolation and structure for the endotoxin from Microcystis aeruginosa NRC-1. Can. J. Biochem., 48, 508-510.

Ostensvik, O., O.M. Skulberg and N.E. Soli (1981). Toxicity studies with blue-green algae from Norwegian inland waters. In W.W. Carmichael (Ed.), The Water Environment: Algal Toxins and Health. Plenum Press, New York. pp. 315-324.

Painuly, P., R. Perez, T. Fukai and Y. Shimizu (1988). The structure of a cyclic peptide toxin, cyanogenosin-RR from Microcystis aeruginosa. Tetrahed. Letters, 29, 11-14.

Persson, P.E., K. Sivonen, J. Keto, K. Kononen, M. Niemi and H. Viljamaa (1984). Potentially toxic blue-green algae (cyanobacteria) in Finnish natural waters. Aqua Fenn., 14, 147-154.

Peterson, J.S., S. Toteberg-Kaulen and H. Rapoport (1984). synthesis of (±)-W-Aza[x.y.1] biocycloalkanes by an intromolecular Mannich reaction. J. Org. Chem., 49, 2948-2953.

Rabin, P. and A. Darbre (1975). An improved extraction procedure for the endotoxin form Microcystis aeruginosa NRC-1. Biochem. Soc. Trans., 3, 428-430.

Rinehart, K.L., K-I. Harada, M. Namikoshi, C. Chen, C. Harvis, M.H.G. Munro, J.W. Blunt, P.E. Mulligan, V.R. Beasley, A.M. Dahlem and W.W. Carmichael (1988). Nodularin, microcystin and the configuration of ADDA. J. Am. Chem. Soc. (in press).

Runnegar, M.T.C., A.R.B. Jackson and I.R. Falconer (1988a). Toxicity to mice and sheep of a bloom of the cyanobacterium (blue-green algae) Anabaena circinalis. Toxicon, 26, 599-602.
Runnegar, M.T.C., A.R.B. Jackson and I.R. Falconer (1988b). Toxicity of the cyanobacterium Nodularia spumigena. Mertens. Toxicon, 26, 143-151.
Runnegar, M.T.C., J. Andrews, R.G. Gerdes and I.R. Falconer (1987). Injury to hepatocytes induced by a peptide toxin from the cyanobacterium Microcystis aeruginosa. Toxicon, 25, 1235-1239.
Runnegar, M.T.C., I.R. Falconer, T. Buckley and A.R.B. Jackson (1986a). Lethal potency and tissue distribution of ^{125}I-labeled toxic peptides from the blue-green alga Microcystis aeruginosa. Toxicon, 24, 506-509.
Runnegar, M.T.C. and I.R. Falconer (1986b). Effect of toxin from the cyanobacterium Microcystis aeruginosa on ultra-structural morphology and actin polymerization in isolated hepatocytes. Toxicon, 24, 105-115.
Runnegar, M.T.C. and I.R. Falconer (1981). Isolation, characterization and pathology of the toxin from the blue-green alga Microcystis aeruginosa. In W.W. Carmichael (Ed.), The Water Environment: Algal Toxins and Health. Plenum Press, New York. pp. 325-342.
Santikarn, S., D.H. Williams, R.J. Smith, S.J. Hammond and H. Botes (1983). A partial structure for the toxin BE-4 from the blue-green algae, Microcystis aeruginosa. J. Chem. Soc. Chem. Commun., 12, 652-654.
Sargunar, H.T.P. and A.A.A. Sargunar (1979). Phycotoxins from Microcystis aeruginosa. Their implication in human and animal health. Proc. 4th Int. IUPAC Symp. - Mycotoxins and Phycotoxins, Lausanne, Switz. (Abstract #610).
Sasner, J.J., Jr., M. Ikawa and T.L. Foxall (1984). Studies on Aphanizomenon and Microcystis toxins. In E.P. Ragelis (Ed.), Seafood Toxins. American Chemical Society Symposium Series 262, Washington, D.C. pp. 391-406.
Sawyer, P.J., J.H. Gentile and J.J. Sasner, Jr. (1968). Demonstration of a toxin from Aphanizomenon flos-aquae (L.) Ralfs. Can. J. Microbiol., 14, 1199-1204.
Schwimmer, M. and D. Schwimmer (1968). Medical aspects of phycology. In D.F. Jackson (Ed.), Algae, Man and the Environment. Syracuse University Press, Syracuse, New York. pp. 279-358.
Shimizu, Y., M. Norte, A. Hori, A. Genenah and M. Kobayushi (1984). Biosynthesis of saxitoxin analogues: The unexpected pathway. J. Am. Chem. Soc., 106, 6433-6434.
Skulberg, O.M., G.A. Codd and W.W. Carmichael (1984). Toxic blue-green algal blooms in Europe: A growing problem. Ambio, 13, 244-247.
Spivak, C.E., J. Waters, B. Witkop and E.X. Albuquerque (1983). Potencies and channel properties induced by semirigid agonists at frog nicotinic acetylcholine receptors. Mol. Pharmacol., 23, 337-343.
Spivak, C.E., B. Witkop and E.X. Albuquerque (1980). Anatoxin-a, a novel, potent agonist at the nicotinic receptor. Mol. Pharmacol., 18, 384-394.
Theiss, W.C., W.W. Carmichael, J. Wyman and R. Bruner (1988). Blood pressure and hepatocellular effects of the cyclic heptapeptide toxin produced by Microcystis aeruginosa strain PCC-7820. Toxicon, 26, 603-613.
Tufariello, J.J., H. Meckler and K.P.A. Senaratne (1985). The use of nitrones in the synthesis of anatoxin-a, very fast death factor. Tetrahedron, 41, 3447-3453.
Tufariello, J.J., H. Meckler and K.P.A. Senaratne (1984). Synthesis of anatoxin-a: Very fast death factor. J. Am. Chem. Soc., 106, 7979-7980.
Wiseman, J.R. and S.Y. Lee (1986). Synthesis of anatoxin-a. J. Org. Chem., 51, 2485-2487.

MYCOTOXINS - AN OVERVIEW

Bruce B. Jarvis

Department of Chemistry and Biochemistry
University of Maryland
College Park, Maryland 20742

ABSTRACT

Mycotoxins are secondary metabolites produced by a variety of filamentous fungi which pose a hazard to the health of both animals and humans. The trichothecene and aflatoxin mycotoxins are the most important members of this very diverse class of toxins. The biological properties of these and other mycotoxins is presented with a special emphasis on those which have been isolated from unusual sources.

KEYWORDS

Aflatoxins, *Aspergillus*, *Baccharis*, fungi, *Fusarium*, *Myrothecium*, *Penicillium*, *Stachybotrys*, tremorgens, trichothecenes.

The dangers of eating poison mushrooms date back to prehistory, but it wasn't until the 18th century that people realized that certain filamentous fungi (molds), associated with plant material were another source of hazard to health. These fungi act as saprophytes and/or plant pathogens and most often belong to the class of *Fungi imperfecti*. The toxins produced by these molds are called mycotoxins, and it is the intent of this chapter to give an overview of this subject.

There is not space enough to delve into this topic in any great detail. Fortunately, there have been a number of reviews, monographs, and treatises written on numerous aspects of mycotoxins since the early 1970's (*inter alia*:: Betina, 1984; Ciegler et al., 1971; Cole, 1986; Cole and Cox, 1981; Lacey, 1985; Mirocha et al., 1980; Rechcigl, 1983; Rodricks et al., 1977; Shank, 1981; Smith and Moss, 1985; Steyn and Vleggaar, 1986; Ueno, 1986), and the reader is encouraged to refer to these reviews for additional information.

The first clearly recognized episodes involving mycotoxins in human toxicoses were those of ergot poisoning, though the relationship between ergotism and the responsible fungus (*Claviceps*) which infected the rye was not recognized until the 18th century. Ergotism has a long and facinating history, (Groger, 1972) - it has even been suggested as a cause of the hysteria that led to the Salem witch trials (Caporael, 1976) and to the public discourse leading up the French revolution (Matossian, 1983) - but, for the most part, as a mycotoxicology problem, it has dissappeared from view in modern time. Although there were reports in the literature of other mycotoxicosis outbreaks during the 19th and early to mid-20th centuries in central and eastern Europe and in Asia (Ciegler et al., 1981), they essentially went unnoticed in the West. That situation came to an abrupt end in 1960, when British turkey farmers lost 100,000 animals, the loss of which was traced to *Aspergillus* fungi contaminating the peanut meal feed imported from Brazil. Subsequent work with *A. flavus* and *A. parasiticus* showed them to be producers of a then new class of mycotoxins called the aflatoxins. A retrospective analysis of the etiology of this so-called turkey "X" disease has suggested that the real culprit may have been cyclopiazonic acid (another mycotoxin produced by Aspergillus) (Cole, 1986a), a tetramic acid derivative related to a class of antibiotics (e.g. streptolydigin) produced by *Streptomyces*. However, aflatoxins have turned out to be among the most important of the mycotoxins, not because of their acute toxicity but because of their potency as carcinogens.

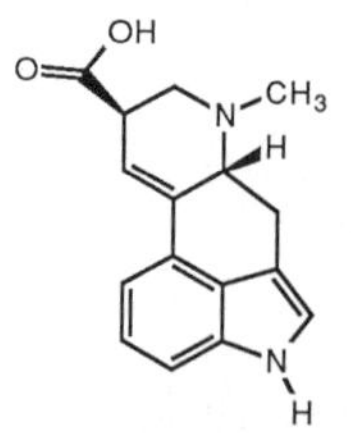

Lysergic Acid
(An Ergot Alkaloid)

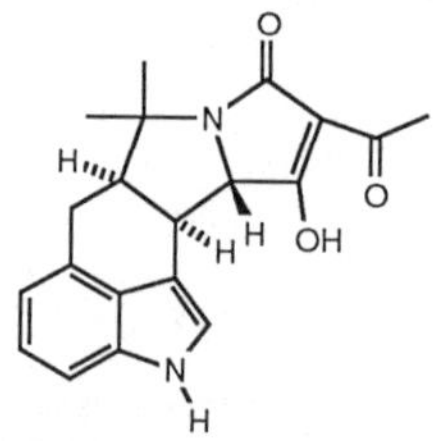

Cyclopiazonic Acid

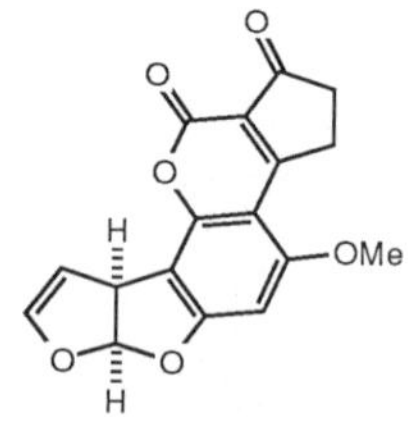

Aflatoxin B_1

Although it is simple to give an operational definition of mycotoxins, the chemists and biologists have no simple way to categorize these substances. There are several hundred different structure types found in the mycotoxins, and each one of these may have up to twenty or more naturally occurring closely related derivatives. The chemical structures of mycotoxins vary tremendously, from simple molecules such as moniliformin to complex polypeptides such as cyclochlorotine; the latter is in fact related to the anticancer nitrogen mustard drugs. Other chlorine-containing mycotoxins include ochratoxin A (*Penicillium islandicum*) which is purported to cause nephrosis in both humans and pigs in Europe (Steyn, 1984) and sporidesmin A (*Pithomyces chartarum*) which causes facial eczema in sheep (Nagarajan, 1984). However, ochratoxin B, which lacks the chlorine atom is considerably less toxic than ochatoxin A. Epoxide functionalities (as in PR toxin from *Penicillium roqueforti* and trichothecenes from *Fusarium* spp.) and highly unsaturated systems (as in citreoviridin from *Penicillium* spp. and *Aspergillus terreus*) also are to be found in several mycotoxins. Rubratoxin B (*Penicillium rubrum* and *P. purpurogenum*), unique in that it contains a nine-membered carbocyclic ring, has been implicated in hemorrhagic disease in various farm animals (Davis and Richard, 1984).

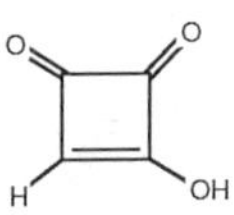

Moniliformin

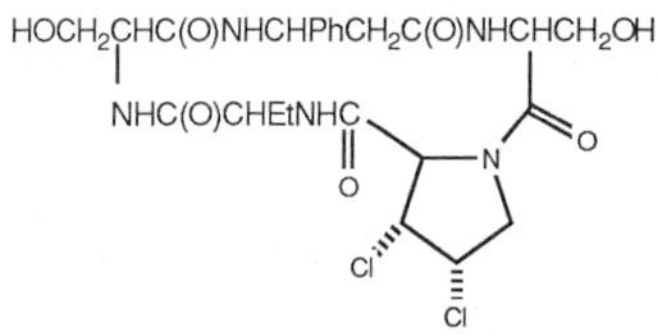

Cyclochlorotine

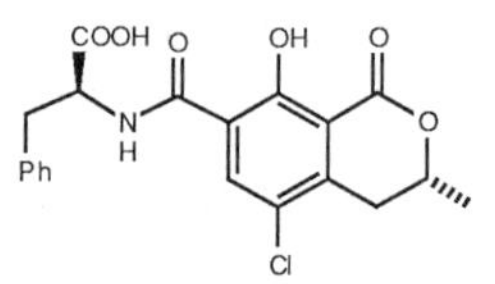

Ochratoxin A

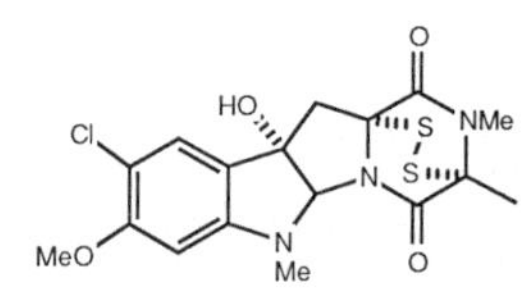

Sprridesmin B

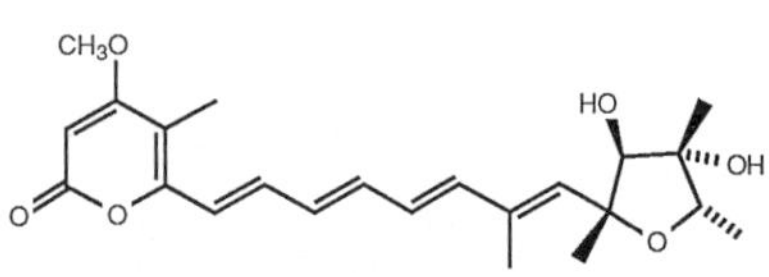

Citreoviridin

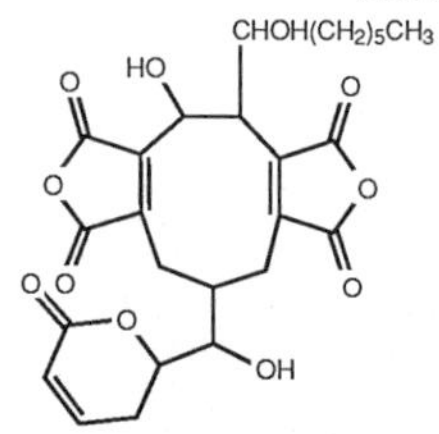

Rubratoxin B

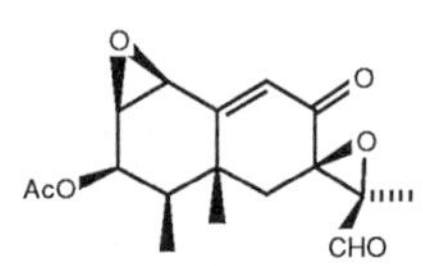

PR Toxin

For the biologist looking for some taxonomically or pathophysiologically recurring theme among the producers of mycotoxins, the situation is formidable. The matter is no better for the toxicologist when he finds that the different types of mycotoxins invariably cause different toxic responses in the target organisms. On the other hand, this diversity of chemical structure and biological activity associated with mycotoxins assures the mycotoxicologist of an unending and fascinating topic for research.

It is worth pointing out how these toxins initially come to the attention of the mycotoxicologist. From a scientific standpoint, the ideal situation would be that when a suspected case of mycotoxicosis has occurred, a team of chemists, microbiologists, and toxicologists would arrive on the scene and find everything intact. The victims would be present (dead or alive) so that they could be studied and analyzed. All of the environmental samples would be present, and upon examination would be found to be contaminated by a monoculture of one species of fungi. There would be sufficient material to do toxicological studies in test animals as well as to yield sufficient amounts of pure toxins for the chemist to characterize.

To my knowledge, such an ideal happenstance has never occurred. The basic reason for this is that by the time the toxic episode is recognized as a possible case of mycotoxicosis, the environmental samples are no longer available. If there is in fact some of the sample remaining (it often has either been used up, destroyed, or diluted -the solution to pollution is dilution), it rarely is sufficient for toxicological or, sometimes even chemical studies. Furthermore, it is almost unheard of to find these samples contaminated with a monculture of a single fungal species. Commonly, they are contaminated by several related and unrelated species of fungi. In the end, the role of mycotoxins in the etiology of many diseases comes down to building a case based on strong circumstantial evidence. For example, one sometimes finds that feed held responsible for an animal toxicosis is heavily contaminated by one fungal species. The fungus may then be grown up, as a single culture on this substrate in the laboratory and fed to test animals. If the disease is then reproduced in the laboratory animals, the culture is grown in sufficient quantity to allow the isolation of pure chemicals in quantities sufficient to characterize (with modern techniques of analysis (Cole, 1986), this is usually not a problem) and test them for toxicity in the animals. Although this may sound straightforward, it is rife with pitfalls, some of which will be discussed later.

In addition to there being a large number of structure types, the system is further complicated by the fact that a given type of mycotoxin can be produced by several different genera of fungi, while any given genera of fungi may be found to produce a wide range of different mycotoxins. Thus, trichothecenes have been reported to be produced by a least ten different genera of fungi (Ichinoe and Kurata, 1983), while the cytochalasans and related congeners have been found in the cultures of nine genera (Busby and Wogan, 1981). The cytochalasins have particularly interesting biological effects, one of which is the inhibition of cell movement. At higher concentrations, cytochalasins and chaetoglobosins cause the ejection of the cell nucleus, a process which is reversible (Tamm, 1980).

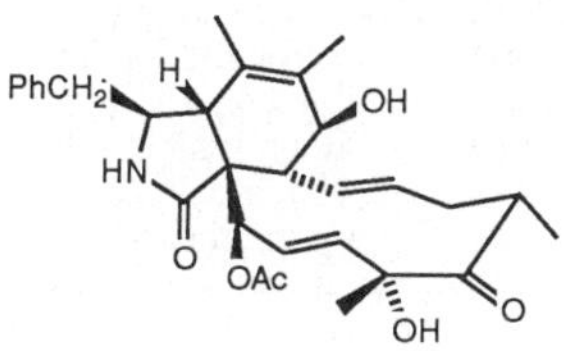

Cytochalasin C

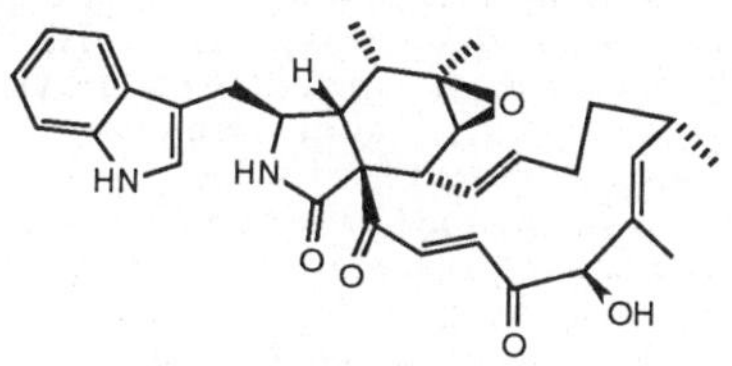

Chaetoglobosin A

Considering the vast amount of literature on mycotoxins generated since 1960 (Hesseltine, 1986), by necessity I will have to restrict this discussion to only a few of the more important mycotoxins. Of course the word "important" implies a value judgement on my part, and certainly does not suggest that those who deal with mycotoxins omitted herein are not involved with "important" mycotoxins.

There is likely to be little disagreement that of the mycotoxins, the aflatoxins and trichothecenes pose the most serious threat to the health of humans and animals. These toxins typically are produced by *Aspergillus* and *Fusarium* species, respectively, though only two species of *Aspergillus* (*A. flavus* and *A. parasiticus*) and a limited number of *Fusarium* species are producers of these particular mycotoxins.

The most common as well as toxic member of the aflatoxins is aflatoxin B_1 (AFB). Its acute toxicity varies a great deal from animal species to animal species, e.g. the $LD_{50's}$ in rabbit and in mice are 0.3 mg/kg and 40 mg/kg, respectively (Busby and Wogan, 1981a). Clearly the most serious problem associated with AFB is its potential as a carcinogen. AFB has induced liver cancer in all species of laboratory animals tested some of whom are equisitely sensitive to this potent hepatocarcinogen (e.g. rainbow trout) (Ayres et al., 1971). The sensible presumption is that AFB is a human carcinogen as well. Since testing can not be carried out in humans, an evaluation of this presumption must be based on a retrospective analysis of the epidemiological data. Indeed such an analysis of the incidence of liver tumors in the populations has shown a high correlation with elevated levels of aflatoxins in the diets. However, these populations also have a high incidence of hepatitis B viral infections which could also be a determining factor. The general consensus now appears to be that both of these factors play roles in the etiology of liver cancers in these areas (Hsieh, 1986). Concern about the carcinogenicity of aflatoxins has led many of the western nations to put a limit on the total concentration of aflatoxins in food and feed which in the United States is 20 ppb for both human food and animal feed (United States Federal Register #39, p. 42748, 1974). The level for aflatoxin M_1 (an AFB metabolite) in milk is set at 0.5 ppb (United States Federal Register #42, p. 61630, 1977).

Much has been published about the mechanism of action of the aflatoxins. AFB first must be metabolically activated to the 2,3-epoxide which then functions as the proximate carcinogen by intercalating into DNA and alkylating the guanine residues (Fig. 1) (Stark, 1986).

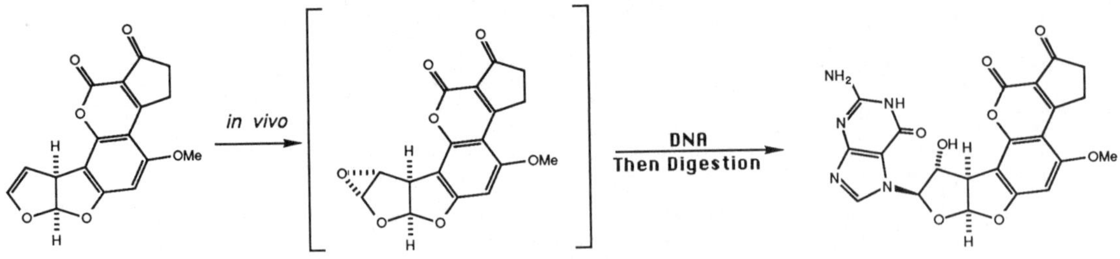

Aflatoxin B_1

Fig. 1. Aflatoxin-guanine adduct formation

Corn, ground nuts, and cottonseed meal are the principal commodities that become contaminated with the aflatoxins. Obviously, the best way to prevent this contamination would be to prevent the growth of the toxigenic strains of *Aspergillus*. However, the environmental factors which control the growth of mycotoxin-producing fungi in the field are quite complex and usually out of our control (Lacey, 1986). High temperatures and drought conditions favor the development of aflatoxin-producing strains of *Aspergillus*, not because these are favorable conditions for toxin production, but because these harsh conditions have a more adverse effect on the other fungi which normally are in competition with *Aspergillus* for the substrate (Dorner et al., 1988). In recent years, commerical processes have been developed to decontaminate animal feeds, which have become spoiled with aflatoxins, by treating the feed with ammonia under heat and pressure (Prevot, 1986). In the United States, our problems with mycotoxins are pretty much divided along the Mason-Dixon line: aflatoxins to the south and trichothecenes to the north. If our changing weather patterns bring increasing high temperatures and drought conditions, this line of division is very likely to move north.

The trichothecene mycotoxins can be divided into two structure types: the simple (e.g. T-2 toxin, diacetoxyscirpenol (DAS), deoxynivalenol (DON), verrucarol, etc.) and the macrocyclic trichothecenes (e.g. roridin E, verrucarin A, satratoxin H, baccharinoid B4, etc.). *Fusarium* is the most important genera of fungi that produces the simple trichothecenes while *Stachybotrys atra* (also known as *S. chartarum*) and *Myrothecium roridum* and *M. verrucaria* are the most important producers of the macrocyclics. The Fusaria must be considered to be among the most important of the toxigenic fungi, not only because of their producing trichothecenes, but also because they produce a variety of other mycotoxins. Furthermore, Fusaria occur worldwide, and nearly every country (especially in the temperate zones) has reported toxicoses cases. However, the taxonomy of the *Fusarium* has presented significant problems with respect to the proper identification of the species under study. An important treatise has been published recently which straightens out much of the confusion that has been generated in the literature concerning the correct identification of toxigenic Fusaria. This text also lists all of the reported toxigenic strains of *Fusarium* along with the mycotoxins produced by these fungi as reported in the literature through 1981 (Marasas et al., 1984).

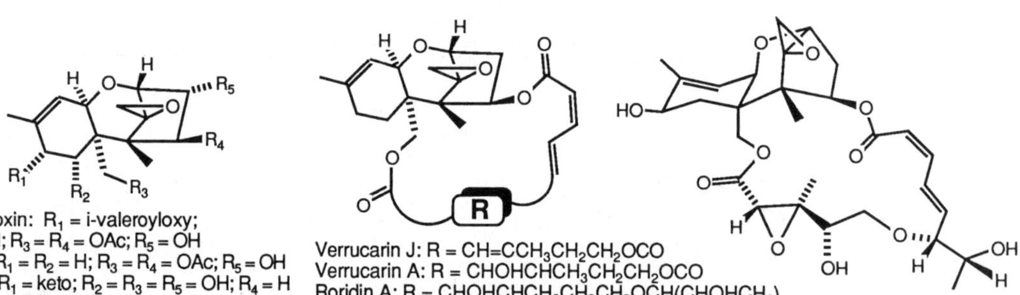

T-2 Toxin: R_1 = i-valeroyloxy; R_2 = H; R_3 = R_4 = OAc; R_5 = OH
DAS: R_1 = R_2 = H; R_3 = R_4 = OAc; R_5 = OH
DON: R_1 = keto; R_2 = R_3 = R_5 = OH; R_4 = H
Verrucarol; R_1 = R_2 = R_5 = H; R_3 = R_4 = OH

Verrucarin J: R = $CH{=}CCH_3CH_2CH_2OCO$
Verrucarin A: R = $CHOHCHCH_3CH_2CH_2OCO$
Roridin A: R = $CHOHCHCH_3CH_2CH_2OCH(CHOHCH_3)$
Roridin E: R = $CH{=}CCH_3CH_2CH_2CH(CHOHCH_3)$

Baccharinoid B4

The number of reported naturally occurring trichothecenes and related biosynthetic metabolites numbers well over 100. In addition, a large number of semisynthetic trichothecenes has been prepared in connection with drug development as anticancer agents (Jarvis et al., 1984; Kaneko et al., 1982; Kaneko et al., 1985). Although some members of the trichothecene complex of antibiotics are considerably more acutely toxic than are the aflatoxins, the trichothecenes are clearly far less carcinogenic (Ohtsubo, 1983). However, like the aflatoxins the trichothecenes are immunosuppresive agents (Pier and McLaughlin, 1985). This means that many cases of trichothecene toxicoses in farm animals may go unrecognized since a veterinarian unfamiliar with such toxicoses will not realize that the secondary opportunistic bacterial infections in the stricken animals are a result of their having ingested these immunosuppresive mycotoxins (Yarom et al., 1984).

The trichothecenes were discovered in the late '40's during a screening program designed to pickup antifungal agents (Freeman and Morrison, 1948). Although they proved to be too toxic to be of value as antifungal agents, interest was renewed in the early '60's because of their potential as anticancer agents (Doyle and Bradner, 1980). Diacetoxyscirpenol (also called anguidine) eventually made it into phase II clinical trails but failed to be carried further because of lack of response in the human subjects and rather severe and unpleasant side effects (Adler et al., 1984).

The biochemical mode of action of the trichothecenes has been extensively studied and found to be that of protein synthesis inhibition. Trichothecenes bind to the 60S subunit of eucaryotic ribosomes and interfere with the peptidyltransferase enzyme. The trichothecenes are the most potent of the small molecule protein synthesis inhibitors (McLaughlin et al., 1977), and do so with all eucaryotic systems except with those organisms which produce the trichothecenes (Hobden and Cundliffe, 1980). A number of structure-activity relationship studies have been carried out with the trichothecenes, but the chemical nature of the trichothecene - ribosome binding is unknown, although it is interesting to note that this binding is reversible with the simple trichothecenes but irreversible with the macrocyclics (Hernandez and Cannon, 1982).

The trichothecenes have been implicated in a number of cases of human toxicoses (Ueno, 1980), the most notorious of which (alimentary toxic aleukia, ATA) occurred in the Orenburg district of western Siberia from 1942 to 1947 (Joffe, 1983). Upwards to 10% of the population was affected with thousands perishing. Although *Fusarium sporotrichioides* was identified early on as the responsible organism which contaiminated the wintered grains, it was not until 30 years later, that workers showed that these Russian isolates of *F. sporotrichiodes* were potent producers of the highly toxic T-2 toxin (Yagen et al., 1977).

Fortunately, few cases of trichothecene toxicoses result in the loss of human life. In general, the most serious problems result from feed refusal in swine where the lack of weight gain translates into the loss of substantial amounts money for the farmers. Similarly, zearalenone, another mycotoxin commonly produced by trichothecene-producing *Fusarium* (principally *F. graminearum*) elicits a hyperestrongenic reponse in swine which also leads to financial loss (Mirocha et al., 1977). The less toxic trichothecenes, such as deoxynivalenol (DON, also known as vomitoxin) are the ones usually involved in these cases (Vesonder, 1983). At the moment, there is no commercially available decontamination process for DON as there is for the aflatoxins, though this one day may become economically feasible (Young et al., 1987). One obvious question in this regard is how much of a mycotoxin survives food processing. Afterall, if processing and cooking destroys the toxins, one would be far less concerned with mycotoxin contamination of food stocks that undergo such treatment. What little has been done in this area (Scott, 1984), suggests that trichothecenes and aflatoxins are fairly stable toward baking and food processing, and so it would appear to be rather important that the quality of our cereals and grains be continually monitored for these toxins.

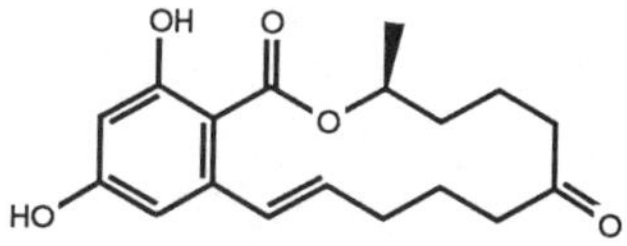

Zearalenone

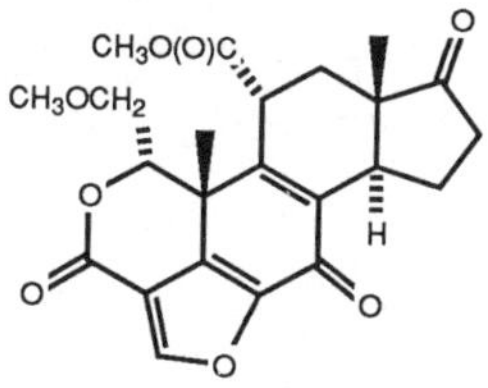

Wortmannin

Although the macrocyclic trichothecenes are more toxic than the simple ones, they appear to come into contact with animals and humans far less often. The most common problems are associated with *Stachybotrys atra (chartarum)* , a fungus commonly found growing on damp materials of high cellulose and low nitrogen content. This fungus tends to grow on substrates, such as straw and hay, where other normally more vigorous organisms can not compete. This characteristically black fungus also grows well on moist paper and debris. Stachybotryotoxicosis (Forgacs, 1972) appears to be relatively common in eastern Europe and the Soviet Union but seems not to be recognized as a general problem elsewhere, though this may be more a matter of ignorance on the part those who come across this disease in the field (Schneider et al., 1979). Horses seem to be particularly sensitive to this disease, and it is an interesting historical note that Stalin was so upset with the loss of Ukranian horses, from what appeared to be this disease (Khrushchev, 1970), he was going to have the veterinarians shot. Toxigenic strains of *S. atra* produce verrucarin J, roridin E, and a series of related derivatives known as the satratoxins (Jarvis et al., 1983). Although these toxins have been found not only in laboratory-grown cultures of *S. atra* associated with animal intoxications (Jarvis et al., 1986), but also from the field samples themselves (Harrach et al., 1983). There is no doubt that the animals have ingested these toxins; however, it is by no means clear that the concentrations of these toxins in the natural samples were sufficient to cause the dramatic effects noted in the animals, particularly the massive hemorrhaging. There may well be other secondary metabolites present in these toxigenic cultures that act synergistically with the trichothecenes to bring about these potent effects. A recent report (Abbas and Mirocha, 1988) determined that the hemorrhagic factor in *Fusarium oxysporum* was due to wortmannin, a toxin known to be produced by *Penicillium wortmannii* (McMillan et al., 1972), *P. funiculosum* (Haefliger and Hanser, 1973), and *Myrothecium roridum* (Petcher et al., 1972). The latter is a well known producer of macrocyclic trichothecenes (Jarvis et al., 1983).

The only report of an apparent case of stachybotryotoxicosis in the United States occurred with humans in a house in suburban Chicago. For five years, the residents of this house had been complaining about various medical problems including headaches, burning skin (trichothecenes are potent skin irritants), diarrhea, intermittent focal alopecia, etc. An investigation of the home revealed several water damaged areas and substantial growth of *S. atra* in various parts of the house including the air ducts. Air samples were shown to contain numerous spores of *S. atra* , and chemical analysis of material taken from the house led to the isolation of several of the macrocyclic trichothecenes (Croft et al. 1986). Since the macrocyclic trichothecenes are concentrated in the spores of this fungus (Sorenson et al., 1987), it is clear that these people had had a long term exposure to these toxins which could explain their medical problems. After the house was rid of the fungus, the occupants no longer complained of the distresses noted above. This, in fact is typical of trichothecene toxicoses: if the animal survives the toxic episode and the offending toxins are removed, the animal recovers completely with no long term ill effects. In otherwords, one manifestation of trichothecene toxicosis is the suppression of the immune system with resultant infections by opportunistic pathogens. If the toxins are removed, the immune system will recover completely. In this regard, one should pay attention to the possible contributions by mycotoxins to our "indoor air pollution" problems. There are an increasing number of complaints from office workers in modern buildings where the turnover in air is held to a minimum to conserve energy. If moisture is present, the dust and debris that accumulate in the air system could act as substrate for mycotoxin-producing fungi resulting in the release of mycotoxins into the rooms (Bissett, 1987; Flannigan, 1987).

Some diseases in humans are linked to mycotoxins only by the epidemiological data. For example, the high rate of esophagal cancer in the Transkei region of South Africa (Marasas et al., 1984a) and Kashin-Beck disease (Marasas et al., 1984b) in eastern Siberia, North Korea and northern China are linked to the *Fusarium* -contaminated food consumed in these regions. This latter disease develops slowly and chronically and affects the growth and development of the growing skeleton. This crippling disease in humans is reminiscent of a disease in chickens called tibial dyschondroplasia (TDP) where the lesions occur in the leg bones. An Alaskan TDP-causing isolate of *F. graminearum* was shown to produce a new mycotoxin called fusarochromanone which when given to chickens reproduced the disease (Pathre et al., 1986). However, a survey of over 100 isolates of *Fusarium* collected from a region of northern China where Kashin-Beck disease is common was negative for the production of fusarochromanone (Mirocha, 1988).

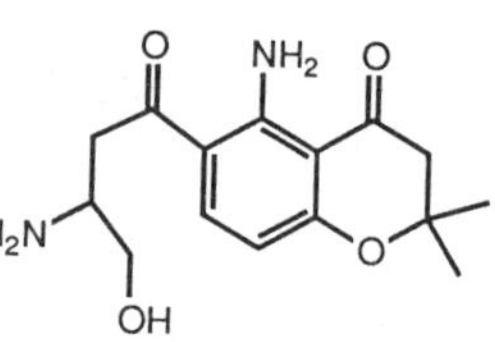

Fusarochromanone

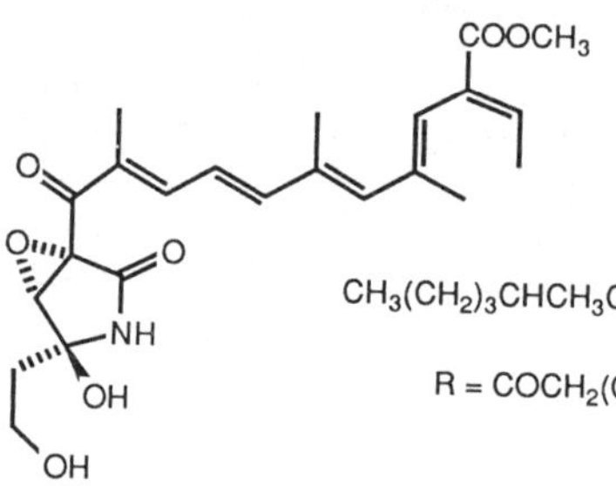

Fusarin C

$CH_3(CH_2)_3CHCH_3CH(OR)CH(OR)CH_2CHCH_3(CH_2)_6CHOHCH_2CHOH$

$\qquad AcNHCHCH_3$ (attached at the CH of CH_2CHOH)

$R = COCH_2(COOH)CH_2COOH$

Fumonisin A_2

The etiology of some diseases associated with fungal contamination can prove maddening. Equine leukoencephalomalacia (LEM) is a particularly vexing problem, apparently unique to equine (horses, mules, and donkeys) (Marasas et al., 1984c). In its later and most severe stages, LEM results in liquefactive necrotic brain lesions; literally gaping holes are generated in the white matter of the cerebral hemispheres. Descriptions of LEM go back to the mid-19th century, and over the years this disease has been reported in many counties. The worst outbreak of LEM in the United States occurred in Illinois in late 1934 early 1935, where an estimated 5,000 horses perished (Schwarte, 1938). It is clear that LEM is associated with *Fusarium moniliforme* (Marasas et al., 1984c); however, it has yet to be established just what mycotoxin(s) produced by *F. moniliforme* is responsible. Studies have established that neither fusaric acid, moniliformin, nor the potent mutagen fusarin C are responsible (Marasas et al., 1984c); perhaps the recently isolated fumonisins (Bezuidenhout et al., 1988) are the caustive agents. A serious problem with the isolation and identification of the mycotoxin(s) responsible for LEM is the fact that horses (or other large and expensive equines) must be employed as bioassays to follow the fractionation of the culture extracts. If a small animal model could be found which would give a reliable assay for LEM, the isolation of LEM-causing mycotoxin would be greatly simplified.

One of the more interesting types of mycotoxicoses arises from animals' eating plants infected with toxigenic endophytes. Endophytes are fungi which actually live inside plants often causing no apparent harm to the plant. In fact, New Zealand perennial ryegrass is considerably less susceptible to Argentine stem weevil predation when the grass is infected by endophytic *Lolium perenne* . Unfortunately, such infected ryegrass poses a serious hazard to grazing animals since *L. perenne* in the infected plant produces a series of potent tremorgens (Cole and Dorner, 1986), lolitrems, which are the cause of ryegrass staggers. It is perhaps a perverse trick of nature to make the toxic endophyte-infected ryegrass more appealing to the animals since the infected grass is protected from weevil attack, and unprotected ryegrass grows poorly in the presence of the insects (Latch, 1985).

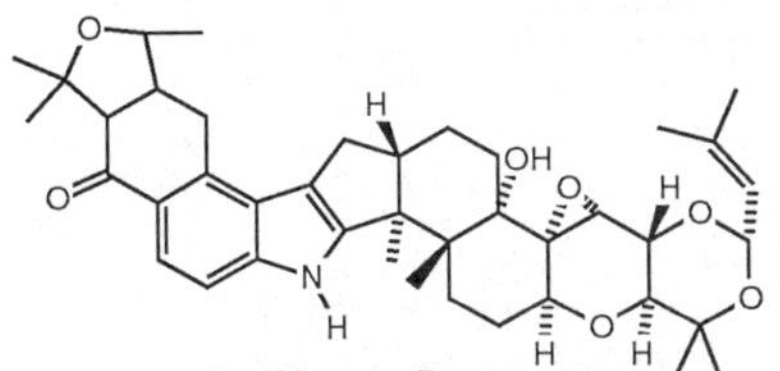

Lolitrem B

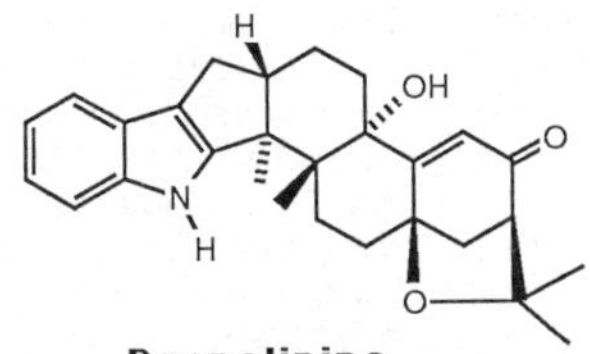

Paspalinine

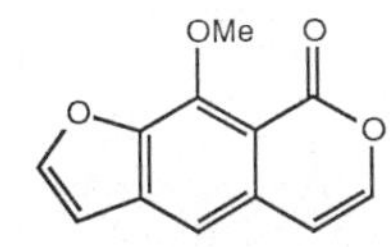

8-Methoxypsoralen

The ergot fungus *Claviceps paspali* infects grasses which when ingested by cattle cause pasalum staggers (Cole and Dorner, 1986). The tremorgenic metabolites isolated from the sclerotia have been identified as the paspaline alkaloids. Tall fescue grass staggers is caused by the endophyte *Acremonium coenophialum* which produces ergot alkaloids resulting in intoxication to those animals which eat this infected grass (Lyons et al., 1986). Actually, it is difficult to prove whether the fungus itself produces the toxins or whether it stimulates the plant to produce the toxin (a phytoalexic response, Keen, 1986) (Putnam and Tang, 1986). It is normally very difficult to work with endophytes outside their host plant since such organisms do not grow well under these conditions (Clay, 1987; Siegel et al., 1985). A similar problem interpreting whether the psoralens isolated from celery infected with the fungus *Sclerotinia sclerotiorum* arise through fungal metabolism or as a metabolic response (phytoalexic) by celery to fungal attack or some complex combination of both (Busby and Wogan, 1981b). In any event, workers handling such infected celery suffer dermatitis following exposure to sunlight. However, psoralen derivatives have proven clinically useful in the treatment of psoriasis (Busby and Wogan, 1981b).

This brings us to the strange case of the presence of macrocyclic trichothecenes in the Brazilian shrub, *Baccharis megapotamica* . During the course of screening plants for anticancer agents, Kupchan et al. (1976) found that a crude extract of *B. megapotamica* exhibited exceptional activity *in vivo* against P388 murine leukemia. The active principles were shown to be the baccharinoids (Jarvis et al., 1987, 1987a; Kupchan et al., 1977), which are closely related in structure to the roridins produced by *Myrothecium* fungi. Inspection of the plant material did not reveal any fungal activity nor are any of the numerous trichothecene-producing fungi known to be endophytic or even reasonably related to fungi which are. The suggestion was made that the baccharinoids were plant-altered fungal toxins which the *Baccharis* plant acquired from an associative fungus. It was shown that *B. megapotamica* grown from seed in a local Maryland greenhouse did not produce the toxins (*N.B.* these plants have never come into flower in the Maryland greenhouse - the importance of this point will soon become evident). Futhermore, when roridin A was injected into the plant, *B. megapotamica* converted it to baccharinoid B7 (Jarvis et al., 1981), a metabolite found in this plant collected from Brazil. This Brazilian plant shows no toxic response to the macrocyclic trichothecenes, whereas all other plants tested, including a local Maryland species, *B. halimafolia,* are extremely sensitive to these highly potent phytotoxins (Jarvis et al., 1988; Culter and Jarvis, 1985). Later, other workers showed that a related Brazilian plant, *B. coridifolia* contained roridins A and E which appeared to account for the death of many cattle in southern Brazil that had ingested this plant (Habermehl et al., 1985). Microbiological examination of plant tissue and surrounding soils yielded isolates of *M. verrucaria* and *M. roridum* (Habermehl et al., 1985; Jarvis et al., 1987b), though there did not appear to be any unusual fungal activity associated with these plants.

On the surface, this system seems to be reminiscent of endophyte-produced mycotoxins, e.g. the lolitrems. However, several observations suggested to us that this system was not your usual endophyte-plant system. One aspect characteristic of endophytes and, in fact, fungi in general is that different isolates of the same species behave quite differently with respect to toxin production. Typically, isolates obtained from different sources have much different patterns of toxin production. It is not uncommon to have one isolate of a fungus be a good toxin producer and another isolate obtained from a similar source be a non-producing strain. In the case of endophytes, there is most often a great variation observed, even in the same field, with respect to which individual plants are infected. What was striking about these Brazilian *Baccharis* was that plants collected from regions separated by 1000 km all had approximately the same levels of toxins and the same distribution of roridins and verrucarins in each plant (Jarvis et al., 1988). Such consistency is certainly not characteristic of fungi.

During the course of a survey of Brazilian *Baccharis* with the objective of uncovering the putative fungus involved with the plants, one of the plant samples analyzed appeared to be devoid of macrocyclic trichothecenes (Jarvis et al., 1987b). This particular sample was that of a male *B. megapotamica. Baccharis* is a dioecious genus with the inflorescences appearing on separate male and female plants. In April of 1987, *B. coridifolia* was collected from two regions of Brazil. Analysis of the plants showed that the macrocyclic trichothecenes (roridins A, D, and E and verrucarins A and J) were only in the female plants; these toxins could not be detected in either the male plants or plants (presumably a mix of males and females) that had yet to come into flower (Jarvis et al., 1988). Furthermore, the toxins were concentrated in the seed heads where they were found almost exclusively in the seeds themselves. Although the seeds of *Baccharis* are tiny (few hundred micrograms each), the seeds were carefully dissected, and analysis showed that the toxins were restricted to the seed coats where their concentrations were measured to be as high as 50,000 ppm! Inspection of these plants for endophytes, by electron microscopy, was negative, and no fungi could be cultured from the seeds.

In May of 1987, *B. coridifolia* which had been grown from seed in our Maryland greenhouse came into flower (*B. megapotamica* has never done so in our greenhouse but has come into flower in one located in Irvine, CA). Three male and three female plants were grown together, and one female plant was segregated and prevented from being pollinated. During the course of the next two months, these plants were monitored for toxin production. None of the males nor the segregated female plant ever produced measurable quantities of the trichothecenes, but all of the female plants which had been pollinated by the males produced the roridins and verrucarins. Again, the toxins were localized in the seeds (Jarvis et al., 1988). In a recent experiment, we have performed the following experiment on a single female plant. Six sets of flowers were treated in the following manner: one set pollinated with the male of her species (*B. coridifolia*), four sets cross pollinated by males of different *Baccharis* species, and the sixth set was left unpollinated. A month later the seeds were harvested and analyzed for the toxins. Only the seeds pollinated by the male of her species contained the toxins; at best, the other seeds (actually unfertilized ova) contained, at best only traces of toxins (Fig. 2).

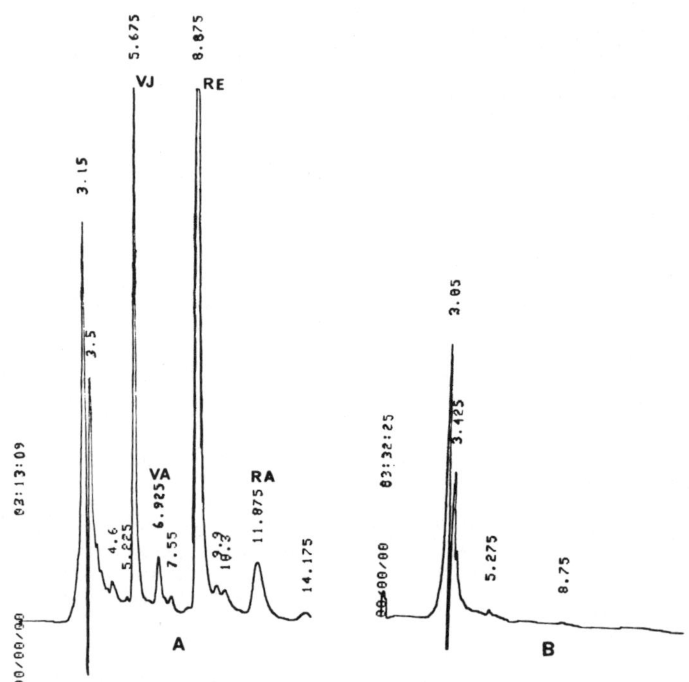

Fig. 2 Hplc trace (60% of 1% 2-propanol in ethyl acetate, 40% hexane, 5 micron silica Zorbax column, flow of 1 ml / min, detector at 265 nm) for extracts of *B. coridifolia* seeds. **A:** pollinated with *B. coridifolia*. **B:** unpollinated or cross pollinated with different *Baccharis* species. VJ, VA, RE, RA = verrucarins J and A and roridins E and A, respectively.

So there you have it. Not only does it appear that it is *B. coridifolia* itself that synthesizes the macrocyclic trichothecenes, but the biosynthesis is coupled to the pollination process, i.e. expression of the genes that control the biosynthesis of these toxins is controlled by the pollination process. We have examined a dozen other Brazilian *Baccharis* species as well as several North American species; with the exception of *B. coridifolia* and *B. megapotamica*, none appears to produce the macrocyclic trichothecenes.

These findings raise a number of intriguing questions most of which are related to chemical ecology. However, by far the most important is the question of how it is that these plants are able to synthesize macrocyclic trichothecenes in the first place. In the case of *B. coridifolia*, one must account for the fact that it produces ***exactly*** the same toxins, and in the same typical ratios, as is produced by *Myrothecium* fungi. The hplc trace shown in Fig. 2**A** could easily pass for that obtained from an extract of a *Myrothecium* culture (Jarvis et al., 1983). There are three possibilities to account for the ability of *Baccharis* to produce these trichothecenes: a) convergent evolution, b) divergent evolution and c) horizontal gene transfer from a fungus (*Myrothecium* is an obvious candidate) to *Baccharis*.[1]

There certainly are some spectacular examples of convergent evolution in nature (e.g. eye development in mammals and cephalopods). However, it is well known that many classes of secondary metabolites are restricted to certain types of organisms (Luckner, 1980). Thus, penicillins have never been found to be produced by higher plants, and with the exception of *Baccharis*, the same holds true for the trichothecenes. There certainly is nothing in theory that prevents higher plants from synthesizing the same secondary metabolites as are synthesized by fungi; it is just that many types of compounds appear to be restricted in their production. Of course, there are some noticeable exceptions: the prostanoids biosynthesized in mammals and soft coral by pathways clearly arrived at by convergent evolution (Corey et al., 1988). However, prostanoids are derived from arachidonic acid, a common fatty acid, by a relatively simple transformation. The molecular events leading from farnesylpyrophosphate to the macrocyclic trichothecenes are considerably more complex (Jarvis et al., 1982; Tamm and Breitenstein, 1980). It certainly would be extraordinary if *Baccharis* has acquired the ability to biosynthesize these toxins through convergent evolution. If this has indeed occurred, it would seem to be beyond the pale for the plant to have evolved the **same** set of genes to carry out the process (Dawkins, 1987). Divergent evolution also strikes me as being most unlikely. One would have to argue that the genes for toxin production have been conserved in *Baccharis* since the time of separation in evolution of the progenators of *Baccharis* and *Myrothecium*.. The fact that other plants, especially other *Baccharis* species do not produce trichothecenes, presumably would be due to their genes being "silent," i.e. not expressed.

The third possibility is that of interspecific gene transfer from a fungus to *Baccharis*. Although such transfers from bacteria and viruses to higher plants are known (Gardner and Houck, 1984), to my knowledge, no such interspecific transfer from a fungus to a higher plant has ever been reported. The number of genes involved in the biosynthesis of these macrocyclic trichothecenes is unknown but certainly must be substantial (Bu'Lock, 1980), and it is difficult to imagine how a large number of genes could be transferred and expressed in the plant host (Eckes et al., 1987; Schell, 1987), although the evolutionary principles of such a transfer have been presented (Lamboy, 1984). Perhaps one could argue that *Baccharis* already has much of the genetic machinery to make these compounds by virtue of its ability to biosynthesize related sesquiterpenes, and all the plant really required were a few critical genes to perfect the transformations; *Baccharis* is is a member of the Asteraceae family which is well known for its ability to produce sesquiterpenes (Herz, 1977).

If indeed *Baccharis* does biosynthesize the macrocyclic trichothecenes, there now appears to be the means to distinguish the above possibilities, i.e. convergent evolution, divergent evolution, or horizontal gene transfer. A critical enzyme, trichodienesynthetase, involved in the biosynthesis of trichothecenes in *Fusarium* has been isolated (Hohn and Vanmiddlesworth, 1986), and its gene cloned (Hohn, 1988). If this gene can be shown through hybridization experiments to be present in *Myrothecium*, it may be used as a probe to find out whether it is present in *Baccharis*. If it is, this would seem to rule out convergent evolution. On the otherhand, if the gene is present only in the two trichothecene producing species of *Baccharis* and not in other species of *Baccharis*, divergent evolution also would seem not to be a viable explanation.

There are other cases of unusual metabolites being found both in microorganisms and in higher plants, and the suggestion has been made that interspecific gene transfer could account for this (Bu'Lock, 1973). Several cases come to mind: the gibberellins and absissic acid (The latter has been reported present in mammalian brain tissue, Chen et al., 1988.), (Smith and Moss, 1985a), the ergot alkaloids being found in morning glory seeds (Groger, 1972), and the maytansinoid ansamitocins found in two families (Celastraceae and Euphorbiaceae) and three genera of higher plants (Smith and Powell, 1984). The latter case is particularly relevant since until the discovery of the maytansinoids in higher plants, the ansamitocins were the exclusive province of microorganisms. Sometime later, Japanese workers showed that an actinomycetes, *Actinosynnema pretiosum* produced compounds of a very similar nature (Asai et al., 1979; Hasegawa et al., 1983). Like our case with the trichothecenes in *Baccharis*, these plant-derived ansamitocins appear to be concentrated in the seeds of the plants (Nettleton et al., 1981; Powell et al., 1983).

[1] Prof. G.G. Habermehl has informed me that his laboratory has cultured *M. verrucaria* from beneath the surface of the roots of *B. coridifolia*. This suggests that the original hypothesis of the involvement of an associative fungus with *Baccharis* (Kupchan et al., 1976) may turn out to be correct. If so, it appears from our experiments that pollination of the flowers in the female plants somehow triggers the release of the toxins from the associative fungus to the plants resulting in their accumulation in the seeds.

One of the aims of this all too brief description of mycotoxins is to convince the reader that this subject is extraordinarily rich and that mycotoxins are not a class of obscure compounds with no relevance to matters outside microbiology. Rather, these fascinating fungal metabolites play roles in our lives that range from affecting the course of historical events to serving as tools in the emerging science of molecular biology. However, the interesting question of why the organisms themselves produce mycotoxins in the first place is fraught with teleological overtones, though it is an important but perhaps unanswerable question (Ciegler, 1983).

REFERENCES

Abbas, H.K. and C.J. Mirocha (1988). Isolation and purification of a hemorrhagic factor (wortmannin) from *Fusarium oxysporum* (N17B). *Appl. Environ. Microbiol.*, 54, 1268-1274.

Adler, S.S., S. Lowenbraum, B. Birch, R. Jarrell and J. Garrard (1984). Anguidine: a broad phase II study of the Southeastern Cancer Study Group. *Cancer Treatment Rep.*, 68, 423-432.

Asai, M., E. Mizuta, M. Izawa, K. Haibara and T. Kishi (1979). Isolation, chemical characterization and structure of ansamitocin, a new antitumor ansamycin antibiotic. *Tetrahedron*, 35, 1079-1085.

Ayres, J.L., D.J. Lee, J.H. Wales and R.O. Sinnhuber (1971). Aflatoxin structure and hepatocarcinogenicity in rainbow trout (*Salmo gairdner*), *J. Natl. Cancer Inst.*, 47, 561-565.

Betina, V., (Ed.) (1984). *Mycotoxins: Production, Isolation, Separation and Purification. Develop. Food Sci.*, Vol. 8. Elsevier, New York.

Bezuidenhout, S.C., W.C.A. Gelderblom, C.P. Gorst-Allman, R.M. Horak, W.F.O. Marasas, G. Spiteller and R. Vleggaar (1988). Structure elucidation of the fumonisins, mycotoxins from *Fusarium moniliforme. J. Chem. Soc. Chem. Commun.*, 743-745.

Bissett, J. (1987). Fungi associated with urea-formaldehyde foam insulation in Canada. *Mycopatholgia,* 99, 47-56.

Bu'Lock, J.D. (1973). In: *Nobel Symposia: Chemistry in Botanical Classification* (G. Bendz and J. Santesson, Eds.), p. 313. Academic Press, New York.

Bu'Lock, J.D. (1980). Mycotoxins as secondary metabolites. In: *The Biosynthesis of Mycotoxins* (P. S. Steyn, Ed.), p. 5. Academic Press, New York.

Busby, W.F., Jr. and G.N. Wogan (1981). Cytochalasins. In: *Mycotoxins and N-Nitroso Compound: Environmental Risks* (R.C. Shank, Ed.), Vol. II, pp. 259-290. CRC Press, Baco Raton, FL.

Busby, W.F., Jr. and G.N. Wogan (1981a). Aflatoxins. In: *Mycotoxins and N-Nitroso Compounds: Evnironmental Risks* (R.C. Shank, Ed.), Vol. II, pp. 3-28. CRC Press, Baco Raton, FL.

Busby, W.F., Jr. and G.N. Wogan (1981b). Psoralens. In: *Mycotoxins and N-Nitrosocompounds: Environmental Risks* (R.C. Shank, Ed.), Vol. II, pp. 105-119. CRC Press, Boca Raton, FL.

Caporael, L.R. (1976). Ergotism: the satan lossed in Salem. *Science* (Washington, D.C.), 192, 21-26.

Chen, F.S.C., J.M. Mactaggar, T., L.C.H. Wang and J. C. Westly (1988). Analytsis of absissic acid in the brains of rodents and ruminants. *Agric. Biol. Chem.*, 52, 1273-1274.

Ciegler, A., S. Kadis, and S.J. Ajl (Eds.) (1971). *Microbial Toxins*, Vols. VI, VII, VIII. Academic Press, New York.

Ciegler, A., H.R. Burneister, R.F. Vesonder and C.W. Hesseltine (1981). Mycotoxins: Occurrence in the environment. In: *Mycotoxin and N-Nitroso Compounds: Environmental Risks,* (R. C. Shank, Ed.), Vol. 1, pp. 1-50. CRC Press, Boca Raton, Fl.

Ciegler, A. (1983). Evolution, ecology and mycotoxins. *Mycol. Ser.*, 5, 429-439.

Clay, K. (1987). Grass endophytes. In: *Microbiology of the Phyllosphere,* (N. J. Fokkema and J. van den Heuvel, Eds.), pp. 189-204. Cambridge University Press, London.

Cole, R.J. and R.H. Cox (Eds.) (1981). *Handbook of Toxic Fungal Metabolites.* Academic Press, New York.

Cole, R.J. (Ed.) (1986). *Modern Methods in the Analysis and Structural Elucidation of Mycotoxins.* Academic Press, New York.

Cole, R.J. (1986a). Etiology of turkey "X" disease in retrospect: case for the involvement of cyclopiazonic acid. *Mycotoxin Res.*, 2, 3-7.

Cole, R.J. and J.M. Dorner (1986). Role of fungal tremorgens in animal diseases. In: *Mycotoxins and Phycotoxins,* (P.S. Steyn and R. Vleggaar, Eds.), pp. 501-511. Elsevier, Amsterdam.

Corey, E. J., S. P. T. Matsuda, R. Nagata and M. B. Cleaver (1988). Biosynthesis of 8-R-HPETE and preclavulone-A from arachidonate in several species of Caribbean coral. A widespread route to marine prostanoids. *Tetrahedron Lett.*, 29, 2555-2558.

Croft, W.A., B.B. Jarvis and C.S. Yatawara (1986). Airborne outbreak of trichothecene toxicosis. *Atmospheric Environ.*, 20, 549-552.

Cutler, H.C. and B.B. Jarvis (1985). Preliminary observations on the effects of macrocyclic trichothecenes on plant growth. *Exper. Environ. Bot.*, 25, 115-128.

Davis, R. M. and J. L. Richard (1984). Rubratoxins and related substances. In: *Mycotoxins: Production, Isolation, Separation and Purification. Develop. Food Sci.* (V. Betina, Ed.), Vol. 8, 315-328. Elsevier, New York.

Dawkins, R. (1987). *The Blind Watchmaker*, pp. 43-74. W. W. Norton & Co., New York.

Dorner, J.M., R.J. Cole, T.H. Sanders and P.D. Blankenship (1988). Interrelationship of kernal water activity, soil temperature, maturity and phytoalexin production in preharvest aflatoxin contamination of drought stressed peanuts. Submitted for publication.

Doyle, T.W. and W.T. Bradner (1980). Trichothecenes. In: *Anticancer Agents Based on Natural Product Models* (J.M. Cassidy and J.D. Douros, Eds.), pp. 43-72. Academic Press, New York.
Eckes, P., G. Donn and F. Wengenmayer (1987). Genetic engineering in plants. *Angew. Chem. Int. Ed. Engl.*, 26, 382-402.
Flannigan, B. (1987). Mycotoxins in the air. *Internat. Biodeterior.*, 23, 73-78.
Forgacs, J. (1972). Stachybotryotoxicosis. In: *Microbial Toxins* (S. Kadis, A.Ciegler and S. J. Ajl, Eds.), Vol. VIII, pp. 95-128. Academic Press, New York.
Freeman, G.G. and R.I. Morrison (1948). Trichothecin: an antifungal metabolic product of *Trichothecium roseum* Link. *Nature* (London), 162, 30.
Gardner, R. C. and C. M. Houck (1984). Development of plant vectors. In: *Plant-Microbe Interactions* (T. Kosuge and E. W. Nester, Eds.), Vol. 1, pp. 146-167. Macmillan Publishing Co., New York.
Gröger, D. (1972). Ergot. In: *Microbial Toxins* (S. Kadis, A. Ciegler and S.J. Ajl, Eds.), Vol. VIII, pp. 321-373. Academic Press, New York.
Habermehl, G.G., L. Busam, P. Heydel, D. Mebs, C.H. Tokarnia, J. Dobereiner and M. Spraul (1985). Macrocyclic trichothecenes: cause of livestock poisoning by the Brazilian plant *Baccharis coridifolia. Toxicon*, 23, 731-745.
Haefliger, W. and D. Hanser (1973). Isolierung und Strukturaufklarung von II-Desacetoxy-Wortmanniin. *Helv. Chim. Acta*, 56, 2901-2904 (In German).
Harrach, B., A. Bata, E. Bajmo'cy and M. Benko (1983). Isolation of satratoxins from the bedding straw of a sheep flock with fatal stachybotryotoxicosis. *Appl. Environ. Microbiol.*, 45, 1419-1422.
Hasegawa, T., S. Tanida, K. Hatano, E. Hagashide and M. Yoneda (1983). *Int. J. Syst. Bacteriol.*, 33, 314.
Hernandez, F. and M. Cannon (1982). Inhibition of protein synthesis in *Saccharomyces cerevisiae* by the 12,13-epoxytrichothecenes trichodermol, diacetoxyscirpenol and verrucarin A. *J. Antibiotics*, 35, 875-881.
Herz, W. (1977). Chemistry of *Baccharis*. In: *The Biology and Chemistry of the Compositae,* (V. H. Heywood, J. B. Harborne and B. L. Turner, Eds.), pp. 567-576. Academic Press, New York.
Hesseltine, C.W. (1986). Global significance of mycotoxins. In: *Mycotoxin and Phycotoxins* (P.J. Steyn and R. Vleggaar, Eds.), pp. 1-18. Elsevier, Amsterdam.
Hobden, A.N. and E. Cundliffe (1980). Ribosomal resistance to the 12,13-epoxytrichothecene antibiotics in the producing organism *Myrothecium verrucaria. Biochem. J.*, 190, 765-770.
Hohn, T. M. and F. Vanmiddlesworth (1986). Purification and chacterization of the sesquiterpene Cyclase Trichodiene Synthetase from *Fusarium sporotrichioides. Arch. Biochem. Biophys.*, 251, 756-761.
Hohn, T. M. (1988). Personal communication.
Hsieh, D.P.H. (1986). The role of aflatoxin in human cancer. In: *Mycotoxins on Phycotoxins* (P.S. Steyn and R. Vleggaar, Eds.), pp. 447-456. Elsevier, Amsterdam.
Ichinoe, M. and H. Kurata (1983). Trichothecene-producing fungi. In: *Trichothecenes-Chemical, Biological and Toxicological Aspects. Develop. Food Sci.* (Y. Ueno, Ed.), Vol 4, pp. 73-82. Kodansha LTD, Tokyo.
Jarvis, B.B., J.O. Midiwo, D.Tuthill and G.A. Bean (1981). Interaction between the antibiotic trichothecenes and the higher plant *Baccharis megapotamica. Science* (Washington, D.C.), 214, 460-462.
Jarvis, B. B., G. P. Stahly, G. Pavanasasivam, J. O. Midiwo, T. DeSilva, C. E. Holmlund, E. P. Mazzola and R. F. Geohegan, Jr. (1982). Isolation and characterization of the trichoverroids and new roridins and verrucarins. *J. Org. Chem.*, 47, 1117-1124.
Jarvis, B.B., R.M. Eppley and E.P. Mazzola (1983). Chemistry and bioproduction of macrocyclic trichothecenes. In: *Trichothecenes - Chemical, Biological and Toxicological Aspects Develop. Food Sci.*, (Y. Ueno, Ed.), Vol. 4, pp. 20-38. Kadansha LTD, Tokyo.
Jarvis, B.B., J.O. Midiwo and E.P. Mazzola (1984). Antileukimic compounds derived by chemical modifications of macrocyclic trichothecenes. 2. Derivatives of roridins A and H and verrucarins A and J. *J. MEd. Chem.*, 27, 239-244.
Jarvis, B.B., Y.-W. Lee, S.N. Çömozoḡlu and C.S. Yatawara (1986) Trichothecenes produced by *Stachybotrys atra* from eastern Europe. *Appl. Environ. Microbiol.*, 51, 915-918.
Jarvis, B.B., S.N. Çömezoḡlu, M.M. Rao, N.B. Pena, F.E. Boettner, Tara, M. Williams, G. Forsyth and B. Epling (1987). Isolation of macrocyclic trichothecenes from a large scale extract of *Baccharis megapotamica. J. Org. Chem.*, 52, 45-56.
Jarvis, B.B., S.N. Çömezoḡlu, H.L. Ammon, C.K. Breedlove, R.F. Bryan, R.W. Miller, M.K. Woode, D.R. Streelman, A.T. Sneden, R.G. Dailey, Jr. and S.M. Kupchan (1987a). New macrocyclic trichothecenes from *Baccharis megapotamica. J. Nat. Prod.*, 50, 815-828.
Jarvis, B.B., K. M. Wells, Y.-W. Lee, G. A. Bean, T. Kommedahl, C.S. Barros and S.S. Barros (1987b). Macrocyclic trichothecenes mycotoxins in Brazilian species of *Baccharis. Phytopathology*, 77, 980-984.
Jarvis, B.B., J.O. Midiwo, G.A. Bean, M.B. Aboul-Nasr and C.S. Barros (1988). The mystery of trichothecene antibiotics in *Baccharis* species. *J. Nat. Prod.*, 51, 736-744.
Joffe, A.Z. (1983). Foodborne diseases: alimentary toxic aleukia. In: *Handbook of Foodborne Diseases* (M. Rechcigl, Jr., Ed.), pp. 353-495. CRC Press, Boca Raton, FL.
Kaneko, T., H. Schmitz, J.M. Essery, W. Rose, H.G. Howell, R.A. O'Herron, S. Nochfolger, J. Huftalen, W.T. Bradner, R.A. Partyka, T.W. Doyle, J. Davies and E. Cundliffe (1982). Structural modifications of anguidine and antitumor activities of its analogues. *J. MEd. Chem.*, 25, 579-589.
Kaneko, T., H. Wong, H.G. Howell, W.C. Rose, W.T. Bradner and T.W. Doyle (1985). Reductive amination of C3-ketoanguidine and antitumor activity of the products. *J. MEd. Chem.*, 28, 958-960.

Keen, N. T. (1986). Phytoalexins and their involvement in plant disease resistance. *Iowa St. J. Res.*, 60, 477-499.

Khrushchev, N. (1970). *Khrushchev Remembers* (S. Talbott, Ed.), pp. 111-113. Little, Brown and Company, Boston.

Kupchan, S.M., B.B. Jarvis, R.G. Dailey, Jr., W. Bright, R.F. Bryan and Y. Shizuri (1976). Baccharin, a novel potent antileukimic trichothecene triepoxide from *Baccharis megapotamica*. *J. Am. Chem. Soc.*, 98, 7092-7093.

Kupchan, S.M., D.R. Streelman, B.B. Jarvis, R. G. Dailey, Jr. and A.T. Sneden (1977). The isolation of potent new antileukemic trichothecenes from *Baccharis megapotaica*. *J. Org. Chem.*, 42, 4221-4225.

Lacey, J. (1986). Factors affecting mycotoxin production. In: *Mycotoxins and Phycotoxins* (P.S. Steyn and R. Vleggaar, Eds.), pp. 65-76. Elsevier, Amsterdam.

Lacey, J. (Ed.) (1985). *Trichothecenes and Other Mycotoxins*. John Wiley & Sons, New York.

Lamboy, W. F. (1984). Evolution of flowering plants by fungus-to-host horizontal gene transfer. *Evolutionary Theory*, 7, 45-53.

Latch, G.C.M. (1985). In: *Trichothecenes and Other Mycotoxins* (J. Lacey, Ed.), pp. 135-140. John Wiley & Sons, New York.

Luckner, M. (1980). Expression and control of secondary metabolism. In : *Secondary Plant Products* (E. A. Bell and B. V. Charlwood, Eds.), pp. 23-63. Springer-Verlag, New York.

Lyons, P.C., R.D. Plattner and C.W. Bacon (1986). Occurrence of peptide and clavine ergot alkaloids in tall fescue grass. *Science* (Washington, D.C.), 232, 487-489.

MacMillan, J., A.E. Vanstone and S.K. Yeboah (1972). Fungal products. 3. Structure of wortmannin and some hydrolysis products. *J. Chem. Soc. Perkins Trans* 1., 22, 2898-2903.

Marasas, W.F.O., P.E. Nelson and T.A. Toussoun (1984). *Toxigenic Fusarium Species*. The Pennsylvania State University Press, University Park and London.

Marasas, W.F.O., P.E. Nelson and T.A. Toussoun (1984a), *ibid.*, p. 220.

Marasas, W.F.O., P.E. Nelson and T.A. Toussoun (1984b), *ibid.*, pp. 76-76.

Marasas, W.F.O., P.E. Nelson and T.A. Toussoun (1984c), *ibid.*, pp. 217-219.

Matossian, M.K. (1983). The time of the great fear. *The Sciences* (New Academy of Sciences), pp. 38-41.

McLaughlin, C.S., M. H. Vanghan, I.M. Campbell, C.M. Wei, M.E. Stafford and B.S. Hansen (1977). Inhibition of protein synthesis by trichothecenes. In: *Mycotoxins in Human and Animal Health* (J.V. Rodricks, C.W. Hesseltine and M.A. Mehlman, Eds.), pp. 263-273. Pathotox Publishers, Park Forest South, IL.

Mirocha, C.J. (1988). Personal communication.

Mirocha, C.J., S.V. Pathre and C.M. Christensen (1977). Zearalanone. In: *Mycotoxins in Human and Animal Health* (J.V. Rodricks, C.W. Hesseltine and M.A. Mehlman, Eds.), pp. 345-364. Pathotox Publishers, Park forest South, IL.

Mirocha, C.J., S.V. Pathre and C.M. Christensen (1980). Mycotoxins. In: *Advances in Cereal Science and Technology* (Y. Pomeranz, Ed.), Vol. 3, pp. 159-225. American Association of Cereal Chemists, Inc., St. Paul, MN.

Nagarajan, R. (1984). Gliotoxin and epipolythiodioxopiperazines. In: *Mycotoxins: Production, Isolation, Separation and Purification., Delelop. Food Sci.* (V. Betina, Ed.), Vol. 8, pp. 351-385. Elsevier, New York.

Nettleton, D. E., Jr., D. M. Balitz, M. Brown, J. E. Moseley and R. W. Myllymaki (1981). Large scale isolation of maytansine and other maytansinoids from the seeds of *Maytenus rothiana* using preparative LC. *J. Nat. Prod.*, 44, 340-347.

Ohtsubo, K. (1983). Chronic toxicity of trichothecenes. In: *Trichothecenes - Chemical, Biological and Toxicological Aspects. Develop. Food Sci.* (Y. Ueno, Ed.), Vol. 4, pp. 171-176. Kodansha LTD, Tokyo.

Pathre, S.V., W.B. Gleason, Y.-W. Lee and C.J. Mirocha (1986). The structure of fusarochromanone: New mycotoxin from *Fusarium roseum*, "Graminearum." *Can. J. Chem.*, 64, 1308-1311.

Petcher, T.J., H.P. Weber and Z. Kis (1972). Crystal structure and absolute configuration of wortmannin and wortmannin p-bromobenzoate. *J. Chem. Soc. Chem. Commun.*, 1061-1062.

Pier, A.C. and M.E. McLoughlin (1985). Mycotoxin suppression of immunity. In: *Trichothecenes and other Mycotoxins.* (J. Lacey, Ed.), pp. 507-519. John Wiley & Sons, New York.

Powell, R.G., C.R. Smith, Jr., R.D. Plattner and B.E. Jones (1983). Additional new maytansinoids from *Trewia nudifolia*: 10-epitrewiasine and nortrewiasine. *J. Nat. Prod.*, 46, 660-666.

Prevot, A. (1986). Chemical detoxification of aflatoxin-contaminated peanut meal. In: *Mycotoxins and Phycotoxins* (P.S. Steyn and R. Vleggaar, Eds.), pp. 34-351. Elsevier, Amsterdam.

Putnum, A. and C.-S. Tang (Eds.), (1986). *The Science of Allelopathy*. John Wiley & Sons, New York.

Rechcigl, M., Jr. (Ed.) (1983). *Handbook of Foodborne Diseases of Biological Origin*. CRC Press, Boca Raton, Fl.

Rodricks, J.V., C.W. Hesseltine and M.A. Mehlman (Eds.) (1977). *Mycotoxins in Human and Animal Health*, Pathotox, Park Forest South, Il.

Schell, J. S. (1987). Transgenic plants as tools to study the molecular organization of plant genes. *Science* (Washington, D. C.), 237, 1176-1183.

Schneider, D.J., W.F.O. Marasas, J.C.D. Kuys, N.P.J. Kriek and G.C. Van Schalkwyk (1979). A field outbreak of suspected stachybotryotoxicosis in sheep. *J. S. Afr. Vet. Assoc.*, 50, 73-81.

Schwarte, L.H. (1938). Moldy corn poisoning in horses. *JARVMA*, 92, 152-158.

Scott, P.M. (1984). Effects of food processing on mycotoxins. *J. Food Protec.*, 47, 489-499.

Shank, R.C. (Ed.) (1981). *Mycotoxins and N-Nitroso Compounds: Environmental Risks*, Vols. I and II. CRC Press, Boca Raton, Fl.

Siegel, M.R., G.C.M. Latch and M.C. Johnson (1985). *Acremonium* fungal endophytes of tall fecue and perennial

rye grass: significance and control. *Plant Disease,* 69, 179-183.
Smith, C.R. and R.G. Powell (1984). Chemistry and pharmacology of maytansinoid alkaloids. In: *Alkaloids: Chemical and Biological Perspectives* (W. S. Pelletier, Ed.), Vol. 2, p.149. John Wiley & Sons, New York.
Smith, J.E. and M.O. Moss (1985). *Mycotoxins: Formation, Analysis and Significance.* John Wiley & Sons, New York.
Smith, J.E. and M.O. Moss (1985a). *Ibid.*, pp. 41-42.
Sorenson, W.G., D.G. Frazer and B.B. Jarvis (1987). Trichothecene mycotoxins in airborne conidia of *Stachybotrys atra. Appl. Environ. Microbiol.*, 53, 1370-1375.
Stark, A.-A. (1986). Molecular aspects of aflatoxin B_1 mutagenesis and carcinogensis. In: *Mycotoxins and Phycotoxins* (P.S. Steyn and R. Vleggaar, Eds.), pp. 435-445. Elsevier, Amsterdam.
Steyn, P. S. (1984). Ochratoxins and related dihydroisocoumerins. In: *Mycotoxins: Production, Isolation, Separation and Purification. Develop. Food Sci.* (V. Betina, Ed.), Vol. 8, pp. 183-216. Elsevier, New York.
Steyn, P.S. and R. Vleggaar (Eds.) (1986). *Mycotoxins and Phycotoxins.* Elsevier, Amsterdam.
Tamm, Ch. (1980). The biosynthesis of the cytochalasans. In: *The Biosynthesis of Mycotoxins* (P.S. Steyn, Ed.), pp. 269-299. Academic Press, New York.
Tamm, Ch. and W. Breitenstein (1980). The biosynthesis of trichothecene mycotoxins. In: *The Biosynthesis of Mycotoxins* (P.S. Steyn, Ed.), pp. 69-104. Academic Press, New York.
Ueno, Y. (1980). Trichothecene mycotoxins: mycology, chemistry, and toxicology. *Adv. Nutr. Sci.*, 3, 301-353.
Ueno, Y. (1986). Toxicology of microbial toxins. *Pure & Appl. Chem* ., 58, 339-350.
Vesonder, R.F. (1983). Natural occurrence in North America. In: *Trichothecenes - Chemical, Biological and Toxicological Aspects Develop. Food Sci.* (Y. Ueno, Ed.), Vol. 4, pp. 210-217. Kodansha LTD, Tokyo.
Yagen, B., A.Z. Joffe, P. Horn, N. Mor and I.I. Lutsky (1977). Toxins from a strain involved in ATA. In: *Mycotoxins in Human and Animal Health* (J.V. Rodricks, C.W. Hesseltine and M.A. Mehlman, Eds.), pp. 329-336. Pathotox Publishers, Park Forest South, IL.
Yarom, R., Y. Sherman, R. Moore, I. Ginsburg, R. Borinski and B. Yagen (1984). T-2 toxin effect on bacterial infection and leukocyte functions. *Toxicol. Appl. Pharmacol.*, 75, 60-68.
Young, J.C., H.L. Trenholm, D.W. Friend and D.B. Prelusky (1987). Detoxification of deoxynivalenol with sodium bisulfite and evaluation of the effects when pure mycotoxin or contaminated corn was treated and given to pigs. *J. Agric. Food Chem.*, 35, 259-261.

THE IDENTIFICATION, METABOLISM AND TOXICITY ASSOCIATED WITH THE MACROCYCLIC PYRROLIZIDINE ALKALOIDS

H. J. Segall, D. W. Wilson, D. S. Griffin, C. K. Winter, D. M. Morin and M. W. Lame'

Department of Veterinary Pharmacology and Toxicology, University of California
Davis, California 95616

Department of Veterinary Pathology, University of California
Davis, California 95616

Environmental Protection Agency, Washington, D. C.

Department of Entomology, University of California
Riverside, California 96521

ABSTRACT

The macrocyclic pyrrolizidine alkaloids (PAs) are phytotoxins produced by numerous plant species worldwide. Many are hepatotoxins or lung toxins which have been responsible for numerous livestock losses and human poisonings. Using PAs derived from *Senecio vulgaris* (common groundsel) and *Crotalaria retusa* (golden yellow sweet pea) and a variety of *in vitro* and *in vivo* techniques, the PAs have been shown to undergo a number of metabolic transformations. Our laboratory used the PA senecionine, mouse hepatic microsomes and appropriate cofactors to identify 4 metabolites. These PA metabolites have been isolated using a number of analytical techniques including HPLC, GC-MS and MS-MS. These techniques have been incorporated in comparative species studies of the hepatic metabolism.

One of the metabolites identified in the mouse hepatic microsomal system was *trans*-4-OH-2-hexenal. Other *trans* alkenals such as *trans*-4-OH-2-nonenal have been identified as major lipid peroxidation products arising due to the toxicity of CCl_4 and $BrCCl_3$. The hepatic pathological changes due to the hydroxyalkenals have been closely correlated to that assigned to senecionine. The *in vitro* formation of cyclic adducts of the alkenals with deoxyguanosine and the *in vivo* covalent binding to rat hepatic macromolecules were isolated. The *in vitro* effects of the alkenals on mouse liver cytochrome P-450 as well as the metabolism by mouse liver aldehyde dehydrogenase were examined. An *in vivo* distribution study of the *trans*-4-OH-2-hexenal recently resulted in the identification of the urinary mercapturic acid of this alkenal.

Further studies have shown the PAs as well as the alkenals exhibit genotoxicity as well as cytotoxicity in isolated hepatocytes. Lipid peroxidation was also examined as a possible mechanism for cell injury. This was followed by treating isolated hepatocytes with the above compounds and examining the role of cellular calcium homeostasis plus the effects of intracellular calcium compartmentation.

It has been estimated that as many as 6000 plant species or 3% of the flowering plants in the world contain PAs (Bull, Culvenor and Dick, 1968). Many are hepatotoxins or lung toxins which have been responsible for numerous livestock poisonings and losses (McLean, 1970; Mattocks, 1972; Culvenor and Smith, 1981; Mattocks, 1986). Grains, bread, milk, honey and herbal teas contaminated with PAs have either caused human poisonings or represent potential sources of human poisonings (Hill and others, 1951; Bras, Jelliffee and Stuart, 1954; Mohabbat and others, 1976; Dickinson and others, 1976; Deinzer and others, 1977; Huxtable, 1980; Culvenor and others, 1980). The macrocyclic PA native to many Senecio species throughout the world, senecionine, is hepatotoxic and has been shown to cause centrilobular hepatocellular necrosis and megalocytosis (McLean, 1970; Allen, Hsu and Carstens, 1975; Petry and others, 1984). Senecionine has been shown to be cytotoxic, mutagenic and genotoxic (Williams and others, 1980; Green, Segall and Byard, 1981; Candrian and others, 1984; Pearson and others, 1984; Mori and others, 1985; Griffin and Segall, 1986) with the toxicity attributed to the formation of reactive pyrroles by the action of hepatic microsomal enzyme systems (Mattocks and White, 1971; White and Mattocks, 1971; Mattocks, 1986).

Much of the metabolism studies of the PAs up to the 1980s had been performed by two groups, Culvenor and his associates at CSIRO and Mattocks with his research group at the MRC. An appreciation of the metabolism of the PAs is important in understanding their varied effects. Evidence has shown that specific PA metabolites originating in the liver rather than the in toto alkaloid were the cause of toxicity (Mattocks, 1986; Mattocks, 1972; Mattocks, 1973). The toxicity of PAs to animals was markedly influenced by the action of compounds that modify the activity of liver metabolizing enzymes. In addition, the major site of damage by the PAs was the liver, which was also the major site of PA metabolism. Finally, the PAs did not produce localized toxicity when applied directly to the skin.

Toxic PAs typically exist as esters of the amino alcohols retronecine or heliotridine (Figure 1) (Mattocks, 1972; Mattocks, 1986). Structural requirements for toxicity are branching of the ester function and unsaturation at the 1-2 position of the pyrrolizidine nucleus (Mattocks, 1973; Culvenor and other, 1976; Mattocks, 1981; Peterson and Culvenor, 1983; Culvenor and others, 1976; Mattocks, 1986).The major pathways for the metabolism of PAs in the liver have been established in laboratory animals and are hydrolysis, N- oxidation and dehydrogenation to pyrrolic derivatives (Figure 2). Both N-oxidation and hydrolysis are believed to be detoxification mechanisms (Mattocks and White, 1971; Mattocks, 1986). Dehydrogenation is thought to represent metabolic activation of the PAs and the majority of PA toxicity has been attributed to the production of toxic pyrrolic metabolites (Mattocks, 1968a; Mattocks and Legg, 1980; Mattocks, 1986).

Mattocks developed a colorimetric method for the analysis of PAs and pyrrolizidine alkaloid N-oxides (Mattocks, 1967b; Mattocks, 1968b) which has recently been improved (Mattocks and Jukes, 1987). In performing the colorimetric test on rat tissues, blood and urine, Mattocks observed that the pyrroles were present in animals provided PAs (Mattocks, 1968a). Pyrroles are formed from PAs through the action of the mixed function oxidase system which are located in the microsomes of a number of organs, but predominantly the liver (Culvenor, Edgar and Smith, 1970; Mattocks and White, 1971; Mattocks, 1973; Mattocks, 1986). Reduced NADP and oxygen are necessary for pyrrole production with recent studies suggesting that cytochrome P-450 monooxygenases may play an important role in pyrrole formation (Buhler and Kedzierski, 1986). The only naturally occurring PA available commercially is monocrotaline and no PA at the present time can be purchased either carbon 14 or tritium radiolabeled. The source of the PAs that we have used has been Senecio vulgaris (common groundsel) and its most abundant PAs are senecionine, seneciphylline and retrorsine. We felt that rapid methods to isolate and identify macrocyclic PAs and their metabolites would facilitate future metabolism studies. The results of these studies were a number of High Performance Liquid Chromatography (HPLC) methods (analytical & preparative) which were adapted for later metabolism studies (Segall, 1979a; Segall, 1979b).

To perform metabolism studies, radiolabeled PAs were obtained by raising S. vulgaris in an enclosed chamber and providing various concentrations and periods of carbon 14 carbon dioxide exposure (Segall, Brown and Paige, 1983). To ensure that fairly uniform labeling was obtained, a carbon 14 and carbon 13 incorporation study was performed. A fairly uniform

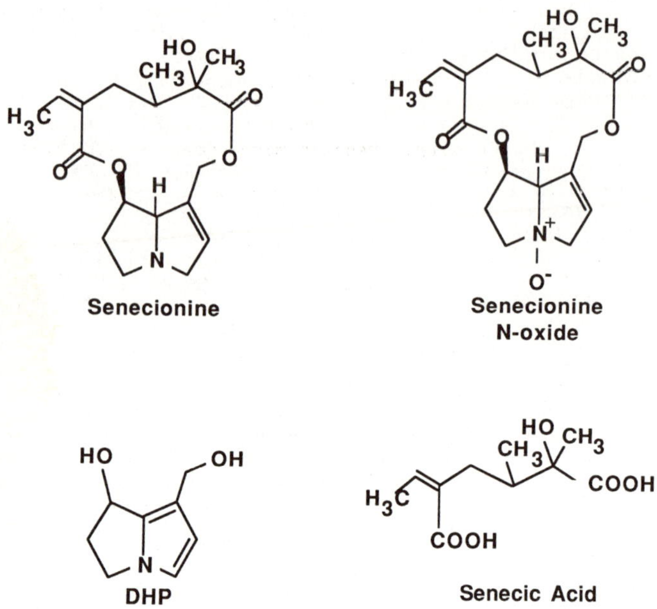

Figure 1 Structures of senecionine, senecionine N-oxide, dihydropyrrole (DHP) and senecic acid.

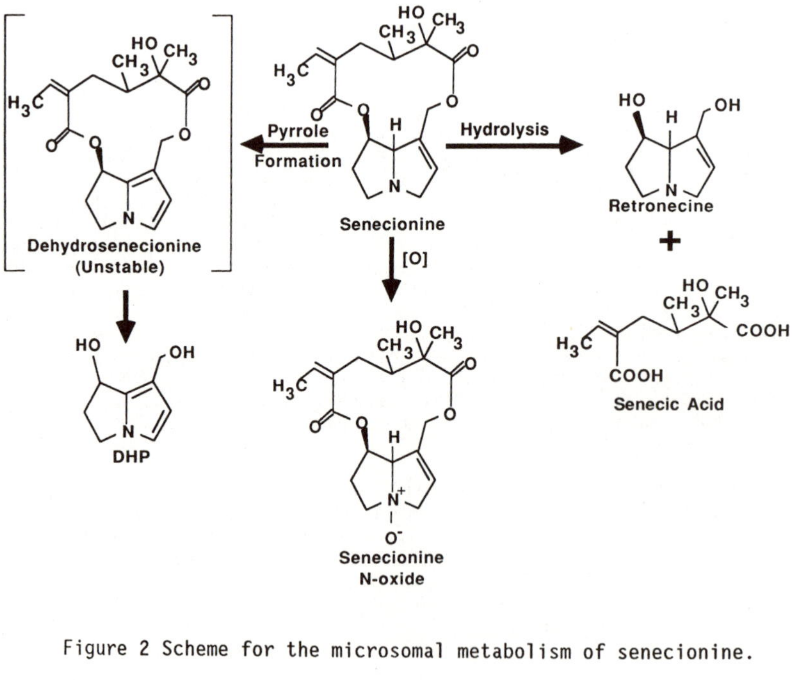

Figure 2 Scheme for the microsomal metabolism of senecionine.

incorporation of carbon 13 was obtained (5.25%-6.25% enrichment) which indicated that carbon 14 would be incorporated in a similar fashion. A follow up experiment using an increased concentration of carbon 14 carbon dioxide yielded the above three alkaloids with specific activities suitable for metabolism studies.

To facilitate the identification of metabolites, the PAs retrorsine, seneciphylline, senecionine and their N-oxides were examined with ^{1}H NMR (Segall and Dallas, 1983). This study plus prior ^{1}H NMR reports aided in the identification of metabolites. To isolate and identify PA metabolites, a rat in vitro hepatic microsomal system, NADPH generating system and the macrocyclic PA senecionine were used. The reactions were stopped 45 minutes later, protein precipitated and the supernatant further purified by a number of chromatography steps that have previously been described (Eastman and Segall, 1982; Segall, Dallas and Haddon, 1983; Segall and others, 1985). The compounds expected in the supernatant based on prior literature reports were senecic acid, senecionine N-oxide, plus unreacted senecionine and these were identified. A number of additional metabolites were identified with the aid of the carbon 14 radiolabeled senecionine. These metabolites were 19-hydroxysenecionine, methoxydehydroretronecine, and hydroxydanaidal which were all pyrrolic compounds. An additional metabolite appeared to rapidly decompose/polymerize, and precipitated with the formation of a dark reddish brown/ purple color during the isolation process. The difficulties in isolating this reactive PA metabolite had been previously described (Butler, Mattocks and Barnes, 1970; Mattocks and Bird, 1983). However, as this metabolite may have originated from either the senecic acid or back portion of senecionine, additional S. vulgaris plants were provided 2-^{14}C ornithine (Green, Segall and Byard, 1981). Prior experiments utilizing Senecio species provided 2-^{14}C ornithine had shown specific incorporation at carbons 7, 8 and 9 of the PA (Bottomley and Geissman, 1964; Hughes, Letcher and Warren, 1964). Separate in vitro mouse hepatic microsomal experiments using ^{14}C senecionine from 2-^{14}C ornithine or $^{14}CO_2$ were performed. This metabolite was determined to be derived from the retronecine portion of senecionine with gas chromatography-mass spectrometry (GC-MS) indicating a molecular weight of 114 with an elemental composition of $C_6H_{10}O_2$ (Segall and others, 1985). An initial proton NMR spectrum indicated that the metabolite was trans-4- hydroxy-2-hexenal (t-4HH, Figure 3). trans-4-Hydroxy-2-hexenal was synthesized according to a literature procedure and the structure confirmed with NMR and MS (Erickson, 1974).

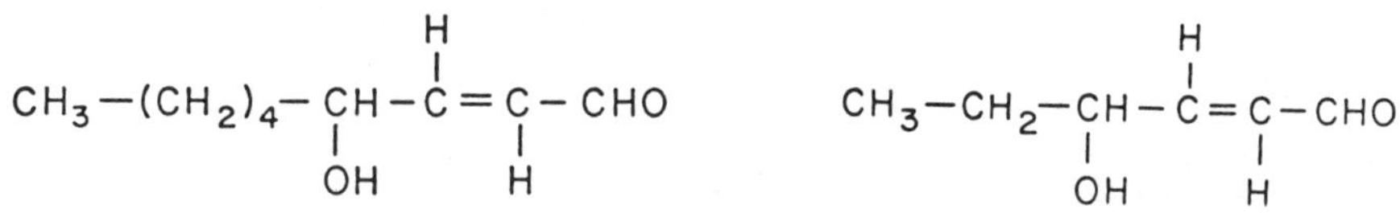

t-4HN **t-4HH**

Figure 3 Structures of t-4HN and t-4HN.

Prior reports have indicated that PA toxicity in vivo was markedly decreased in mice and rats by increasing glutathione and cysteine levels (White, 1976; Miranda and others, 1983). In addition, sulfhydryl groups of low molecular weight thiols (cysteine, glutathione) and proteins will react with 4-hydroxyalkenals to initially form a saturated aldehyde with the first SH group and then react with a second SH group to form a cyclic hemiacetal (Esterbauer, Ertl and Scholz, 1976; Esterbauer, Zollner and Scholz, 1975).

The nonenzymatic autoxidation of polyunsaturated fatty acids is known to cause increased formation of alkenals, alk-2-enals, malonaldehyde and 4-hydroxy alkenals (Schauenstein, 1967; Schaenstein, 1977; Lowry, 1973). A number of alkenals are formed during microsomal lipid peroxidation and some of these alkenals, such as the hydroxyalkenals, are effective nonradical products which could be responsible for part of the effects associated with lipid peroxidation (Casini and others, 1978; Benedetti, Comporti, Esterbauer, 1980; Ferrali, Fulceri, Benedetti, Comporti, 1980; Benedetti and others, 1981; Benedetti and others, 1981; Esterbauer, 1982; Esterbauer and others, 1982). Benedetti, Comporti and Esterbauer, 1980 and Esterbauer and others, 1982 have demonstrated that alkenals are produced during stimulated (ADP-Fe^{+2} or NADPH-Fe^{+2}) microsomal lipid peroxidation and that these alkenals (in particular 4-hydroxyalkenals) could be responsible for part of the destructive effects caused by lipid peroxidation on cells and cell constituents. Senecionine and t-4HH both cause hepatic necrosis when injected as a lipid suspension into the portal vein of rats. The distribution of the necrosis suggests that senecionine requires metabolic activation while t-4HH appeared to be a direct acting hepatotoxin (Wilson, Segall and Lame', 1986). Cytotoxic alkenals originating due to lipid peroxidation were shown to damage cellular membranes of red blood cells, inhibit protein synthesis, and decreased the activity of membrane bound enzymes such as microsomal glucose-6-phosphatase, cytochrome P-450, and aminopyrine N-demethylase (Benedetti, Casini, Ferrali, 1977; Roders, Glende, Recknagel, 1977; Casini and others, 1978; Ferrali, Fulceri, Benedetti, Comporti, 1980; Benedetti and others, 1981 and Benedetti and others, 1981). Further investigations have determined that alkenal compounds may play an important role in liver injury caused by CCl_4 and $BrCCl_3$ (Benedetti and others, 1982a; Benedetti and others, 1982b). Alkenal groups are formed in phospholipids of liver microsomes as a consequence of the peroxidative cleavage of phospholipids-bound unsaturated fatty acids after in vivo intoxication with CCl_4 and $BrCCl_3$ (Benedetti and others, 1982). This article will discuss the metabolism of the PAs and the toxicity/relationship exhibited by the PAs and the alkenals.

Tritiated t-4HH was synthesized with the reaction facilitated by initially tritiating propanal (Erickson, 1974). The in vivo binding of [^{3}H]t-4HH to rat liver DNA, RNA and protein was investigated with the results indicating that no significant binding to hepatic DNA or RNA could be detected (Grasse, Lame' and Segall, 1985). Levels of 429 + 139 pmol/mg were found covalently bound to hepatic proteins 16 h following exposure with levels as high as 916 pmol/mg protein 2 h after administration via the hepatic portal.

The distribution of [^{3}H]t-4HH was examined following the injection into the hepatic portal vein of male Sprague-Dawley rats (Winter, Segall and Jones, 1987). Less than 3% of the tritium label remained in the liver 24 hr following administration, with levels in the other major organs appropriately lower. The majority of recovered radioactivity appeared in the urine with 60-69% appearing within 8 hr after administration. Most of the urinary radioactivity (75%) was recovered in an acidic fraction following acid/base extraction. A tandem mass spectrometry technique using negative fast atom bombardment (FAB) ionization in combination with Mass analyzed Ion Kinetic Energy Spectrometry verified that a C-3 mercapturic acid conjugate of t-4HH was produced as a urinary metabolite. This compound presumably forms via a Michael addition of glutathione at C-3 of t-4HH followed by hydrolysis of glutamate and glycine and acetylation to yield the mercapturic acid (Figure 4). While Michael additions of glutathione to t-4HH related compounds have been observed in vitro, these results provided in vivo evidence of this mechanism.

Another approach we have taken in examining t-4HH and the alkenal commonly isolated from lipid peroxidation studies, trans-4-hydroxy-2-nonenal (t-4HN, Figure 3), has been to react them in vitro with deoxyguanosine at pH 7.4 at 37° (Winter, Segall and Haddon, 1986). Each compound yielded two pairs of diastereomeric adducts which were isolated using HPLC and characterized by their mass spectra and proton magnetic resonance spectra (Figure 5). Adducts 1 and 2 from t-4HH were assigned the structures 3-(2-deoxy-B-D-erythro-pentofuranosyl)-5,6,7,8-tetrahedro-8R-hydroxy-6S[1-(R and S) hydroxypropyl] pyramidol[1,2-a] purine-10-(3H)one. Similar 6-hydroxyhexyl adducts were isolated in the reaction of deoxyguanosine with t-4HN. The reactions appear to involve Michael additions of the N^2 amino acid of deoxyguanosine followed by cyclization at the 1-N site. This reaction mechanism is similar to that reported for deoxyguanosine adduct formation with the nonhydroxylated a,B-unsaturated aldehydes crotonaldehyde and acrolein. Total adduct formations following 16 hr incubations were 0.91% for t-4HH and 0.85% for t-4HN. These results demonstrated that t-4HH and t-4HN possess the ability to alkylate deoxyguanosine in vitro and suggest possible mechanisms for 4-hydroxyalkenal and PA genotoxicity.

To demonstrate similarities in the toxicities of the alkenals and the PAs, genotoxicity and cytotoxicity were examined in primary cultures of rat hepatocytes (Griffin and Segall, 1986). A positive cytotoxic response was exhibited by senecionine, retrorsine, seneciphylline, 19-OH-senecionine, t-4HH, t-4HN, and nonenal as measured by the release of LDH. A weaker response was elicited by hexenal. All of the above compounds exhibited a positive, dose-related genotoxic response as measured by autoradiographic detection for both the PAs and the alkenals. This suggested similarities in the mechanism of action of the PAs and alkenals and supports the role of t-4HH as an important toxic metabolite of the PAs.

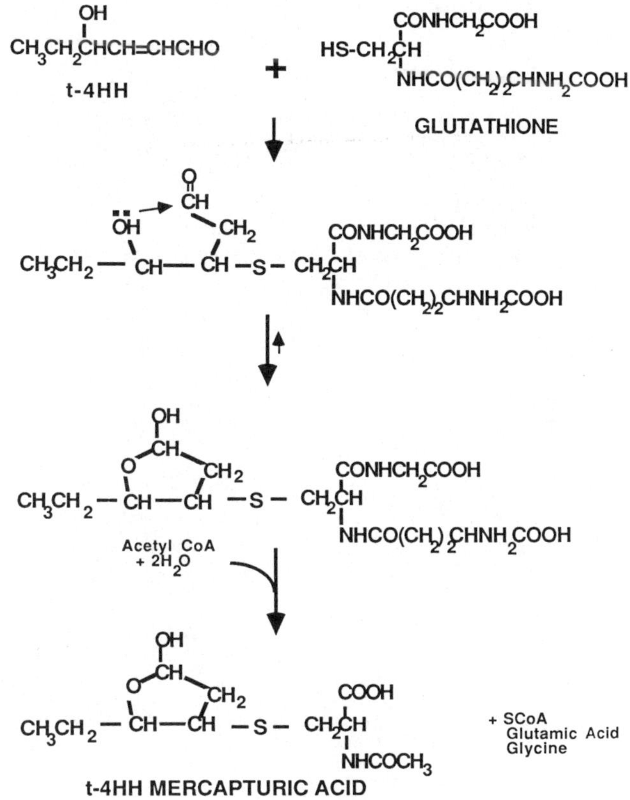

Figure 4 Proposed mechanism for the in vivo formation of t-4HH mercapturic acid.

In a followup study, lipid peroxidation was examined as a possible mechanism for cell injury by t-4HH, related alkenals and the PA senecionine in isolated rat hepatocytes (Griffin and Segall, 1987a). Each of the compounds elicited a positive dose response for peroxidation of cellular lipids as measured by the formation of thiobarbituric acid-reactive products. The addition of the anti-oxidant N,N'-diphenyl-p-phenylenediamine to the hepatocyte suspensions inhibited the production of thiobarbituric acid-reactants. However, the presence of the anti-oxidant had no protective effects on the cell membrane integrity as evidenced by the leakage of lactate dehydrogenase from the cells into the surrounding media. These results suggested that lipid peroxidation which occurs in the presence of senecionine, t-4HH or related alkenals is not entirely responsible for the cellular damage in isolated hepatocytes. A further study using the same compounds examined the role of calcium homeostasis in isolated rat hepatocytes (Griffin and Segall, 1987b). Hepatocytes treated with senecionine and t-4HH demonstrated greater cytotoxicity (leakage of lactate dehydrogenase) when incubated in the absence of extracellular Ca^{2+} than in its presence. Both compounds elicited an increase in cytosolic Ca^{2+} levels of isolated hepatocytes in the presence of extracellular Ca^{2+}. In a related study, senecionine and t-4HH depleted intracellular glutathione levels and induced lipid peroxidation and cytotoxicity in isolated hepatocytes (Griffin and Segall, 1987b). Pretreatment with the thiol reducing agent dithiothreitol prevented depletion of intracellular glutathione and protected hepatocytes against senecionine and t-4HH-induced lipid peroxidation and cytotoxicity. Both compounds also depleted intracellular ATP and NADPH levels. These results suggest that hepatoxicity

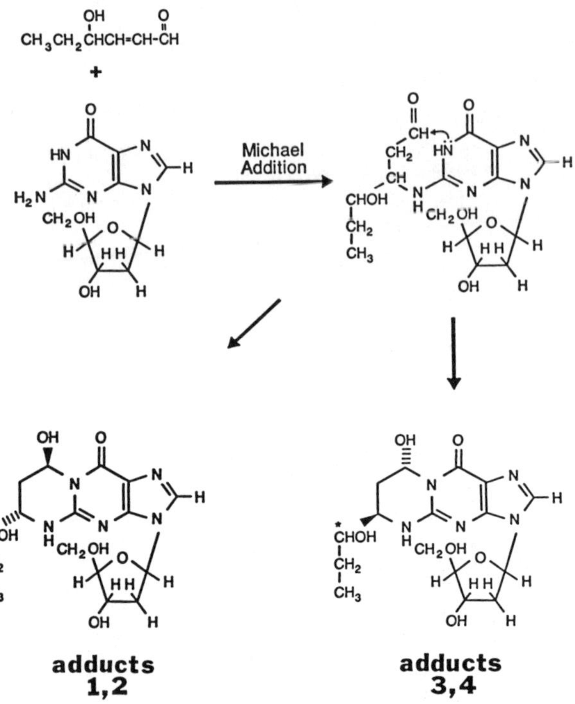

Figure 5 Proposed reaction mechanism for formation of t-4HH deoxyguanosine adducts.

induced by senecionine and t-4HH is not dependent on the influx of extracellular Ca^{2+}; however, alterations in intracellular Ca^{2+}, possibly associated with depletion of intracellular glutathione, NADPH, and ATP, may play a critical role. A related study examined the effects of senecionine, t-4HH and t-2H on the sequestration of Ca^{2+} in mitochondrial and extramitochondrial compartments in isolated hepatocytes. Each of the test compounds elicited a decrease in the available extramitochondrial Ca^{2+} stores which was inhibited by pretreatment with dithiothreitol. Senecionine and t-4HH decreased the level of Ca^{2+} sequestered in the mitochondrial compartment of the hepatocytes while the presence of the nucleotide reducing agent, B-hydroxybutryrate, inhibited this reduction. These results suggested that both senecionine and t-4HH inhibit the sequestration of Ca^{2+} in extramitochondrial and mitochondrial compartments possibly by inactivating free sulfhydryl groups and oxidizing pyridine nucleotides, respectively.

An additional protective measure against PA toxicity may be an increase in aldehyde dehydrogenase. Pregnant mice exhibit a three-fold increase in cytosolic aldehyde dehydrogenase levels and appear to have an increased resistance to PAs (Smolen, Petersen and Collins, 1981). The isolation of trans-4-hydroxy-2-hexenal may provide a partial explanation for this situation.

The in vitro effects of t-4HH, propionaldehyde (PAL) and trans-2-hexenal (t-2H) was examined by mouse liver cytochrome P-450 (Lame' and Segall, 1986). Kinetic experiments with hepatic cytosol as a source for aldehyde dehydrogenase(s) resulted in linear Lineweaver-Burk plots for both t-4HH and t-2H, while PAL produced biphasic plots. Values of 43 and 3 uM were obtained for the apparent Km values for t-4HH and t-2H, respectively, with the two apparent Kms for PAL being 5 uM and 0.8 mM. DEAE-cellulose chromatography of cytosol isolated two peaks capable of oxidizing PAL, but only one peak was able to metabolize t-4HH. Unlike cytosol, mitochondria produced biphasic Lineweaver-Burk plots for t-4HH with two estimated Kms of 52 uM and 0.2mM. The majority of activity for the oxidation of t-4HH, like PAL, was localized in the cytosolic fraction.

Recent studies have produced a rapid sensitive identification and quantification of important PA metabolites using MS/MS and GC/MS (Winter, Segall and Jones, 1988). Identification of N-oxide and hydrolytic metabolites of the PAs senecionine and monocrotaline in extracts of mouse hepatic microsomal incubations were accomplished by comparing collisionally activated decomposition/mass-analyzed ion kinetic energy spectra of specific ions from microsomal extracts with spectra obtained from synthetic standards of suspected metabolites. Trace amounts of the toxic metabolite dihydropyrrolizine (DHP) were observed by GC/MS of trimethylsilyl (TMS) derivatives, but the amount present in hepatic microsomal extracts were far below the MS/MS limit of detection. Quantitative determinations of senecionine N-oxide were performed by fast atom bombardment MS/MS with suppression of N-oxide ionization by other substances in the extract judged to be minimal. The TMS derivatives of the metabolites senecic acid, monocrotalic acid and DHP were quantified using capillary GC/MS. Results from the study demonstrate that the relative contributions of the three major pathways of PA metabolism (N-oxidation, hydrolysis and oxidation to pyrrolic compounds) can be assessed using a single analytical instrument and minimal sample preparation.

The comparative in vitro metabolism of the senecionine was studied in five animal species (Winter, Segall and Jones, 1988a). Senecionine was incubated with microsomes obtained from livers of three species known to be susceptible to PA poisoning (rat, cow and horse) and two resistant species (guinea pig, sheep). Microsomal extracts were analyzed for DHP, N-oxide (senecionine-oxide) and hydrolytic metabolite (senecic acid) using the above MS/MS and GC/MS methods. Levels of the toxic pyrrolic metabolite DHP were higher from guinea pig microsomal incubations (39.9 nmol/mg protein) than from other species (range 0.07 to 7.5 nmol/mg). These results disagree with those of prior studies which reported that pyrrole formation from the guinea pig was low relative to other species. These findings suggest that the resistance of the guinea pig to certain PAs may be due to the guinea pig's resistance to pyrrole toxicity rather than from low levels of pyrrole formation. Minor differences in senecionine N-oxide and senecic acid formation existed between the various species and it was concluded that species differences in hepatic microsomal N-oxidation and hydrolysis may not play a major role in determining species susceptibility to PA poisoning.

Allen, J. R., I. C. Hsu and L. A. Carstens (1975). Dehydroretronecine-induced rhabdomyosarcomas in rats. *Cancer Research*, 35, 997-1002.

Benedetti, A., L. Barbieri, M. Ferrali, A. F. Casini, R. Fulceri and M. Comporti (1981). Inhibition of protein synthesis by carbonyl compounds (4-hydroxyalkenals) originating from the peroxidation of liver microsomal lipids. *Chem. Biol. Inter.*, 35, 331-340.

Benedetti, A., A. F. Casini and M. Ferrali (1977). Red cell lysis coupled to the peroxidation of liver microsomal lipids. Compartmentalization of the hemolytic system. *Res. Commun. Chem. Pathol. Pharmacol.*, 17, 519-528.

Benedetti, A., A. F. Casini, M. Ferrali and M. Comporti (1979). Extraction and partial characterization of dialysable products originating from the peroxidation of liver microsomal lipids and inhibiting microsomal glucose 6-phosphatase activity. *Biochem. Pharmacol.*, 28, 2909-2918.

Benedetti, A., A. F. Casini, M. Ferrali, R. Fulceri and M. Comporti (1981). Cytotoxic effects of carbonyl compound (4-hydroxyalkenals) originating from the peroxidation of microsomal lipids. In: *Recent Advances in Lipid Peroxidation and Tissue Injury*. T. F. Slater and A. Garner, Eds., pp. 56, Brunel Printing Services, Uxbridge.

Benedetti, A., M. Comporti and H. Esterbauer (1980). Identification of 4-hydroxynonenal as a cytotoxic product originating from the peroxidation of liver microsomal lipids. *Biochem. Biophys. Acta*, 620, 281-296.

Benedetti, A., H. Esterbauer, M. Ferrali, R. Fulceri and M. Comporti (1982). Evidence for aldehydes bound to liver microsomal protein following CCl_4 or $BrCCl_3$ poisoning. *Biochem. Biophys. Acta.*, 711, 345-356.

Benedetti, A., R. Fulceri, M. Ferrali, L. Cicoli, H. Esterbauer and M. Comporti (1982). Detection of carbonyl function in phospholipids of liver microsomes in CCl_4 and $BrCCl_3$ poisoned rats. *Biochem. Biophys. Acta.*, 712, 628-638.

Bras, G., D. B. Jellifee and K. L. Stuart (1954). Venoocclusive disease of liver with non-portal type of cirrhosis occurring in Jamaica. *Arch. Path.*, 57, 285-300.

Bottomley, W. and T. A. Geissman (1964). Pyrrolizidine alkaloids. The biosynthesis of retronescine. *Phytochemistry*, 3, 357-360.

Buhler, D. R. and B. Kedzierski. Biological Reactive Intermediates of Pyrrolizidine Alkaloids. In: *Biological Reactive Intermediates III*, edited by Kocsis, J. J., Jollow, D. J., Witmer, C. M., Nelson, J. O. and Snyder, R. New York: Plenum Press, 1986, p. 611-620.

Bull, L. B., C. C. J. Culvenor and A. T. Dick. The Pyrrolizidine Alkaloids, In: *Frontiers of Biology,* Amsterdam: North-Holland, 1968.

Butler, W. H., A. R. Mattocks and J. M. Barnes (1970). Lesions in the liver and lungs of rats given pyrrole derivatives of pyrrolizidine alkaloids. *J. Pathol.,* 100, 169-175.

Candrian, U., J. Luthy, Y. Graf and C. Schlatter (1984). Mutagenic activity of the pyrrolizidine alkaloids seneciphylline and senkirkine in drosophila and their transfer into rat milk. *Food Chem. Toxicol.,* 22, 223-224.

Casini, A. F., A. Benedetti, M. Ferrali, R. Fulceri and M. Comporti (1978). Estrazione di prodotti tossici dializzabili originatisi dalla perossidazione dei lipidi microsomali epatici, *Bull. Soc. Ital. Biol. Sper.,* 54, 893-899.

Culvenor, C. C. J., J. A. Edgar, M. V. Jago, A. Outteridge and J. E. Peterson (1976). Hepato-and pneumotoxicity of pyrrolizidine alkaloids and derivatives in relation to molecular structure. *Chem.-Biol. Interactions,* 12, 299-324.

Culvenor, C. C. J., M. Clarke, J. A. Edgar, J. L. Frahn, M. V. Jago, J. E. Peterson and L. W. Smith (1980). Structure and toxicity of the alkaloids of russian comfrey (Symphytum x uplandicum Nyman), a medicinal herb and item of human diet. *Experientia,* 36, 377-379.

Culvenor, C. C. J., J. A. Edgar and L. W. Smith (1970). Metabolic conversion of heliotridine-based pyrrolizidine alkaloids to dehydroheliotridine. *Molecular Pharmacology,* 6, 402-406.

Culvenor, C. C. J. and L. W. Smith (1981). Plant sources of hepatotoxic pyrrolizidine alkaloids. *Journal of Natural Products,* 44, 129-152.

Deinzer, M. L., P. A. Thomson, D. M. Burgett and D. L. Isaacson (1977). Pyrrolizidine alkaloids: their occurrence in honey from tansy ragwort (Senecio jacobaea L.). *Science,* 195, 497-499.

Dickinson, J. O., M. P. Cooke, R. R. King and P. A. Mohamed (1976). Milk transfer of pyrrolizidine alkaloids in cattle. *J. A. V. M. A.,* 169, 1102-1196.

Eastman, D. F. and H. J. Segall (1982). A new pyrrolizidine alkaloid metabolite, 19-hydroxysenecionine isolated from mouse hepatic microsomes in vitro. *Drug Metabolism & Disposition,* 10, 696-699.

Erickson, B. W. (1974). γ-Hydroxy-a,B-unsaturated aldehydes via 1,3-bis(methylthio)allyllithium: trans-4-hydroxy-2-hexenal, *Org. Synth.,* 54, 19-27.

Esterbauer, H. (1982). Aldehydic products of lipid peroxidation. In: *"Free Radicals, Lipid Peroxidation and Cancer,"* D. C. H. McBrien and T. F. Slater, Eds. pp. 101, Academic Press, Lond.

Esterbauer, H., K. H. Cheeseman, M. U. Dianzani, G. Poli and T. F. Slater. (1982). Separation and characterization of the aldehydic products of lipid peroxidation stimulated by ADP-Fe^{+2} in rat liver microsomes. *Biochem. J.,* 208, 129-140.

Esterbauer, H., A. Ertl and N. Scholz (1976). The reaction of cysteine with a,B-unsaturated aldehydes. *Tetrahedron,* 32, 285-289.

Esterbauer, H., H. Zollner and N. Scholz (1975). Reaction of glutathione with conjugated carbonyls. *Z. Naturforsch. Teil C Biochem. Biophys. Biol. Virol.,* 30, 466-473.

Ferrali, M., R. Fulceri, A. Benedetti and M. Comporti (1980). Effects of carbonyl compounds (4-hydroxyalkenals) originating from the peroxidation of liver microsomal lipids on various microsomal enzyme activities of the liver. *Res. Commun. Chem. Pathol. Pharmacol.,* 30, 99-112.

Grasse, L. D., M. W. Lame' and H. J. Segall (1985). In vivo covalent of trans-4-hydroxy-2-hexenal to rat liver macromolecules. *Toxicology Letters,* 29, 43-49.

Green, C. E., H. J. Segall and J. L. Byard (1981). Metabolism, cytotoxicity, and genotoxicity of the pyrrolizidine alkaloid senecionine in primary cultures of rat hepatocytes. *Toxicol. Appl. Pharmacol.,* 60, 176-185.

Griffin, D. S. and H. J. Segall (1986). Genotoxicity and cytotoxicity of selected pyrrolizidine alkaloids, a possible metabolite of the alkaloids, and related alkenals. *Toxicol. Appl. Pharmacol.,* 86, 227-234.

Griffin, D. S. and H. J. Segall (1987a). Lipid peroxidation and cellular damage caused by pyrrolizidine alkaloid senecionine, the alkenal trans-4-hydroxy-2-hexenal, and related alkenals. *Cell Biology and Toxicology,* 3, 379-390.

Griffin, D. S. and H. J. Segall (1987b). Role of cellular calcium homeostasis in toxic liver injury induced by the pyrrolizidine alkaloid senecionine and the alkenal trans-4-OH-2-hexenal. *J. Biochem. Toxicol.,* 2, 155-167.

Hill, K. R., K. Rhoades, J. L. Stafford and R. Aub (1951). Liver disease in Jamaican children (Serous Hepatosis). *West Indian Med. J.,* 1, 49-63.

Hughes, C. A., R. Letcher and F. L. Warren (1964). The biosynthesis of the "necine" bases from carbon-14 precursors. *J. Chem. Soc.,* 4974-4977.

Huxtable, R. J. (1980). Herbal teas and toxins: novel aspects of pyrrolizidine poisoning in the united states. *Perspectives in Biology and Medicine,* 24, 1-14.

Lame', M. W. and H. J. Segall (1986). Metabolism of the pyrrolizidine alkaloid metabolite trans-4-hydroxy-2-hexenal by mouse liver aldehyde dehydrogenase. *Toxicol. Appl. Pharmacol.*, 82, 94-103.

Lowry, M. (1973). Possible mechanisms of autoxidative rancidity. *Lipids*, 7, 671-675.

Mattocks, A. R. (1967). Spectrophotometric determination of unsaturated pyrrolizidine alkaloids. *Analytical Chemistry*, 39, 443-447.

Mattocks, A. R. (1968a). Toxicity of pyrrolizidine alkaloids. *Nature*, 217, 723-728.

Mattocks, A. R. (1968b). Spectrophotometric determination of pyrrolizidine alkaloids-some improvements. *Analytical Chemistry*, 40, 1749-1750.

Mattocks, A. R. (1972). Toxicity and metabolism of senecio alkaloids. *Phytochemical Ecology, Proceedings of the Phytochemical Society Symposium*, 8, 179-200.

Mattocks, A. R. and I. N. H. White (1971). The conversion of pyrrolizidine alkaloids to N-oxides and to dihydropyrrolizine derivatives by rat-liver microsomes in vitro. *Chem.-Biol. Interactions*, 3, 383-396.

Mattocks, A. R. Mechanisms of pyrrolizidine alkaloids toxicity. In: *Pharmacology and the Future of Man*, Vol. 2, edited by Acheson, G. H. New York: S. Karger, 1973, p. 114-123.

Mattocks, A. R. and R. F. Legg (1980). Antimitotic activity of dehydroretronecine, a pyrrolizidine alkaloid metabolite, and some analogous compounds, in a rat liver parenchymal cell line. *Chem. -Biol. Interactions*, 30, 325-336.

Mattocks, A. R. (1981). Relation of structural features to pyrrolic metabolites in livers of rats given pyrrolizidine alkaloids and derivatives. *Chem.-Biol. Interactions*, 35, 301-310.

Mattocks, A. R. and I. Bird (1983). Alkylation by dehydroretronecine, a cytotoxic metabolite of some pyrrolizidine alkaloids: an in vitro test. *Toxicology Letters*, 16, 1-8.

Mattocks, A. R. *Chemistry and Toxicology of Pyrrolizdine Alkaloids*, New York: Academic Press, 1986.

Mattocks, A. R. and R. Jukes (1987). Improved field tests for toxic pyrrolizidine alkaloids. *Journal of Natural Products*, 50.

McLean, E. K. (1970). The toxic actions of pyrrolizidine (Senecio) alkaloids. *Pharmacological Reviews*, 22, 429-483.

Miranda, C. L., M. C. Henderson, J. A. Schmitz and D. R. Buhler (1983). Protective role of dietary butylated hydroxyanisole against chemical-induced acute liver damage in mice. *Toxicol. Appl. Pharmacol.*, 69, 73-80.

Mohabbat, Q., M. S. Younos, A. A. Merzad, R. N. Srivastava, G. G. Sediq and G. N. Aram (1976). An outbreak of hepatic veno-occlusive disease in northwestern Afghanistan. *Lancet*, 2(7980), 269-271.

Mori, H., S. Sugie, N. Yoshimi, Y. Asada, T. Furuya and G. Williams (1985). Genotoxicity of a variety of pyrrolizidine alkaloids in the hepatocyte primary culture-DNA repair test using rat, mouse and hamster hepatocytes. *Cancer Res.*, 45, 3125-3129.

Pearson, m N., J. J. Karchesy, A. O'C. Deeney, M. L. Deinzer and G. S. Beaudreau (1984). Induction of endogenous avian tumor virus gene expression by pyrrolizidine alkaloids. *Chem.-Biol. Interactions*, 49, 341-350.

Peterson, J. E. and Culvenor, C. C. J. Hepatotoxic pyrrolizidine alkaloids. In: *Handbook of Natural Toxins*, Vol. 1, edited by Keeler, R. F. and Tu, A. T. New York: Marcel Dekker, 1983, p. 637-671.

Petry, T. W., G. T. Bowden, R. J. Huxtable and I. G. Sipes (1984). Characterization of hepatic DNA damage induced in rats by the pyrrolizidine alkaloid monocrotaline. *Cancer Research*, 44, 1505-1509.

Schauenstein, E. (1967). Autoxidation of polyunsaturated esters in water: chemical structure and biological activity of the products. *J. Lipid Res.*, 8, 417-428.

Schauenstein, E., H. Esterbauer and H. Zolner (1977). *"Aldehydes in Biological Systems"*, Pion Limited, London.

Segall, H. J. (1979a). Reverse phase isolation of pyrrolizidine alkaloids. *J. Liquid Chromatography*, 2, 429-436.

Segall, H. J. (1979b). Preparative isolation of pyrrolizidine alkaloids derived from Senecio vulgaris. *J. Liquid Chromatography*, 2, 1319-1323.

Segall, H. J., C. H. Brown and D. F. Paige (1983). The biosynthesis of three macrocyclic pyrrolizidine alkaloids, retrorsine, seneciphylline and senecionine using Senecio vulgaris. *J. Labelled Compds.*, 20, 671-689.

Segall, H. J., J. L. Dallas and W. F. Haddon (1983). Two dihydropyrrolizine alkaloid metabolites isolated from mouse hepatic microsomes in vitro. *Drug Metabolism & Disposition*, 12, 68-71.

Segall, H. J. and J. L. Dallas (1983). ^{1}H NMR spectroscopy of pyrrolizidine alkaloids. *Phytochemistry*, 22, 1271-1273.

Segall, H. J., D. W. Wilson, J. L. Dallas and W. F. Haddon (1985). trans-4-Hydroxy-2-hexenal: A reactive metabolite from the macrocyclic pyrrolizidine alkaloid senecionine. *Science*, 229, 472-475.

Smolen, A., D. R. Petersen and A. C. Collins (1981). Liver cytosolic aldehyde dehydrogenase activity in the pregnant mouse. *Dev. Pharmacol. Thera.*, 3, 31-49.

White, I. N. H. and A. R. Mattocks (1971). Some factors affecting the conversion of pyrrolizidine alkaloids to N-oxides and to pyrrolic derivatives in vitro. *Xenobiotica*, 1, 503-505.

White, Ian N. H. (1976). The role of liver glutathione in the acute toxicity of retrorsine to rats. *Chem.-Biol. Interactions*, 13, 333-342.

Williams, G. M., H. Mori, I. Hirono and M. Nagao (1980). Genotoxicity of pyrrolizidine alkaloids in the hepatocyte primary culture/DNA repair test. *Mutat. Res.*, 79, 1-5.

Wilson, D. W., Segall H. J. and Lame', M. W. Hepatic pathological changes due to hydroxyalkenals. In: *Biological Reactive Intermediates III*, edited by Kocsis, J. J., Jollow, D. J., Witmer, C. M., Nelson, J. O. and Snyder, R. New York: Plenum Publishing Corporation, 1986, p. 853-860.

Winter, C. K., H. J. Segall and W. F. Haddon (1986). Formation of cyclic adducts of deoxyguanosine with the aldehydes trans-4-hydroxy-2-hexenal and trans-4-hydroxy-2-nonenal in vitro. *Cancer Research*, 46, 5682-5686.

Winter, C. K., H. J. Segall and A. D. Jones (1987). Distribution of trans-4-hydroxy-2-hexenal and tandem mass spectrometric detection of its urinary mercapturic acid in the rat. *Drug Metabolism and Disposition*, 15, 608-612.

Winter, C. K., H. J. Segall and A. D. Jones (1988). Determination of pyrrolizidine alkaloid metabolites from mouse liver microsomes using tandem mass spectrometry and gas chromatography/mass spectrometry. *Biomedical and Environmental Mass Spectrometry*, 15, 265-273.

Winter, C. K., H. J. Segall and A. D. Jones (1988a). Species differences in the hepatic microsomal matabolism of the pyrrolizidine alkaloid senecionine. *Comparative Biochemistry and Physiology*, 90C, 429-433.

II. Interaction of Toxins with Ion Channels

THE MOLECULAR PHARMACOLOGY OF TOXINS THAT MODIFY VOLTAGE-GATED SODIUM CHANNELS

G.R. Strichartz

Anesthesia Research Laboratories, Brigham and Women's Hospital
and
Department of Biological Chemistry and Molecular Pharmacology
Harvard Medical School
Boston, MA 02115

ABSTRACT

The voltage-gated sodium channel is the essential entity supporting impulse generation in many excitable cells. A plethora of naturally-occurring plant and animal toxins bind to this glyco-proteinaceous channel and modify its normal behavior. This chapter reviews the separate and interactive affects of these different toxins.

KEYWORDS

Sodium channel; neurotoxin; veratridine; saxitoxin; scorpion toxins.

THE PHYSIOLOGICAL ROLE OF SODIUM CHANNELS

Sodium channels permit the influx of Na^+ that produces the rapid depolarizing phase of action potentials. These channels have a complex physiology that is altered by neurotoxins acting at many different binding sites. A short review of electrophysiology, with some definitions will aid the subsequent description of toxin actions.

Membrane potential is the voltage of the inside of the cell (or organelle) relative to the outside and is most often dominated by the K^+ diffusion potential; typical values range from -90 to -40 mV (negative inside) and result from the selective permeability to K^+ of the resting membrane. Treatments that reduce outward K^+ current at rest (e.g. K^+ channel blockers) tend to depolarize cells, as do treatments that increase inward Na^+ currents (e.g. Na^+ channel activators). Such treatments are often small toxin ligands that bind to the channel macromolecule. From a biochemical perspective, it is useful to consider ion channels as enzymes that catalyze the reactions of passive ion transport. Indeed, these enzymes have turned out to be proteins, and they express the classical enzyme attributes of substrate specificity (ion selectivity), ligand inhibition, and "subunit" regulation. That many of the toxins to be described here act as inhibitors or regulators of ion channel activities further consolidates this analogy.

Channels open, or "gate", in response to a range of "stimuli", variables that perturb the population distribution among a set of possible channel conformations (Hille, 1984). Recognized perturbations include changes in membrane potential, ions themselves, and a range of "regulatory" substances which modify the response to other perturbations through covalent or non-covalent association with the channel. Thus, a channel performs the operations of ion <u>conductance</u> when it is "open", of <u>gating</u> between open and closed states (of which there are often several), and of <u>regulating</u> between "activatable" (gateable = openable) states and other, non-activatable (non-gateable or "inactivated") states.

Ions may carry current through the channel's "pore" (Chandler et al., 1965; Hille, 1972), bind in the channel's pore and <u>occlude</u> it (Woodhull, 1973), bind to or associate with structural features beyond the pore and thereby modify gating (Oxford and Yeh, 1985), and alter the actions of other ligands (Henderson et al., 1974). Although certain quantitative physiological and pharmacological properties of Na^+ channels differ among neuronal, skeletal muscular and myocardial Na^+ channels, we will treat them here as a single entity, with exceptions as noted. The channel possesses an elaborate and well-documented toxinology. Many animals have evolved toxins as offensive or defensive weapons that are directed, respectively, against their prey's or predator's Na^+ channels, and these have been characterized extensively (Catterall, 1980; Strichartz et al., 1987).

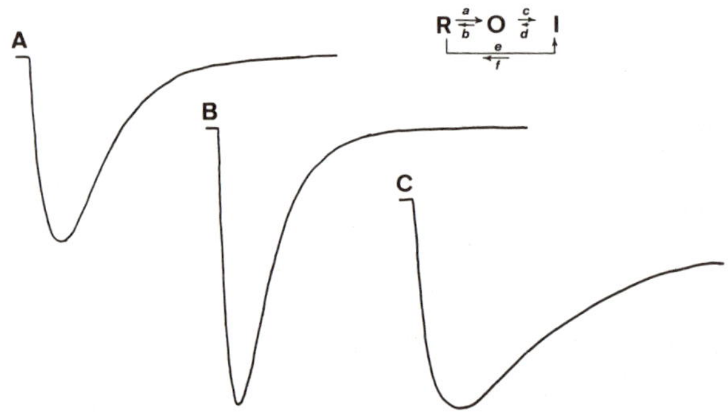

Fig. 1. Simulation of Na^+ current kinetics using a three-state model (upper right diagram). The resultant Na^+ current is graphed as the curves A-C, for comparison with experimental figures presented later. The activation (a,b) and inactivation (c,d) rates (in units $msec^{-1}$) are set to simulate currents in (A) normal channels, (B) channels with accelerated activation and (C) channels with slowed inactivation.

The toxinology of Na^+ channels is best understood in the context of the normal physiology. Sodium channels exist in several different conformations or states, most of which do not conduct ions across the membrane (i.e. are "closed") and some which do conduct ions (i.e. are "open"). Transitions among these different states are termed "gating" reactions. A very simple scheme for Na channel gating and its resultant kinetic output is diagrammed in figure 1. The channel has two non-conducting states - one existing primarily in resting membranes (R, resting) and one primarily in membranes held depolarized (I, inactivated) - as well as one conducting state (O, open). In normal, toxin-free channels responding to membrane depolarization, the R → O process, called "activation", is markedly faster than inactivation (O → I) and is moderately reversible; if inactivation did not occur, 98% of the channels would populate O at equilibrium. Normally, inactivating channels close almost totally irreversible, 99.9% of the channels populating the I state at the end of long depolarizations. The transient population of O is proporational to the inward sodium current shown by the curves in figure 1, which graphs the time course of Na^+ channels in state O during a 5 msec long depolarizing step in membrane potential. For a toxin-free channel, the first opening occurs shortly after depolarization; temporary reversal of opening ("deactivation") accounts for many of the early closings, but eventually the virtually irreversible O → I reaction traps the channel in the inactivated state. Inactivation must also be occurring directly from the resting state (i.e. R → I, in order to assure microscopic reversibility), but normally that process is slow and competes ineffectively with the rapid activation gating. Examples of channels with modified activation (B) and inactivation (C) reactions are also shown in figure 1.

A real protein underlies these kinetic abstractions. Sodium channels are large (ca. 200 kdaltons) glyco-peptides (Miller et al., 1983), heavily acylated with fatty acids (Levinson et al., 1986) and carrying a net charge or dipole moment (Armstrong and Bezanilla, 1974). Anchored within the plasma membrane by hydrophobic, electrostatic, and covalent bonding, the channel protein's electrically charged regions will respond to changes of the membrane potential by conformational changes to the most stable, energetically accessible disposition. These changes constitute the gating reactions we have simplified for figure 1. Binding of toxins to the channels modifies these conformational changes, altering the energetics and changing the apparent gating kinetics.

CLASSIFICATION OF TOXIN ACTIONS

It is not my intention to compile an exhaustive survey, but rather to categorize and to organize toxins into functionally identifiable classes. At first this seems a simple task, but the complexity of actions soon emerges. From the present understanding of ion channel function, no single toxin appears to exert only one simple action. One of the reasons for this is that ion channels are complex proteins whose functions involve subtle, concerted conformational changes, and, at present, our understanding of the structural basis for these functions is inadequate for a proper, molecular description of toxin-induced phenomena. Nevertheless, the observed effects are important to describe and understand, for our comprehension of channel mechanics is paralleled by our evolving knowledge of their molecular toxinology.

The actions of toxins may be classified according to the our current perspective of ion channel function. The known toxinology of the Na^+ channel classifies compounds into three broad categories: <u>activators</u>, <u>stabilizers</u>, and <u>occluders</u>. Although these terms describe the apparent <u>major</u> effect of the toxin, it should be realized that multiple effects are more often the rule than the exception.

<u>Activators</u>.

These toxic agents increase the probability that Na^+ channels will open at membrane potentials where such openings are usually quite rare. As noted above, the normal, voltage-gated process of opening is called "activation", thus the title of this class of drugs. Many of the known activators are alkaloids extracted from terrestrial plants or amphibians, e.g. aconitine, veratridine (VTD: veratrum spp.) or batrachotoxin (BTX), respectively (figure 2; Catterall, 1975). These relatively lipophilic organic molecules, typically of mass less than 10^3 daltons, produce their full pharmacological effects whether applied intracellularly or from without the cell, and probably act from within the membrane. The effects are inhibited non-competitively by occluder toxins (e.g. tetrodotoxin, see below), and result from binding at a specific site on the channel (Catterall, 1980; Lazdunski et al., 1980).

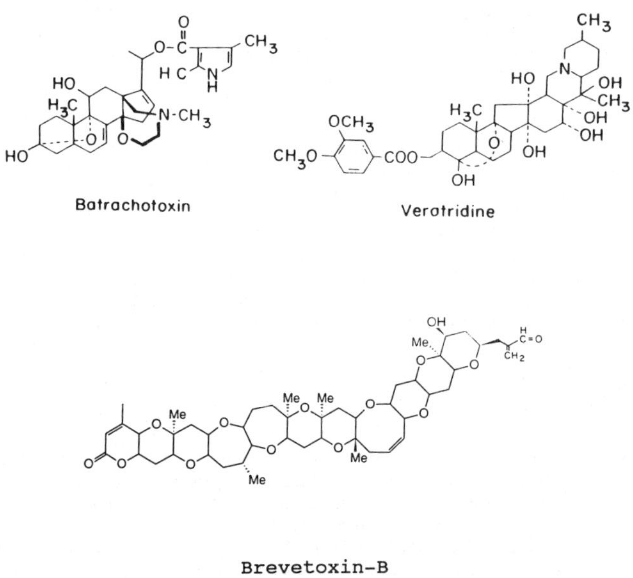

Fig. 2. Structure of three "activators": the alkaloid batrachotoxin, from frog skin; the steroidal activator veratridine, from plants (<u>Melanthacae</u>); the cyclic polyether brevetoxin, from the marine dinoflagellate <u>Gymnodinium breve</u>.

Activators alter the opening and the closing probability of Na^+ channels, tending to activate channels at voltages near the cell's resting potential and to prevent their normal, complete inactivation. The result is a long-lasting increase in Na^+ permeability and a corresponding depolarization from the steady inward Na^+ current (Ulbricht, 1972). But if the membrane potential is held constant by laboratory manipulations (voltage-clamp), then the drug modified channel's activation and inactivation kinetics may be examined under more controlled conditions (Sutro, 1986; Leibowitz et al., 1986; Rando, 1989).

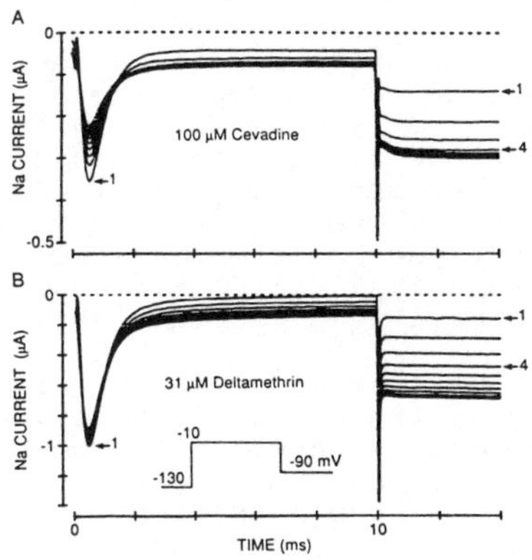

Fig. 3. Kinetic modifications of Na^+ currents by the veratrum alkaloid, cevadine (A) and the pyrethroid, deltamethrin (B). Currents are shown for 10 sequential pulses of the voltage pattern shown at the bottom, applied every 272 msec. Numerals to the right of the arrows indicate the current traces during the first and fourth pulse in that sequence. Time zero marks the beginning of the depolarization to -10 mV, time 10 msec marks the time of repolarization. (from Leibowitz et al. 1987)

Examples of the actions of activators is shown in figure 3, where the responses of Na^+ channels to repetitive depolarization in the presence of one veratridine alkaloid (cevadine) and one pyrethroid are compared. The currents from 0 to 10 msec flow during a depolarization, those after 10 msec during membrane repolarization. For both drugs, the inactivation (declining) phase of the currents is slowed, and a persistent inward current appears after the membrane is repolarized. This "tail" current grows in size with each repeated depolarization and corresponds to the incremental conversion of toxin-free to activator-modified channels, channels which remain open at potentials where the activation "gate" normally rapidly "closes", i.e. where O rapidly reverses to R. With repeated depolarizations the cevadine-modified peak currents decrease incrementally, as if the activatable pool of channels is being reduced in parallel with the growth of modified channels. This behavior is not seen with detamethrin at this stimulation frequency. Some activators have stronger actions than others in altering ion selectivity and open channel conductance, and the details of these modifications are being related to the toxin structures in ongoing studies (cf. Leibowitz et al., 1987).

Repetitive depolarization accelerates the pharmacological modification by toxins because activated channels react more rapidly with the toxins and appear to have a higher affinity for them than do the closed resting or inactivated states (Sutro, 1986; Rando et al., 1986).

This behavior is characteristic of "modulated receptor" models, described later in this chapter. When open, the drug-modified channels have a lower conductance and a different ion selectivity compared to unmodified channels, i.e. the detailed energetics of ion transport are altered (Khodorov, 1985; Garber and Miller, 1987; Rando, 1989). Finally, modified channels may close and re-open many times in a depolarized membrane, in contrast to normal channels which rapidly inactivate (Quandt and Narahashi, 1982). This accounts for the persistent current during a prolonged depolarization.

One activator molecule binding to a Na^+ channel influences its total function, including all the gating and the ion permeation. It is noteworthy that these lipophilic ligands, of a modest size compared to the large channel protein, exert such extensive influence. Either the structural features subserving channel functions are localized in a small, central domain of the protein, or concerted, channel-wide structural changes attending these functions can be affected through one integrative site, or the activator molecule can move in milliseconds among multiple points on the Na^+ channel, which seems unlikely.

The summed effects of activators are to increase the population of open channels (albeit of reduced Na^+ conductance) over a broad range of membrane potentials. Under normal conditions this results in slow depolarization of the membrane attended by a transient period of rapid, spontaneous impulse firing. Nerve, muscle and heart all appear to be sensitive to activators, which probably also penetrate the blood brain barrier, affecting the central nervous system. The pathophysiology of activator intoxication is extensive and interactive.

Stabilizers.

A second category of toxins has an apparently simple action. These drugs prolong and inhibit the inactivation phase of Na^+ currents during depolarization, thereby stabilizing channels in the open state without affecting the activation process (figure 4). The best examples of such toxins are small peptides isolated from scorpion venom (Meves et al., 1982; Wang and Strichartz, 1982,83), from nematocysts of a variety of anemones (Ulbricht and Schmidtmayer, 1981; Schweitz et al., 1981) and larger proteins found in venoms of Conidae (Gonoi et al., 1987). While some of these toxins at high concentrations do reduce the amplitude of Na^+ currents, the more typical effect is prolongation of the period of high Na^+ conductance. In non-voltage clamped membranes, the effect of such stabilizers is to greatly prolong the action potential, generating a "plateau" depolarization lasting from tenths of seconds to seconds (Wang and Strichartz, 1981).

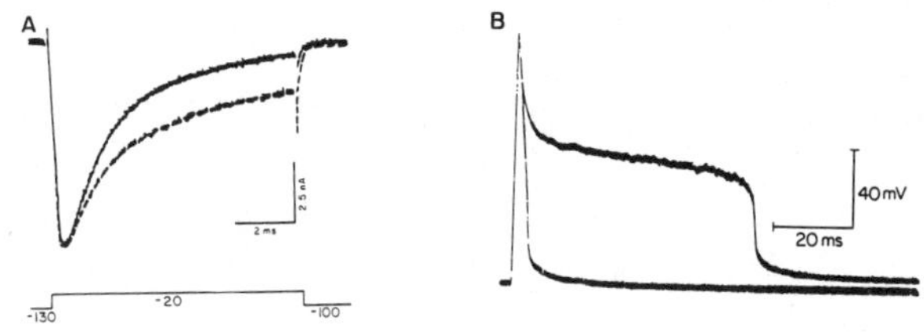

Fig. 4. Modifications of Na^+ currents (A) and action potentials (B) in myelinated nerve by purified α-toxin of <u>Leiurus quinquestriatus</u> scorpion venom. A) Control (solid line) and toxin-treated (broken-line, 200 nM) Na^+ currents in a voltage-clamped fiber. Note the specific effect on inactivation kinetics (cf. Fig. 1, this paper). B) The normally brief action potential, here broadened to 4 msec by TEA^+ blockade of K^+ channels, is extended by a 75 msec plateau through the action of <u>Leiurus</u> α-toxin. (from Wang and Strichartz, 1982)

Stabilizers bind at a site separate from those of traditional activators but they exert a synergistic action on them (Catterall, 1977; Rando et al., 1986). This action potentiates the activators and generally increases their efficacy, yielding larger depolarizations at lower doses.

The actions of stabilizers present one of the classic voltage-dependent toxin effects. Depolarizations of the membrane sufficient to energetically drive stabilizer-bound channels to an inactivated conformation also lead to dissociation of the stabilizer (Mozhayeva et al., 1980; Warashina et al., 1981; Strichartz and Wang, 1986). The energetics of this process are related to its kinetics and to the toxin's affinity. For a tightly binding stabilizer toxin, of $K_D \sim 10^{-8}$M, small depolarizations (e.g. to -20 mV) result only in slow dissociations that require minutes to complete, whereas large depolarizations (e.g. to + 50 mV) result in complete dissociation within 10 milliseconds. Stabilizers that bind less strongly, with $K_D \sim 10^{-6}$M, reverse more rapidly at lower depolarizations. Toxin dissociation results not from a direct effect of the membrane potential on the binding reaction <u>per se</u>, but on a voltage-dependent modulation of the toxin binding site from a high to a low affinity form. Apparently the inactivated state has an affinity for stabilizers that is at least an order of magnitude less than that of the resting or open states. Sufficiently positive potentials force the stabilizer-bound channel into an inactivated conformation, leading to rapid relaxation of toxin binding to the new equilibrium corresponding to the low affinity, inactivated conformation.

Occluders.

Tetrodotoxin (TTX) and the saxitoxins (STX) are classic examples of toxins acting as the third class of agents, occluders. These small (300-450 daltons), organic cations act only from the external surface of Na^+ channels to produce a readily reversible, yet usually high affinity (K_D ~ 10^{-9}M) block of the channel (see figure 5). This block is antagonized by Na^+, Ca^+ and H^+ (Henderson et al., 1974; Strichartz, et al., 1986) and was originally thought to correspond to a "plugging" of the channel's pore (Kao and Nishiyama, 1965). The rapid kinetics of

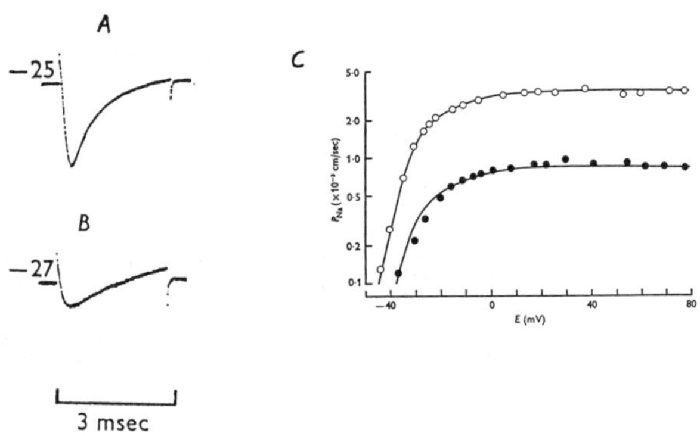

Fig. 5. Reduction of Na^+ current in frog nerve by tetrodotoxin (TTX). A. Currents in toxin-free solution in response to a 3 msec pulse to -25 mV. B. Currents in the same preparation bathed by 9.3 nM TTX. C. The peak sodium permeability at different membrane potentials in control (o) and 9.3 nM TTX-containing (o) solutions. The curve through the control points is multiplied by 0.245 to give the curve through TTX-reduced data. Neither kinetics nor voltage-dependence of Na^+ channel activation appears to be altered by the toxin. (from Ulbricht and Wagner, 1975)

activation and inactivation of conducting channels are unaffected by TTX/STX, and the movement of charge associated with activation remains unchanged (Armstrong and Bezanilla, 1974). The overall effect appears equivalent to reducing, reversibly, the number of channels that have patent conductance pathways (Hille, 1968). However, more recent evidence garnishes this simple plugging model. For one, the structural dependence of toxin activity is more complicated than can be explained by simple pore blockade (Kao, 1983), and the physiological behavior extends beyond simple occlusion (Strichartz et al., 1986). In mammalian cardiac Na^+ channels, an unusually low affinity for TTX ($K_D \approx 10^{-6}$M) is accompanied by an apparent "voltage-dependent" action - the toxin block is altered by the membrane potential, probably through some conformational change of the channel (Cohen et al., 1981). Channel gating is also subtly modified by these toxins; in both cardiac (Burnashev et al., 1984) and neuronal (Strichartz et al., 1986) tissue the tendency, after long ($\geq$ 1 sec) depolarizations, of the channels to dwell in a state from which they can only be slowly made activatable (i.e. a "slow inactivated state"), is furthered by TTX and STX (figure 7). The underlying mechanism for this gating modulation is completely unknown.

Certain occluders also discriminate among Na^+ channels from neuronal and skeletal muscle. But in this case the blocking ligands are small peptides, the μ-conotoxins from the mollusc <u>Conus geographus</u>. This molecule binds tightly to muscle Na^+ channels, effectively reducing Na^+ current (Cruz et al., 1985; see figure 5A), and also can displace bound radiolabelled STX, showing that it acts at the same site (Moczydlowski et al., 1986; Yanagawa et al., 1986). Reversible blockade of single muscle channels resembles that by saxitoxin (figure 5B); although the potency of μ-conotoxins is lower, the dissociation rate is also smaller. In neuronal and cardiac Na^+ channels, the blockade of Na currents and the inhibition of STX binding are far weaker, thus μ-conotoxins discriminate between channels that bind TTX and STX about equally.

The results from such occluders show that Na^+ channels differ in structure between their internal and external surfaces, that they have binding sites for a variety of monovalent and divalent cations, and that thus are pharmacologically different despite very similar physiological actions in nerve, muscle and mammalian cardiac cells. We await the elucidation of the structural features that underlie these chemical differences.

<u>The Na^+ channel is a modulated receptor</u>.

In all of the examples cited above, changes in the states of the channel are affected by toxin action. Reciprocally, the binding and actions of the toxins are changed by voltage-driven gating among different channel conformations. Such a dynamic interaction has been termed the "modulated receptor" model, and was originally proposed as an explanation for effects of local anesthetics on Na^+ channels (see review by Hondeghem and Katzung, 1984). For the toxin classes reviewed here, stabilizers have a selective affinity for resting and activated channels over inactivated channels, occluders seem to react slowly with inactivated states to increase the tendency of channels to enter the "slow inactivated" state, and the activators bind more tightly and certainly more rapidly to an activated state of the Na^+ channel than to resting or inactivated forms. These state-dependent actions may result from a truly high affinity (equilibrium) or from variations in accessibility of constant affinity sites (kinetics) as elaborated recently by C.F. Starmer and colleagues (Starmer and Grant, 1985).

A second aspect of the modulated receptor is the interaction among toxins of different classes. We noted above that activators were potentiated by stabilizers. In addition, the binding of the activator brevetoxin is slightly enhanced by occluders (Poli et al., 1986), occluder binding is modulated by activators (Strichartz et al., 1986) and the blocking action of occluders (STX and TTX) becomes voltage-dependent in activator (BTX)-modified channels (Krueger et al., 1983), whereas it normally exhibits no voltage-dependent action (Rando and

Strichartz, 1986). Thus, the Na^+ channel has multiple, separate, yet interactive binding sites for several types of toxins. Taken together with the broad effects of membrane potential on individual toxin actions, it seems probable that structural changes ripple through extensive domains of the channel during normal physiological gating.

REFERENCES

Armstrong, C.M. and F. Bezanilla (1974). Charge movement associated with the opening and closing of the activation gates of the Na channels. J. Gen. Physiol., 63, 533-552.

Cohen, C.J., B.P. Bean, T.J. Colatsky, and R.W. Tsien (1981). Tetrodotoxin block of sodium channels in rabbit Purkinje fibers. J. Gen. Physiol., 78, 383-411.

Garber, S.S. and C. Miller (1987). Single Na^+ channels activated by veratridine and batrachotoxin. J. Gen. Physiol., 89, 459-480.

Henderson, R., J.M. Ritchie, and G.R. Strichartz (1974). Evidence that tetrodotoxin and saxitoxin act at a metal cation binding site in the sodium channels of nerve membrane. Proc. Nat. Acad. Sci. USA, 71, 3936-3940.

Hille, B. (1968). Pharmacological modifications of the sodium channels of frog nerve. J. Gen. Physiol., 51, 199-219.

Hille, B. (1984). Ionic channels of excitable membranes. Sinauer Associates, Sunderland, MA, USA.

Hondeghem, L.M. and B.G. Katzung (1984). Antiarrhythmic agents: the modulated receptor mechanism of action of sodium and calcium channel-blocking drugs. Ann. Rev. Pharmacol. Toxicol., 24, 387-423.

Kao, C.Y. (1983). New perspectives on the interactions of tetrodotoxin and saxitoxin with excitable membranes. Toxicon, 21 (Suppl. 3), 211-219.

Kao, C.Y. and A. Nishiyama (1965). Actions of saxitoxin on peripheral neuromuscular systems. J. Physiol. (London) 180, 50-66.

Khodorov, B.I. (1985). Batrachotoxin as a tool to study voltage-sensitive sodium channels of excitable membranes. Prog. Biophys. Molec. Biol., 45, 57-148.

Krueger, B.K., J.F. Worley, and R.J. French (1983). Single sodium channels from rat brain incorporated into planar lipid bilayer membranes. Nature, 303, 172-175.

Leibowitz, M.D., J.R. Schwarz, G. Holan, and B. Hille (1987). Electrophysiological comparison of insecticide and alkaloid agonists of Na channels. J. Gen. Physiol., 90, 75-93.

Moczydlowki, E., B.M. Olivera, W.R. Gray and G.R. Strichartz (1986). Discrimination of muscle and neuronal Na-channel subtypes by binding competition between eH-saxitoxin and μ-conotoxins. Proc. Natl. Acad. Sci. USA, 83, 5321-5325.

Mozhayeva, G.N., A.P. Naumov, E.D. Nosyreva, and E.V. Grishin (1980). Potential-dependent interaction of toxin from venom of the scorpion Buthus eupeus with sodium channels in myelinated fibre. Voltage clamp experiments. Biochim. Biophys. Acta, 591, 587-602.

Poli, M.A., T.J. Mende, D.G. Baden (1986). Brevetoxins, unique activators of voltage-sensitive sodium channels, bind to specific sites in rat brain synaptosomes. Mol. Pharmacol., 30, 129-135.

Rando, T.A. (1989). Rapid and slow gating of veratridine modified sodium channels in frog myelinated nerve. J. Gen. Physiol. (in press)

Schweitz, H., J.P. Vincent, J. Barhanin, C. Frelin, G. Linden, M. Hugues, and M. Lazdunski (1981). Purification and pharmacological

properties of eight sea anemone toxins from Anemonia sulcata, Anthopleura xanthogrammica, Stoichactis giganteus, and Actinodendron plumosum. Biochem., 20, 5245-5252.
Starmer, C.F. and A.O. Grant (1985). Phasic ion channel blockade. A kinetic model and parameter estimation procedure. Mol. Pharm., 28, 348-356.
Strichartz, G., T. Rando, and G.K. Wang (1987). An integrated view of the molecular toxinology of sodium channel gating in excitable cells. Ann. Rev. Neurosci., 10, 237-267.
Strichartz, G.R. and G.K. Wang (1986). Rapid voltage-dependent of scorpion α-toxins coupled to Na channel inactivation in amphibian myelinated nerves. J. Gen. Physiol. 88, 413-435.
Ulbricht, W. (1969). The effect of veratridine on excitable membranes of nerve and muscle. Ergeb. Physiol., 61, 18-71.
Ulbricht, W. (1972). Rate of veratridine action on the nodal membrane. II. Fast and slow phase determined with periodic impulses in the voltage clamp. Pflugers Archiv, European J. Physiol., 336, 201-212.
Ulbricht, W. and J. Schmidtmayer (1981). Modification of sodium channels in myelinated nerve by Anemonia sulcata toxin II*. J. Physiol., Paris, 77, 1103-1111.
Ulbricht, W. and H.H. Wagner (1975). The influence of pH on equilibrium effects of tetrodotoxin on myelinated nerve fibres of Rana Esculenta. J. Physiol., 252, 159-184.
Wang, G.K. and G.R. Strichartz (1982). Simultaneous modifications of sodium channel gating by two scorpion toxins. Biophys. J., 40, 182-179.
Woodhull, A.M. (1973). Ionic blockage of sodium channels in nerve. J. Gen. Physiol., 61, 687-708.

INSIGHTS ON THE VOLTAGE-SENSITIVE SODIUM CHANNEL: THE BATRACHOTOXIN CONNECTION

George B. Brown

The Neuropsychiatry Research Program and the Department of Psychiatry
University of Alabama at Birmingham, Birmingham, AL 35294

ABSTRACT

Batrachotoxin (BTX), the prototype of the so-called "lipid-soluble" class of Na^+ channel neurotoxins, binds selectively to a single site on voltage-sensitive sodium channels of excitable membranes, causing the channels to open and remain open for extended times at normal resting membrane potentials. Direct ligand binding experiments using the tritiated derivative batrachotoxinin-A benzoate ([^{3}H]BTX-B) show that the BTX site is coupled to at least five other distinct sodium channel ligand binding domains. The fluorescent derivative batrachotoxinin-A N-methylanthranilate (BTX-NMA) exhibits significant changes in fluorescence parameters upon binding specifically to the BTX site, suggesting that this site lies at the interface of protein and lipid. Resonance energy transfer measurements with this derivative have added to the demonstration that various allosterically-coupled toxin binding domains on the sodium channel are separated from each other by tens of Angstroms. Further insights into the nature of the BTX receptor are being developed with photoaffinity labeling approaches using the photoactivatable and radioactive derivative batrachotoxinin-A o-azidobenzoate ([^{3}H]BTX-OAB). These studies are also suggestive of a binding site at the interface of protein and lipid. The accumulated data thus describe a batrachotoxin "connection", as it were, that is impressively broad, extending functionally to all aspects of channel activity and physically to multiple domains of the channel protein and the membrane environment. Further studies of this key neurotoxin binding site will contribute to a better understanding of the voltage-sensitive sodium channel at the molecular level.

KEYWORDS

Batrachotoxin; sodium channel; ligand binding; photoaffinity labeling; allosteric interactions; lipids.

INTRODUCTION

The voltage-sensitive sodium channel is perhaps the best understood example of the important general class of voltage-gated ion channels, membrane-spanning proteins that mediate ionic fluxes underlying the electrical activity of excitable cells in response to changes in transmembrane potential. Historically, this understanding has grown from elegant phenomenological descriptions of channel function based upon electrophysiological measurements. Even at this level naturally-occurring neurotoxins with specific effects on the voltage-sensitive sodium channel have been important tools, serving to perturb channel function in a variety of ways that facilitated the electrophysiological analysis of that function and mechanisms of action. In the last five years this research has entered a new and exciting phase with the purification, characterization and sequencing of the sodium channel protein(s) from several sources (Moore and coworkers, 1982; Hartshorne and Catterall, 1984; Roberts and Barchi, 1987). We now face the challenge of developing an understanding of the sodium channel in which structure is related to function at the molecular level. In this new arena, specifically acting neurotoxins take on an increasingly important role by providing the tools necessary to probe discrete regions of the channel structure that serve as neurotoxin binding sites. Inasmuch as neurotoxin binding at these sites results in altered channel function, information concerning their structural elements should contribute signficantly to a molecular understanding of the relationship between channel structure and function. Among all voltage-gated channels, the sodium channel

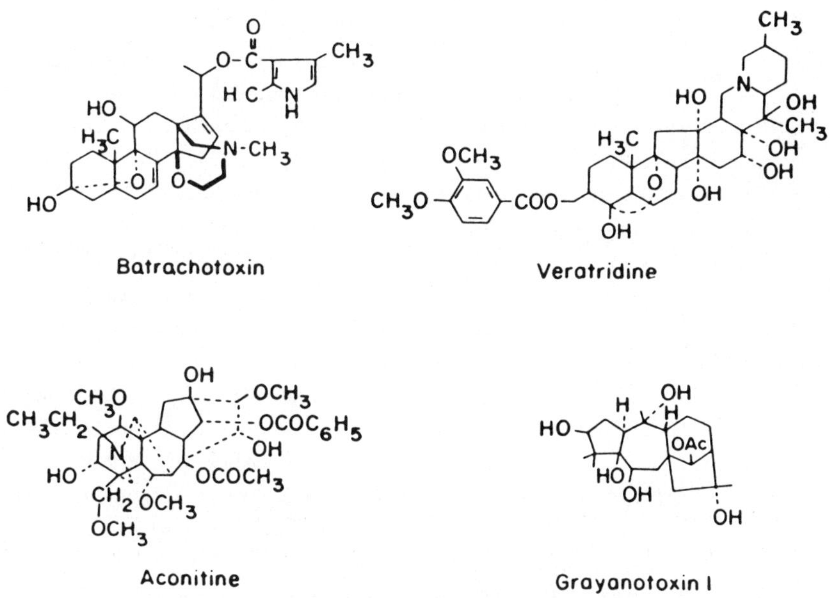

Fig. 1. The structures of the "lipid soluble" sodium channel neurotoxins.

enjoys a distinct advantage here as a target for study because of the impressively large number of naturally-occurring neurotoxins that act specifically and with high affinity at different sites on this channel protein. These toxins include, but are not limited to, the channel blockers tetrodotoxin (TTX) and saxitoxin (STX), the channel activators batrachotoxin (BTX), veratridine and aconitine, the polypeptide α-toxins from scorpion and sea anemone that slow the process of channel inactivatino in contrast to the scorpion β-toxins that affect channel activation, and the polyether brevetoxins isolated from the dinoflagellate *Ptychodiscus brevis*. Each of these toxin groups is known to have a different binding site on the sodium channel. This report will focus on the steroidal alkaloid batrachotoxin, the prototypical and most potent member of the so-called "lipid soluble" group of neurotoxins shown in Fig. 1. One of the most interesting aspects of the action of BTX and its congeners is that every functional property of the sodium channel is altered upon binding to a single site (reviewed in Brown, 1988b). BTX is known to simultaneously shift the voltage dependence for channel activation to more negative membrane potentials, block the inactivation process and associated gating charge movement, and increase the apparent physical dimensions of the selectivity filter with concomittant changes in channel conductance and relative ion permeability. This observation suggests that the BTX binding site lies in a key region of the sodium channel that is connected to other domains through significant conformational dynamics underlying channel function. The work presented here underscores this concept and presents data relating to the nature of the BTX binding site.

METHODS

Specific binding of BTX and its congeners on the sodium channel as well as the effects of other sodium channel neurotoxins and ligands on that binding has been measured in standard radioligand binding assays with mammalian brain synaptoneurosomes and synaptosomes using the biologically active derivative [^{3}H]batrachotoxinin-A benzoate (BTX-B) as described (Catterall and coworkers, 1981a; Brown and Daly, 1981; Creveling and coworkers, 1983; Brown and coworkers, 1988a). Additional BTX derivatives, including the fluorescent batrachotoxinin-A N-methylanthranilate (BTX-NMA) and the photoactivatable compound batrachotoxinin-A o-azidobenzoate (BTX-OAB), were synthesized by selective mixed anhydride esterification of the 20-α hydroxy group of batrachotoxinin-A and the structures (Fig. 2) confirmed by mass spectrometry. For the photolabeling experiments, rat brain synaptoneurosomes were equilibrated in the dark with [^{3}H]BTX-OAB under standard binding conditions with the exception that calcium was omitted and a cocktail of protease inhibitors was included in the incubation buffer. Paired control samples contained excess veratridine or other manipulations to block specific binding. The samples were then irradiated for 1 min at a distance of 3-5 cm using a 30 watt Cole Palmer 3815 UV light, filtered and then washed on GF/C filters. To prepare samples for gel electrophoresis the filters were macerated in 0.5 ml sample buffer (0.1M Tris, pH 6.8, 2% SDS, 10% sucrose, 2% mercaptoethanol and bromphenol blue tracking dye), boiled for 3 min, and the solubilized sample collected by centrifugation. Polyacrylamide gel electrophoresis of 20-40 μl aliquots was carried out on 7.5 - 15% SDS gels as described by Laemmli (1970) using a minigel apparatus. The distribution of radioactivity in the completed gel was determined by liquid scintillation counting of sequential 2 mm gel slices. Alternatively, the filters were repeatedly treated with $CHCl_3$/MeOH 2:1 to extract the lipid like material. Aliquots of the extracts were counted to assess the amount of specifically bound label associated with this fraction and the distribution of that radioactivity following silica gel TLC with the solvent system $CHCl_3$/MeOH/HOAc/H_2O, 50:25:8:4, was determined with a Berthold TLC scanner.

RESULTS

Allosteric Interactions at the BTX Binding Site

With the availability of the biologically active and radioactive BTX analog [^{3}H]BTX-B (Brown and coworkers, 1981) has come the opportunity to investigate the BTX binding site of voltage-sensitive sodium channels with direct radioligand binding techniques. Over the last several years work from this laboratory and others has shown that this site is allosterically coupled

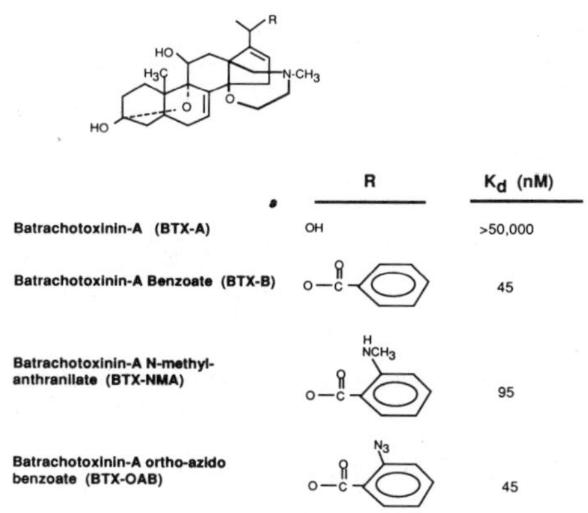

Fig. 2. Structures of synthetic batrachotoxin congeners.

to at least five other distinct domains of the channel protein. Binding of various ligands or toxins to their specific receptors in these domains is thus accompanied by an increase or decrease in BTX-B binding affinity with no change in B_{max} for BTX-B binding. These effects are summarized in Table 1. Such an extensive system of interactions is consonant with the observed multiplicity of BTX effects on channel function and suggests that conformational changes subsequent to BTX binding are distributed broadly to a variety of channel protein domains. Conversely, conformational perturbations initiated at a number of sites that may be molecularly remote are reflected back onto a sensitive, key region of the sodium channel that includes the BTX-B binding site. Direct support of this view has been obtained from fluorescence resonance energy transfer estimates of the distances separating fluorescent neurotoxin derivatives when bound to their respective sodium channel sites. Angelides and his colleagues have found that the separation between such TTX and Leiurus quinquestriatus toxin V derivatives increases by 20% from 35 Å to 42 Å upon binding of BTX (Angelides and Nutter, 1983). The separation between BTX-NMA and the L. quinquestriatus toxin bound to their sodium channel site is approximately 37 Å, showing that these changes must involve major portions of the channel's overall tertiary structure (Angelides and Brown, 1984).

Recently, practical advantage of the extensive allosteric connectivity of the BTX site has been taken in the development of a rapid screening procedure for the detection of compounds active at the voltage-sensitive sodium channel (Brown and Gaupp, 1987). The procedure is based on the standard [^{3}H]BTX-B binding assay, but binding is equilibrated in the presence of several unlabeled effectors, including TTX, the pyrethroid deltamethrin, and L. quinquestriatus scorpion venom, each at approximately half-maximal concentration.

Under these conditions, the specific binding of BTX-B is delicately balanced by the influence of both allosteric inhibition and enhancement, and is poised to respond sensitively to changes in that balance induced by test agents acting at any of at least five distinct channel sites. Active agents are identified either by an observed increase or decrease in specific BTX-B binding. The assay has the utility of casting a rather broad net in a single procedure, but once a test compound has been flagged as being active on the sodium channel, further biochemical and/or electrophysiological tests are required to determine the site and mechanism of action.

Table 1. Allosteric Modifiers of BTX-B Binding

Compound	Effect	Reference
α-Scorpion toxin, sea anemone toxin	Increase affinity	Catterall and coworkers, 1981a
Local anesthetics	Decrease affinity	Creveling and coworkers, 1983, Postma and Catterall, 1984
Diphenylhydantoin and carbamazepine (anticonvulsants)	Decrease affinity	Willow and Catterall, 1982
α-Cyano pyrethroid insecticides	Increase affinity	Brown and coworkers, 1988b
TTX and STX	Decrease affinity	Brown, 1986
Ciguatoxin	Increase affinity (?)	Gonoi and coworkers, 1986
Ptychodiscus brevis toxin	Increase affinity	Catterall and Risk, 1981b Sharkey and coworkers, 1987

This procedure can be quite useful in a variety of circumstances, such as the screening of a panel of monoclonal antibodies raised against channel epitopes, the testing of chromatographic fractions of toxic venoms, or the screening of potential therapeutic compounds resulting from a program of synthesis (G.B. Brown, J.E. Gaupp and R.J. Bradley, unpublished work, in publication).

Nature of the BTX Binding Site

Given these rather distinguishing features of BTX interaction with the sodium channel, it becomes important to learn something more about this unique binding site. What is the environment like? Where is it located with respect to the overall channel structure? How is it related topographically to other channel protein domains? While all of the answers are not known, progress is being made in defining important features of the BTX binding site. The experiments discussed below contribute to a model suggesting that the binding site lies at an interface of protein and lipid in a relatively sequestered fold of the structure, probably at the level of the lipid hydrocarbon chains. Both hydrophilic and hydrophobic mechanisms apparently contribute to the binding interaction.

Not surprisingly, the lipid soluble BTX can access its binding site from either side of the cell membrane, indicating a capacity to permeate the lipid bilayer (Narahashi and coworkers, 1971). Paradoxically, it is a charged, protonated form of BTX that is the active species. By virtue of the slightly basic (pK_a = 8.2) homomorpholino ring nitrogen, BTX (and its congeners) exists as a mixture of protonated and nonprotonated forms at physiological pH (Brown and Daly, 1981). Originally it was thought that the nonprotonated form was the active species (Warnick and coworkers, 1975), but the observation of Bartels-Bernal et al (Bartels-Bernal and coworkers, 1977) that a permanently charged methiodide derivative retained some biological activity forced a more vigorous test of this hypothesis. The specific binding of $[^3H]$BTX-B to mouse brain synaptoneurosomes was therefore measured as a function of pH inthe range 6.0 - 9.0.

As seen in Fig. 3A, the profile is described by a bell-shaped curve with a binding maximum at pH 7.5. Deconvolution of this curve using methods developed by Cleland (1979) show it to be the result of two titratable residues with pK_a's of 7.2 and 8.2 corresponding to the left and right arms of the curve, respectively. Since the pK_a for BTX-B is 8.2, the most parsimonious explanation is that [H+]BTX-B is active and deprotonation of BTX-B with increasing pH leads to decreased binding. The left arm of the curve must then be ascribed to titration of a sodium channel residue of pK_a 7.2, protonation of which blocks toxin binding. The only other possibility is

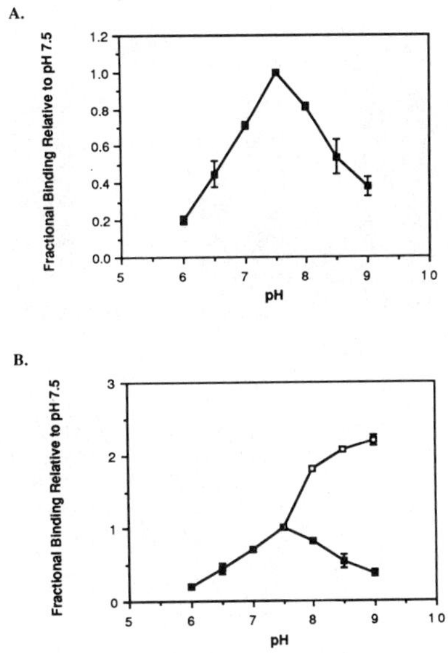

Fig. 3. The pH dependence of BTX-B binding. (A) Mouse brain synaptoneurosomes were equilibrated with 15 nM [^{3}H]BTX-B at the indicated pHs. The resulting specific binding at each pH is expressed as a fraction of that found at pH 7.5 where specific binding is maximal. (B) The normal titration curve shown in (A) for specific BTX-B binding (filled squares) is compared to the superimposed condition where the concentration of the protonated form of BTX-B is held constant at the pH 7.5 level as the pH is varied between 7.5 and 9.0 (open squares).

that both forms of BTX-B are active, and two titratable sodium channel residues are determinants of binding. The experiment illustrated in Fig. 3B was carried out to eliminate this latter possibility. Here, as the pH was varied from 7.5 - 9.0, the total concentration of [^{3}H]BTX-B in the assay mixture was increased as dictated by the Henderson-Hasselbalch equation so that the concentration of the protonated from was constant at each pH. On the other hand, the concentration of nonprotonated BTX-B was 30-fold greater at pH 9.0 than at pH 7.5. If non-protonated BTX-B were an active species one would therefore expect to find a dramatic increase in specific binding across pH range. The result shown in the figure is incompatible with this expectation, but the small two-fold increase in binding actually observed is nicely accounted for by residual deprotonation of the channel pK_a 7.2 residue across this pH range assuming protonated BTX-B to be the active species.

These findings immediately raise a question of the identity of the titratable sodium channel residue responsible for inhibition of BTX-B binding. Although pK_a's for a given protein amino acid residue may vary greatly depending upon the environment, a value of 7.2 focusses attention on weakly basic amino, sulfhydryl or histidyl moieties. Selected group specific chemical modification reactions were therefore carried out as shown in Fig. 4. Rat brain synaptoneurosomes were pre-equilibrated under the indicated conditions, washed, and then resuspended in reagent-free assay buffer for measurement of specific [^{3}H]BTX-B binding. The lack of effect of acetic

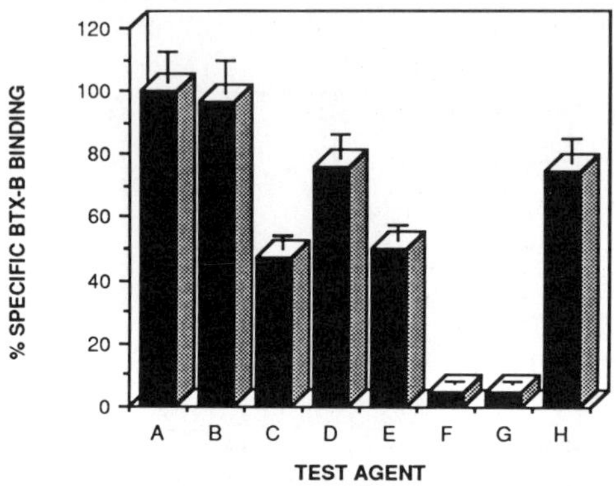

Fig. 4. Effects of amino acid modification reactions on BTX-B binding. Specific [^{3}H]BTX-B binding was determined following pretreatment of synaptoneurosomes with the following reagents as described in the text: (A) Control, sham treated; (B) Acetic anhydride, 85 mM, 1 hr; (C) p-Chloromercuribenzenesulfonic acid, 1 mM, 1 hr; (D) N-Ethylmaleimide, 10 mM, 1 hr; (E) N-Ethylmaleimide, 10 mM, 2 hr; (F) Mercuric chloride, 1 mM, 15 min; (G) Rose bengal-sensitized photooxidation, 10 min; (H) Diethylpyrocarbonate, 0.75 mM, 1 hr.

anhydride argues against the involvement of an accessible amino group, but reagents reacting with cysteinyl and/or histidyl residues all lead in inhibition of BTX-B binding. It is sometimes difficult to distinguish these two possibilities because of overlap in reaction specificities, but the weight of evidence would seem to favor the cysteinyl residue. N-ethylmaleimide and the mercurials are generally quite specific for sulfhydryl groups, but dye-sensitized photooxidation does not discriminate well between the two (Means, and Feeney, 1971). Diethylpyrocarbonate is reasonably specific for the imidazole moiety of histidine, and this treatment does have a significant effect. However, it is possible that this is not specific, since diethylpyrocarbonate slowly hydrolyzes in water yielding two moles of ethanol and ethanol has been reported to inhibit BTX-stimulated sodium flux (Mullin and Hunt, 1985). If, as the data suggest, a cysteinyl group is responsible for inhibition of binding at low pH, then this moiety is likely to be in a rather hydrohilic environment considering the relative sensitivity to mercuric chloride as compared to the less polar p-chloromercuribenzenesulfonic acid and N-ethylmaleimide. It would be premature, however to make this assignment to the BTX binding site. Given the demonstrated conformational connectivity of that site, it is entirely possible, even likely, that the suspected cysteinyl residue is significantly removed from the binding site proper.

Although the above results may not speak directly to the nature of the BTX binding site, other experiments do support the notion that at least part of the binding site microenvironment is relatively polar, consistent with the protonated toxin being the active species. The fluorescent

BTX analog, BTX-NMA, has been particularly useful as a sensitive reporter of the binding site microenvironment (Brown and Bradley, 1984; Angelides and Brown, 1984). When mixed with synaptosomes in the absence of α-scorpion toxin, the emission maximum of BTX-NMA undergoes a blue shift from 425 nm to 405 nm indicating a redistribution from the bulk aqueous phase into a region of greater hydrophobicity. Since this signal could not be blocked by the addition of an excess of nonfluorescent BTX, it was ascribed to nonspecific binding, presumably through intercalation into the synaptosomal membrane interior. However, upon incubation with the allosteric binding enhancer α-scorpion toxin V from L. quinquestriatus, a dramatic 30 nm shift to the red was observed along with an 8-fold increase in fluorescence intensity, showing that under these conditions the fluorophore was situated in a relatively hydrophilic environment. That the shifted signal was due to specifically bound BTX-NMA was demonstrated by the fact that more than 70% of the signal could be blocked by excess BTX.

Further information concerning the BTX binding site could be obtained by application of the photoactivatable BTX derivative $[^3H]$BTX-OAB to covalently label specific elements of that site. Preliminary experiments have been carried out in rat brain cortical synaptosomes and synaptoneurosomes with similar results for both preparations. The basic approach has been to equilibrate tissue with $[^3H]$BTX-OAB in the dark under various experimental and control conditions, irradiate the preparation either prior to or after removal of free $[^3H]$BTX-OAB filter and wash on glass fiber filters, macerate the filters in a minimal volume of SDS sample solution for polyacrylamide gel electrophoresis (PAGE), boil, and finally collect the solubilized samples by filtration or centrifugation for analysis. The finding mentioned above that ligand binding is blocked at this site at pH below 6 has been used to assess the proportion of specific binding that is covalently incorporated. Thus, 30 min incubation in buffer that has been acidified with HCL results in complete dissociation of all noncovalently-bound label, both specific and nonspecific, and the label can easily be removed from the tissue upon filtration. When this procedure is applied to irradiated preparations, 10-30%, depending on conditions, of specifically bound label is irreversibly incorporated into the tissue. Specifically bound label has been defined in numerous controls, including incubations containing excess unlabeled BTX-OAB, BTX-B or veratridine to displace specifically bound label, incubations without scorpion toxin, and incubations using pre-irradiated BTX-OAB. To summarize, all procedures that block specific binding of BTX-OAB also block in a corresponding manner covalent incorporation of label upon photolysis. There is thus every confidence that the data reflect specific covalent labeling of the binding site within the normal constraints of photoaffinity labeling procedures. The initial analysis of photoaffinity labeled samples has been carried out by SDS polyacrylamide gel electrophoresis. Following electrophoresis the gel lanes are sliced, incubated for 5 days in a 1% Triton X-100 solution to leech out the components and then counted by liquid scintillation spectroscopy. Three examples of the results are shown in Fig. 5.

As can be seen, the hallmark of these gels is the major incorporation of specifically bound label into low molecular weight components. The apparent molecular weights, estimated from protein standards on the 15% gels, are <3000 Da. Additional experiments indicate that these components are "lipid-like". Vigorous extraction of the samples with $CHCl_3$/MeOH 2:1 prior to preparation for gel electrophoresis results in the absence of these peaks on the gel. The organic extracts have been analyzed in a preliminary manner by TLC on silica gel plates developed in $CHCl_3$/MeOH/HOAc/H_2O 50:25:8:4, a typical solvent system for separation of phospholipids. One

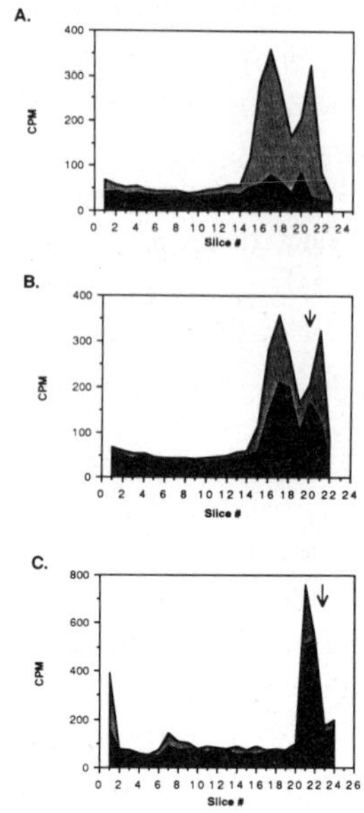

Fig. 5. SDS polyacrylamide gel electrophoresis of photoaffinity-labeled rat brain synaptoneurosomes. (A) A 15% gel comparing incorporation of 20 nM labeled BTX-OAB in the presence and absence of 250 μM veratridine. (B) A 15% gel in which the control was run in the absence of scorpion toxin, resulting in lower affinity BTX-OAB binding, but not in block of binding. (C) A 7.5% gel with veratridine control showing incorporation into protein components. The concentration of BTX-OAB in this experiment was 200 nM. The arrows indicate the dye front of the gels.

broad band of radioactivity is found centered at $R_f = 0.82$. Essentially no radioactivity remains at the origin as would be expected if the sample contained labeled proteinaceous material. When the organic extraction is carried out in a quantitative manner to assess the proportion of covalently bound label in this fraction, 80% of the total specific counts appear in the extract. Similarly, only 10-15% of the total specific counts are precipitable from the SDS sample solution by trichloroacetic acid. Thus, the available data indicate that about 80% of the specifically-incorporated label is found in association with what in all likelihood is lipid. It is interesting to note the significant overall covalent incorporation of label that is obtained (10-30%). Such a large percentage is the exception rather than the rule in these types of studies, and reinforces the hypothesis that the binding site lies in a rather inaccessible fold at a protein-lipid interface. It is as if the bound ligand is "caged" so that ample opportunity exists for the irradiation-induced nitrene to react with its neighbors.

The specific incorporation is not quite so favorable for the proteinaceous components as indicated in Fig. 5C. Here can be seen significant labeling of a protein component in slice 1, corresponding to a M.W. >220,000 Da on this 7.5% gel. This peak can be moved into the gel with a lower crosslinking (5%), but it becomes difficult to analyze because of the low counts distributed over a broad band. This band presumably corresponds to the 260,000 Da α-subunit of the rat brain sodium channel, although there is currently no independent evidence that this is the case other than the fact that its labeling is blocked under conditions that block specific binding of the toxin. The extent of labeling is significantly less than that with the "lipid-like" components, and the concentration of labeled BTX-OAB used for this sample was 200 nM, 10 times higher than that used for labeling in panels A and B. Bands at M.W. ≈ 150 kDa (slice 7 in panel C) and at 45 kDa are sometimes seen in these gels, but due to the paucity of counts it is difficult to ascribe much significance to them at the moment. It is possible they are proteolytic fragments of the larger component, although a cocktail of protease inhibitors is routinely included in all buffers.

CONCLUSION

Data from both electrophysiological and biochemical studies of the effects of BTX and its congeners on the voltage-sensitive sodium channel are consistent in the evocation of a channel model involving extensive conformational interactions between various domains that may be separated by tens of Angstroms. The BTX binding site is somehow central to these interactions, as radioligand binding measurements of the "batrachotoxin connection" demonstrate, and additional information concerning this site promises to provide useful insights on the relationship between sodium channel structure and function. To date, several experimental approaches with radioactive, fluorescent, and/or photoactivatable BTX derivatives have contributed to the working hypothesis that the binding site lies at the interface of lipid and the α-subunit sodium channel polypeptide at the level of the cell membrane interior. It will be of interest to determine the identity of the lipid-like material specifically labeled by the photoactivatable probe BTX-OAB, as other data suggest a close relationship between lipid and channel topology or function (reviewed in Brown, 1988b). Biochemical studies of the α-subunit purified from electric eel have shown that fully 3% of the mass is comprised of lipid that is covalently attached to the protein, and at least an equivalent amount is so tightly associated with the purified protein that it cannot be dissociated by detergent, but requires vigorous extraction with chloroform/methanol mixtures for its removal (Levinson and coworkers, 1986). The covalently attached lipid corresponds to an unprecedented 25 fatty acyl chains per α-subunit, and the function of such extensive acylation is currently unknown.

Ultimately, assignment of the BTX binding site will require knownledge of the specific amino acid segments of the primary channel sequence that interact with the bound neurotoxin. In a major advance, the complete amino acid sequence(s) of the α-subunit from several sources has now been deduced using the techniques of modern molecular biology (Noda and coworkers, 1984; Noda and coworkers, 1986; Salkoff and coworkers, 1987). Based upon the preliminary results of photolabeling experiments with BTX-OAB, it should eventually be possible to isolate and sequence the relevant peptide segments so that they may then be mapped to the known primary sequence. This work is currently in progress. Coupled with similar data for other neurotoxins and a knowledge of the molecular distances between bound neurotoxins as determined from resonance energy transfer measurements, this information will be critically important for the developing understanding of the sodium channel tertiary structure and for understanding the relationship between that structure and function.

ACKNOWLEDGEMENT

Aspects of this work were supported by NIH grant NS-15617 and a US Army Medical Research Acquisition Activity Contract DAMA17-86-C-6057.

REFERENCES

Angelides, K.J., and G.B. Brown (1984). Fluorescence resonance energy transfer on the voltage-dependent sodium channel. Spatial relationship and site coupling between the batrachotoxin and Leiurus quinquestriatus alpha-scorpion toxin receptors. J. Biol. Chem., 259, 6117-6126.

Angelides, K.J., and T.J. Nutter (1983). Mapping the molecular structure of the voltage-dependent sodium channel. Distances between the tetrodotoxin and Leiurus quinquestriatus quinquestriatus scorpion toxin receptors. J. Biol. Chem., 258, 11958-11967.

Angelides, K.J., S. Terakawa, and G.B. Brown (1986). Spatial relations of the neurotoxin binding sites on the sodium channel. Ann. N.Y. Acad. Sci., 479, 221-237.

Bartels-Bernal, E., T. Rosenberry, and J.W. Daly (1977). Effect of batrachotoxin on electroplax of electric eel: Evidence for a voltage-sensitive interaction with sodium channels. Proc. Natl. Acad. Sci. U.S.A., 74:951-955.

Brown, G.B. (1986). Batrachotoxinin A benzoate binding to voltage-sensitive sodium channels: Inhibition by the channel blockers tetrodotoxin and saxitoxin. J. Neurosci., 6, 2064-2070.

Brown, G.B., and R.J. Bradley (1984). Batrachotoxinin A N-methylanthranilate, a new fluorescent ligand for voltage-sensitive sodium channels. J. Neurosci. Meth., 13, 119-129.

Brown, G.B., and J.W. Daly (1981). Interaction of batrachotoxinin A benzoate with voltage-sensitive sodium channels: The effects of pH. Cell Molec. Neurobiol., 1, 361-371.

Brown, G.B., and J.E. Gaupp (1987). A rapid screening procedure for the detection of compounds active at the voltage-sensitive sodium channel. Soc. Neurosci. Abstracts, 13, 147-147.

Brown, G.B., S.C. Tieszen, J.W. Daly, J.E. Warnick, and E.X. Albuquerque (1981). Batrachotoxinin A 20-alpha-benzoate: A new radioactive ligand for voltage-sensitive sodium channels. Cell Molec. Neurobiol. 1, 19-40.

Brown, G.B., J.E. Gaupp, and R.W. Olsen (1988a). Pyrethroid insecticides: Stereospecific, allosteric interaction with the batrachotoxinin A benzoate binding site of voltage-sensitive sodium channels. Mol. Pharmacol., (In Press).

Brown, G.B. (1988b). Batrachotoxin: A window on the allosteric nature of the voltage-sensitive sodium channel. Int. Rev. Neurobiol., 29, 77-116.

Catterall, W.A., C.S. Morrow, J.W. Daly, and G.B. Brown (1981a). Binding of batrachotoxinin A 20-alpha-benzoate to a receptor site associated with sodium channels in synaptic nerve ending particles. J. Biol. Chem., 256, 8922-8927.

Catterall, W.A., and M. Risk (1981b). Toxin T46 from Ptychodiscus brevis (formerly Gymnodinium breve) enhances activation of voltage-sensitive sodium channels by veratridine. Mol. Pharmacol., 19, 345-348.

Cleland, W.W. (1979). Statistical analysis of enzyme kinetic data. Meth. Enzymol., 63A, 103-138.

Creveling, C.R., E.T. McNeal, J.W. Daly, and G.B. Brown (1983). Batrachotoxin-induced depolarization and 3H-batrachotoxinin-A 20-alpha-benzoate binding in a vesicular prepartion from guinea pig cerebral cortex: Inhibition by local anesthetics. Cell Molec. Neurobiol., 23, 350-358.

Gonoi, T., K. Ashida, D. Feller, J. Schmidt, M. Fujiwara, and W.A. Catterall (1986). Mechanism of action of a polypeptide neurotoxin from the coral Goniopora on sodium channels in mouse neuroblastoma cells. Mol. Pharmacol., 29, 347-354.

Hartshorne, R.P., and W.A. Catterall (1984). The sodium channel from rat brain. Purification and subunit composition. J. Biol. Chem., 259, 1667-1675.

Laemmli, U.K. (1970). Cleavage of structural proteins during the assembly of the head of bacteriophage T4. Nature, 227, 680-685.

Levinson, S.R., D.S. Duch, B.W. Urban, and E. Recio-Pinto (1986). The sodium channel from Electrophorus electricus. Ann. N.Y. Acad. Sci., 479, 162-178.

Means, G.E., and R.E. Feeney (1971). Chemical Modification of Proteins, Holden-Day, San Francisco.

Moore, A.C., W.S. Agnew, and M.A. Raftery (1982). Biochemical characterization of the tetrodotoxin binding protein from Electrophorus electricus. Biochem. USA, 21, 6212-6220.

Mullin, M.J., and W.A. Hunt (1985). Actions of ethanol on voltage-sensitive sodium channels: Effects on neurotoxin-stimulated sodium uptake in synaptosomes. J. Pharmacol. Exptl. Therap., 232, 413-419.

Narahashi, T., E.X. Albuquerque, and T. Deguchi (1971). Effects of batrachotoxin on nerve membrane potential and conductance of squid giant axon. J. Gen. Physiol., 58, 54-70.

Noda, M., et al., and S. Numa (1984). Primary sequence of the sodium channel. Nature, 312, 121-125.

Noda, M., T. Ikeda, T. Kayano, J. Suzuki, H. Takashima, M. Kurasaki, H. Takahashi, and S. Numa (1986). Existence of distinct sodium channel messenger RNAs in rat brain. Nature, 320, 118-192.

Postma, W.W., and W.A. Catterall (1984). Inhibition of binding of [3H]batrachotoxinin A 20-alpha-benzoate to sodium channels by local anesthetics. Mol. Pharmacol., 25, 219-227.

Roberts, R.H., and R.L. Barchi (1987). The voltage-sensitive sodium channel from rabbit skeletal muscle. Chemical characterization of subunits. J. Biol. Chem., 262, 2298-2303.

Salkoff, L., A. Butler, A. Wei, N. Scararda, K. Baker, D. Pauron, and C. Smith (1987). Molecular biology of the voltage-gated sodium channel. TINS, 10, 522-527.

Sharkey, R.G., E. Jover, F. Courad, D.G. Baden, and W.A. Catterall (1987). Allosteric modulation of neurotoxin binding to voltage-sensitive sodium channel by *Ptychodiscus brevis* toxin 2. Mol. Pharmacol., 31, 273-278.

Warnick, J.E., E.X. Albuquerque, R. Onur, S.E. Jansson, J.W. Daly, T. Tokuyama, and B. Witkop (1975). The pharmacology of batrachotoxin. VII. Structure-activity relationships and the effects of pH. J. Pharmacol. Exptl. Therap., 193, 232-245.

Willow, M., and W.A. Catterall (1982). Inhibition of binding of [3H]batrachotoxinin A 20 alpha-benzoate to sodium channels by the anticonvulsant drugs diphenylhydantoin and carbamazepine. Mol. Pharmacol., 22, 627-635.

CONOTOXINS: BIOCHEMICAL PROBES FOR ION CHANNELS AND RECEPTORS

Lourdes J. Cruz

Department of Biochemistry and Molecular Biology, College of Medicine, University of the Philippines, P.O. Box 593, Manila, Philippines and Department of Biology, University of Utah, Salt Lake City, UT 84112, USA

ABSTRACT

Conotoxins are a group of neurotoxic peptides found in the venom of marine snails of the genus *Conus*. Currently in use as tools in neurobiology are the major paralytic toxins from fish-hunting species: α-conotoxins which inhibit the acetylcholine receptor at the postsynaptic terminus, ω-conotoxins which block the voltage-sensitive calcium channels at nerve endings, and μ-conotoxins which block muscle voltage-sensitive sodium channels. Although μ-conotoxins have so far been purified only from *C. geographus* venom, α and ω-conotoxins have been isolated from different fish-hunting cone snails. Representatives of each class have been chemically synthesized and radioiodinated for use in examining properties of the target molecules. Our recent data suggest that the various forms and derivatives of conotoxins will be useful in distinguishing channel/receptor subtypes and examining phylogenetic specificities. Many other biologically active peptides have been isolated not only from *C. geographus* and other piscivorous species but also from mollusc-eating and worm-hunting cone snails. These peptides are potentially useful as biochemical probes for the examination of ion channels and receptors which participate in specific behavioral circuits of the brain.

KEYWORDS

Conotoxin; *Conus* venom; snail toxin; conopeptide; conopressin; ion channel; acetylcholine receptor; sodium channel; calcium channel.

INTRODUCTION

For the past several years, the venom of marine snails in the genus *Conus* has provided an increasing number of peptides now used as tools in neurobiology (Gray *et al*., 1988; Olivera *et al*., 1988). Since the first report on the isolation of a paralytic toxin from *Conus geographus* in 1978 (Cruz *et al*., 1978), more than 50 biologically active peptides have been isolated and sequenced (Cruz *et al*., 1985; Gray *et al*., 1988; Hillyard *et al*., 1988; Olivera *et al*., 1985; Zafaralla *et al*., 1988; Corpuz and Ramilo, unpublished data, Zafaralla and Abogadie, unpublished data). In this paper, the biochemistry of the major paralytic toxins and their use as probes for ion channels will be discussed. Examples of other biologically active peptides will be given to illustrate the variety of peptides from *Conus* venom which can be developed as probes for ion channels and receptors. Possible biological reasons for the existence of these numerous peptides in *Conus* venom will be presented.

Most of the peptides so far reported are from a fish-hunting cone snail, *C. geographus*, the most dangerous species. Careless handling of the cone shell by divers and collectors has resulted in human fatalities; over 20 fatal stinging cases are reported in the literature (reviewed in Cruz *et al*., 1985). Among the symptoms observed in man are numbness at the site of stinging which spreads to the upper part of the limb and to the rest of the body.

Blurring of vision, impaired speech and muscle paralysis precedes death (Clench and Kondo, 1943; Lyman, 1948) which is believed to be due to asphyxiation by paralysis of the diaphragm muscles (Endean and Rudkin, 1963).

The venom is used by *Conus* mainly for catching and paralyzing prey (Kohn *et al*., 1960). It is synthesized in a long venom duct and injected into the prey by means of a disposable harpoon/tooth which comes from a radula sac adjacent to the pharynx; numerous harpoons at different stages of formation are contained in the sac. When ready to sting, a harpoon is positioned at the end of a distensible proboscis and used like a hypodermic needle. The fish gets paralyzed and rapidly engulfed by the cone snail. Although the major venom peptides, ω, α and μ-conotoxins can all paralyze fish, only α and μ-conotoxins are paralytic to mice and most probably humans.

α-CONOTOXINS

The α-conotoxins are a group of homologous basic peptides which inhibit the acetylcholine receptor (Gray *et al*., 1981). Several peptides belonging to this toxin class have been isolated from fish-hunting species. Comparison of the amino acid sequences of α-conotoxins from *C. geographus* (Gray *et al*., 1981) and *C. magus* (McIntosh *et al*., 1982) indicates a high degree of homology (see Table 1). The peptides shown contain 13 to 15 amino acid residues of which four are cysteine residues participating in disulfide bonds (Gray *et al*., 1983, 1984; Nishiuchi and Sakakibara, 1982) as indicated. All four toxins can cause paralysis in fish and mice when injected intraperitoneally (ip).

Table 1. α-Conotoxins: Inhibitors of nicotinic acetylcholine receptors

Species	α-Conotoxin	Sequence[a]	Charge[b]
C. geographus	GI	E C C N P A C G R H Y S C *	+1.5
	GIA	E C C N P A C G R H Y S C G K *	+2.5
	GII	E C C H P A C G K H F S C *	+2
C. magus	MI	G R C C H P A C G K N Y S C *	+3.5
Disulfide bridges		- C C - - - C - - - - - - C - (C1–C3, C2–C4)	

[a]Symbols are standard one-letter code for amino acids; *, amidated carboxy-terminal.
[b]Net ionic charge at neutral pH.

α-Conotoxin GI has been shown to compete with d-tubocurarine and α-bungarotoxin for the acetylcholine (ACh) receptor (McManus *et al*., 1981, 1985). One of the proposed molecular models for GI shows a similarity in the orientation of side groups with that of the active loop of a snake α-neurotoxin, erabutoxin (Gray *et al*., 1985). Radiolabeled derivatives of synthetic α-conotoxins have been prepared and used for studies of their crosslinking with the ACh receptor. In membrane preparations from *Torpedo* electric organ, ^{125}I α-conotoxin MI labels the γ and β subunits of the ACh receptor (Myers, unpublished data). Since the binding of snake α-neurotoxins are mainly with the α subunits, the crosslinking data together with competition data could suggest the location of MI binding sites close to the α-β and α-γ subunit boundaries of the receptor.

Recently three other α-conotoxins have been isolated from another fish-hunting species, *C. striatus*. With the chemical synthesis of α-conotoxin SI, enough material has become available for comparison of its activities with those of conotoxins from *C. geographus* and *C. magus* as indicated in Table 2 (Zafaralla *et al*., 1988). The relative activities shown for *Torpedo* and chick are based on the competition of GI, MI and SI with α-bungarotoxin for sites on membrane preparations from *Torpedo* electric organ and chick optic lobe, respectively.

Although the three peptides have similar activities in Torpedo electroplax, MI differs from the other two with respect to its very high activity in chick optic lobe. In contrast to GI and MI, α-conotoxin SI does not paralyze mice when injected ip. However, SI is paralytic to fish, the natural prey. Comparison of the amino acid sequences of the peptides suggest that the replacement of Glu-1 in α-conotoxin GI by Gly-Arg in α-conotoxin MI may be responsible for the activity difference of the two peptides in chick brain; the inability of SI to paralyze mice may be due to the replacement of Arg-His in positions 9-10 of GI or Lys-Asn in positions 10-11 of MI by Pro-Lys in positions 9-10 of SI.

Table 2. Structure-activity relationshps of α-conotoxins

α-Conotoxin	Relative Activity		
	Torpedo electric organ	Chick optic lobe	Mouse ip injection
GI	0.6	<< 0.1	~ 1
MI	1.0	1.0	~ 1
SI	0.8	< 0.01	< 0.02

α-Conotoxin	Amino acid sequence
GI	E C C N P A C G R H Y S G - NH_2
MI	**G R** C C H P A C G K N Y S C - NH_2
SI	I C C N P A C G **P K** Y S C - NH_2

The availability of several α-conotoxins with different phylogenetic specificities provides a set of useful tools for the study of the structure of ACh receptors from different organisms. One of the other peptides recently isolated from C. striatus presents an even more novel α-conotoxin structure containing six Cys residues, three of which are contiguous (Zafaralla et al., unpublished data). This should provide valuable information on the interaction of α-conotoxins with ACh receptor variants.

ω-CONOTOXINS

One family of Conus peptides, the ω-conotoxins has been shown to block the voltage-sensitive calcium channel at nerve terminals (Feldman et al., 1987; Kerr and Yoshikami, 1984). The peptides were first isolated as components of C. geographus venom which induce "shaking" in mice when injected intracranially (Olivera et al., 1984). They paralyze fish and so far ω-conotoxins have been found in all fish-hunting Conus species examined including C. geographus (Olivera et al., 1985), C. magus (Olivera et al., 1987), C. striatus (Zafaralla and Cruz, unpublished data) and C. tulipa (Haack and Olivera, unpublished data). Structures published to date are shown in Table 3. The toxins contain 24-29 amino acid residues, three disulfide bridges and a charge of +4 to +6. The peptides are amidated at the C-terminal and on the average, one out of every three amino acids are hydroxylated. The original grouping of ω-conotoxins into the VI and VII series was based on the ability of GVIA but not of MVIIA to block calcium channels at the frog neuromuscular junction (Olivera et al., 1985). Succeeding peptides isolated were assigned to a particular series depending on their structural similarity to either peptide. Slight differences among GVIA, B and C are probably due to processing variation at the carboxyl end; divergence between peptides within the VII series is much greater. Representatives of the VI and VII series have been chemically synthesized (Olivera et al., 1987; Sakakibara et al., 1986).

Monoiodinated derivatives of ω-conotoxin GVIA are biologically active (Cruz et al., 1986, 1987) and have been used as biochemical probes for neuronal calcium channels (reviewed in Gray et al., 1988). Autoradiographic techniques to determine the site of binding of GVIA in rat brain slices indicate binding to practically all portions of the brain but with insignificant labeling of corpus callosum and some regions of the cerebellum (Kerr et al., 1988). Physiological and pharmacological studies suggest, however, a multiplicity of neuronal calcium channels. Gel patterns obtained after crosslinking of two different radioiodinated derivatives of GVIA with membrane preparations from chick brain apparently supports this (Cruz *et al.*, 1987b; Imperial *et al.*, unpublished data). Using ^{125}I photo-activatable derivatives of GVIA, major specifically labeled bands were obtained at 93 K, 240 K and 300 K daltons. With ^{125}I-GVIA crosslinked to the membrane preparation by the bivalent crosslinker disuccinimidyl suberate, two major bands at 135 K and 195 K were obtained. Three minor bands were also evident at 160 K, 220 K and 300 K daltons. Although some of the bands may correspond to different subunits of the same channel, there is evidence that at least other bands may be due to different channels or receptors. In *Torpedo* electric organ, it does not matter which GVIA derivative is used; a band at 150 K daltons is always obtained. This may indicate the presence of only one major calcium channel type in the tissue.

Table 3. ω-Conotoxins: Blockers of neuronal voltage sensitive calcium channels

Species	ω-Conotoxin	Sequence[a]	Charge[b]
C. geographus	GVIA	C K S P̲ G S S C S P̲ T S Y N C C R S C N P̲ Y T K R C Y *	+5
	B	- Y G	(+4)
	C	- -	(+4)
	GVIIA	C K S P̲ G T P̲ C S R G M R D C C T S C L L Y S N K C R R Y	(+5)
	B	- S - - - - - - - - -	(+5)
C. magus	MVIIA	C K G K G A K C S R L M Y D C C T G S C R S G K C *	+6
	MVIIB	C - - - - - S C H - T S - - C C - - - C N R - - C *	+5½
Disulfide Bridges		C - - - - - - C - - - - - - - C C - - - C - - - - - C -	

[a]Symbols as in Table 1, plus: P̲, hydroxyproline; -, same residue as in peptide immediately above.
[b]Net ionic charge. Values in parentheses based on assumption of free carboxy-terminus.

Until recently, synthetic drugs such as dihydropyridines, phenylalkylamines and benzothiazepines were the only major probes used for studying voltage-sensitive calcium channels; dihydropyridines have been used to isolate calcium channels from T-tubules (Curtis and Catterall, 1984; Borsotto *et al.*, 1985). With the introduction of ω-conotoxins as probes, researchers are now looking at the properties of neuronal calcium channels. These structurally related peptides from venom of fish-hunting species specifically inhibit voltage-sensitive neuronal calcium channels thus preventing the release of neurotransmitters from nerve endings (Dooley *et al.*, 1987; Reynolds *et al.*, 1986; Yeager *et al.*, 1987). Calcium channels from heart and skeletal muscles are apparently insensitive to these toxins (Cruz *et al.*, 1987). In chick dorsal root ganglion (DRG), McCleskey *et al.* (1987) demonstrated GVIA to irreversibly block the L type and N type calcium channels but not T type channels. There is evidence that ω-conotoxin GVIA differs from MVIIA with respect to their interaction with calcium channels from different organisms (Cruz *et al.*, 1987c; Olivera *et al.*, 1987). ω-Conotoxin variants from different *Conus* species and their derivatives are very promising as potential biochemical probes for distinguishing subtypes of neuronal calcium channels.

μ-CONOTOXINS

The μ-type of *Conus* peptides cause paralysis in fish and mice by blocking the voltage-sensitive sodium channels in skeletal muscle (Cruz *et al.*, 1985a) So far μ-conotoxins have only been isolated from *C. geographus*. The primary structures of the known variants are shown in Table 4. The peptides have 22 amino acid residues, 3 disulfide bonds and 2 to 3 residues of hydroxyproline. Like the two other types of paralytic toxins, μ-conotoxins are positively charged (+6 to +7) and are amidated at the C-terminal. Although the disulfide bonding pattern of μ-conotoxins has not yet been determined, GIIIA has already been chemically synthesized (Cruz et al., 1988).

Table 4. μ-Conotoxins: Blockers of muscle voltage-sensitive sodium channels

μ-Conotoxin	Sequence[a]	Charge[b]
GIIIA	R D C C T P̲ P̲ K K C K D R Q C K P̲ Q R C C A *	+6
[Pro^6] GIIIA	- - - - - P - - - - - - - - - - - - - - - -	
[Pro^7] GIIIA	- - - - - - P - - - - - - - - - - - - - - -	
GIIIB	R D C C T P̲ P̲ R K C K D R R C K P̲ M K C C A *	+7
[Pro^6] GIIIB	- - - - - P - - - - - - - - - - - - - - - -	
[Pro^7] GIIIB	- - - - - - P - - - - - - - - - - - - - - -	
GIIIC	R D C C T P̲ P̲ K K C K D R R C K P̲ L K C C A *	+7

[a]Symbols as in Tables 1 and 3.
[b]Net ionic charge at neutral pH.

μ-Conotoxins compete with saxitoxin and tetrodotoxin for Site 1 on the sodium channel but not with batrachotoxin or Leiurus scorpion toxin which bind at other sites (Ohizumi et al., 1986, 1986a; Yanagawa et al., 1987). However, they differ from the guanidinium toxins in being very selective for the muscle type channel versus the neuronal sodium channel by about 1000-fold discrimination (Moczydlowski et al., 1986, 1986a). Cardiac muscle sodium channels are insensitive to μ-conotoxins. A ^{125}I-(4-hydroxyphenyl) propionyl derivative of GIIIA has been prepared and used for examining binding of the toxin to membrane preparations from electric eel. The labeled toxin is specifically competed out by unlabeled GIIIA and tetrodotoxin but not by α and ω-conotoxins (Cruz et al., 1988). Preliminary crosslinking studies revealed a specifically labeled band in the size region for sodium channels (Olivera and LeCheminant, unpublished data). μ-Conotoxins are potentially useful probes for the biochemical dissection of muscle voltage-sensitive sodium channels.

OTHER BIOLOGICALLY ACTIVE PEPTIDES OF CONUS VENOM

In addition to the 24 paralytic toxins of the ω, μ and α types, about 30 other peptides have been isolated and sequenced from various Conus species (see Fig. 1) including mollusc-hunters such as C. textile and C. marmoreus (Corpuz et al., unpublished data) and worm-eaters such as C. quercinus (Abogadie et al., unpublished data). The conopeptides induce a spectrum of behavioral symptoms when injected intracranially in mice. One of the more interesting peptides isolated from C. geographus induces young mice to sleep but causes hyperactivity in older animals (McIntosh et al., 1984; Rivier et al., 1987). The peptide (designated as GV) has 5 residues of an unusual amino acid, γ-carboxyglutamate (Gla) out of 17 amino acids; no cysteines are present. Recently another "sleep-inducing" peptide has been isolated from C. tulipa (designated as TV); among its amino acids, four of the Gla residues are conserved (J. Haack and B.M. Olivera, unpublished data). Gla has been found only in few proteins including blood clotting proteins and bone proteins where they play an important role in protein interaction with calcium ions (Hauschka et al., 1982; Poser et al., 1980; Stenflo and Suttie, 1977).

A couple of vasopressin analogs (Table 5) have also been isolated from C. geographus and C. tulipa as peptides which cause mice to scratch when injected ic (Cruz et al., 1987a). Both conopressin G from C. geographus and conopressin S from C. striatus have arginine at position 4 instead of the glutamine present in vasopressin and oxytocin resulting in an additional positive charge. All other substitutions are relatively conservative.

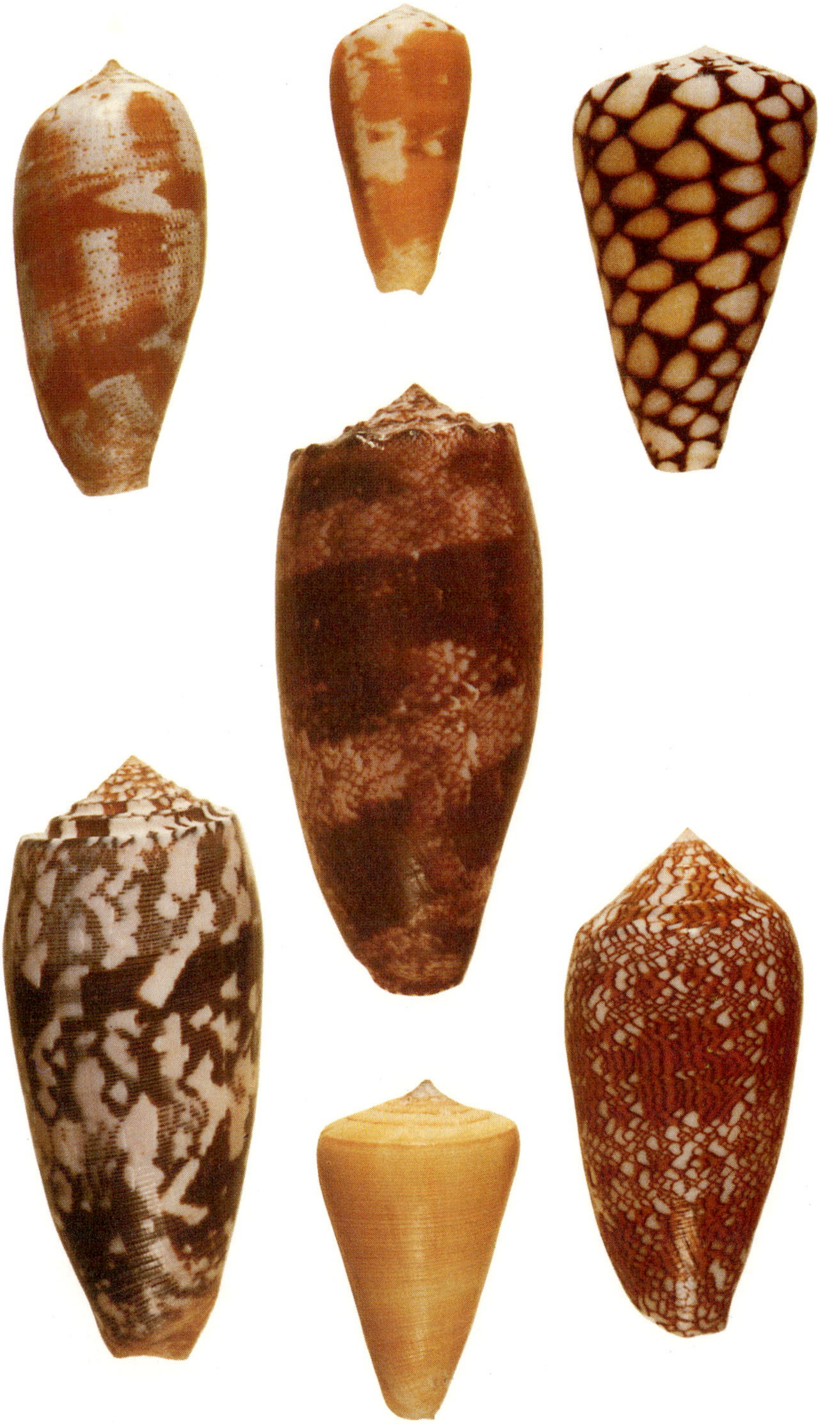

Fig. 1. Shells of several *Conus* species. Center: the geography cone, *Conus geographus* Linné. From top clockwise: *Conus magus* Linné, *Conus marmoreus* Linné, *Conus textile* Linné, *Conus quercinus* Solander, *Conus striatus* Linné, *Conus tulipa* Linné. All specimens were obtained from the Philippines. *C. textile* and *C. marmoreus* are molluscivorous; all other specimens shown are piscivorous.

Table 5. Primary structure of conopressins and related peptides

Species or Animal Group	Peptide	Sequence	Charge
C. geographus	Conopressin G	C F I R N C P K G *	+3
C. striatus	S	C I I R N C P R G *	+3
Vertebrates	Arg-Vasotocin	C Y I Q N C P R G *	+2
Mammals	Arg-Vasopressin	C Y F Q N C P R G *	+2
Mammals	Oxytocin	C Y I Q N C P L G *	+1

Examination of venom from molluscivorous and vermivorous Conus species reveals numerous other peptides not found in fish-hunting species. Among these is a peptide from C. textile which is not active in mice or fish but causes periodic convulsion-like motion in garden snails. When injected into lobsters, the peptide induces a dominant posture never observed in small lobsters in the presence of a bigger lobster in the same aquarium, thus the name "King-Kong peptide" (Hillyard et al., 1988).

The availability of numerous peptides affecting behavior will be a boon to neurobiology by providing possible tools for the examination of ion channels and receptors which participate in specific behavioral circuits in the brain.

WHY SO MANY PEPTIDES IN CONUS VENOM?

The variety of peptides found in Conus venom is staggering. One would think that a single lethal or paralytic component might be sufficient to subdue the prey. Instead, in C. geographus venom alone, three types of paralytic peptides blocking successive steps in impulse transmission are found, and each type is represented by several homologous peptides. In addition, there are many other peptides such as conotoxin GV and conopressin G which are not strongly paralytic to fish.

The range of situations encountered by cone snails in their habitat may provide the key to the existence of a variety of peptides in Conus venom (Olivera et al., 1985). In the case of fish-hunting species, it is necessary to very rapidly paralyze a much more mobile prey to ensure its capture and to prevent the attraction of predators. Even in aquaria, cones bury under the gravel or hide in corners and crevices right after catching a fish, most probably as a safety measure to prevent attack at the time when they are most vulnerable. The simultaneous blockade of three key elements involved in the transmission of impulses will ensure rapid paralysis and may provide a wider spectrum of susceptible prey types. Some peptides may play accessory roles to facilitate the effect of paralytic toxins in fish perhaps by promoting rapid transport of paralytic toxins to their targets. Such a role may be played by peptides like conopressin G and S. Still other conopeptides may function in defense mechanisms against predators such as crabs which can crush thin-shelled Conus species such as C. geographus and C. tulipa. These peptides may target toward ion channels and receptors of the predator neuromuscular system.

The existence of as many active components has not yet been demonstrated for other venoms. Although the situation could be unique to Conus species, a more detailed examination of minor venom components in other animals may reveal more complex mixtures than what is currently apparent.

ACKNOWLEDGMENTS

The work described here was done mainly in collaboration with B.M. Olivera of the Dept. of Biology, University of Utah, and with J.R. Rivier of the Peptides Biology Laboratory, The Salk Institute and W.R. Gray of the Dept. of Biology, University of Utah. Since the Conus project started 18 years ago, it has been supported at one time or another by grants to the author from the National Research Council of the Philippines, Marine Science Institute of the University of the Philippines, Miles Laboratories Inc., U.S.A. and the International Foundation for Science, Stockholm, Sweden, and by grants to Dr. B.M. Olivera from the National Institutes of Health, U.S.A.

REFERENCES

Archer, R. (1980). Molecular evolution of biologically active polypeptides. Proc. R. Soc. Lond. B. Biol. Sci., 210, 21-45.

Borsotto, M., J. Barhanin, M. Fosset and M. Lazdunski (1985). The 1,4-dihydropyridine receptor associated with the skeletal muscle voltage-dependent Ca^{++} channel. J. Biol. Chem., 260, 14255-14263.

Clench, W.J. and Y. Kondo (1943). The poison cone shell. Amer. J. Trop. Med., 23, 105-120.

Cruz, L.J., W.R. Gray and B.M. Olivera (1978). Purification and properties of a myotoxin from Conus geographus venom. Arch. Biochem. Biophys., 190, 539-548.

Cruz, L.J., W.R. Gray, D. Yoshikami and B.M. Olivera (1985). Conus venoms: A rich source of neuroactive peptides. J. Toxicol.-Toxin Reviews, 4, 107-132.

Cruz, L.J., W.R. Gray, B.M. Olivera, R.D. Zeikus, L. Kerr, D. Yoshikami and E. Moczydlowski (1985a). Conus geographus toxins that discriminate between neuronal and muscle sodium channels. J. Biol. Chem., 260, 9280-9288.

Cruz, L.J. and B.M. Olivera (1986). Calcium channel antagonists. ω-Conotoxin defines a new high affinity site. J. Biol. Chem., 261, 6230-6233.

Cruz, L.J., D.S. Johnson and B.M. Olivera (1987). A characterization of the ω-conotoxin target. Evidence for the tissue-specific heterogeneity in Ca channel types. Biochemistry, 26, 820-824.

Cruz, L.J., V. de Santos, G.C. Zafaralla, C.A. Ramilo, R. Zeikus, W.R. Gray and B.M. Olivera (1987a). Invertebrate and vasopression/oxytocin homologs. Characterization of peptides from Conus geographus and Conus striatus venoms. J. Biol. Chem., 262, 15821-15824.

Cruz, L.J., J.S. Imperial, D.S. Johnson and B.M. Olivera (1987b). Crosslinking by ^{125}I-ω-conotoxin: Evidence suggesting multiple neuronal calcium channel subtypes. Abstr. Soc. Neurosci., 13, 1011.

Cruz, L.J., D.S. Johnson, J. Imperial, D. Griffin, G.W. LeCheminant, G.P. Miljanich and B.M. Olivera (1987c). ω-Conotoxins and voltage sensitive calcium channel subtypes. Current Topics in Membranes and Transport, 33, 417-429.

Cruz, L.J., G. Kupryszewski, G.W. LeCheminant, W.R. Gray, B.M. Olivera and J. Rivier (1988). μ-Conotoxin GIIIA, a peptide ligand for muscle Na channels: Chemical synthesis, radiolabeling and receptor characterization. Biochemistry, Accepted for publication.

Curtis, B.M. and W.A. Catterall (1984). Purification of the calcium antagonist receptor of the voltage-sensitive calcium channel from skeletal muscle transverse tubules. Biochemistry, 23, 2113-2118.

Dooley, D.J., A. Lupp and G. Hertling (1987). Inhibition of central neurotransmitter release by ω-conotoxin GVIA, a peptide modulator of the N-type voltage-sensitive calcium channel. Naunyn-Schmiedeberg's Arch. Pharmacol., 336, 467-470.

Endean, R. and C. Rudkin (1963). Studies of the venoms of some Conidae. Toxicon, 1, 49-64.

Feldman, D.M., B.M. Olivera and D. Yoshikami (1987). Omega Conus geographus toxin: A peptide that blocks Ca channels. FEBS. Lett., 214, 295-300.

Gray, W.R., A. Luque, B.M. Olivera, J. Barrett and L.J. Cruz (1981). Peptide toxins from Conus geographus venom. J. Biol. Chem., 256, 4734-4740.

Gray, W.R., J.E. Rivier, R. Galyean, L.J. Cruz and B.M. Olivera (1983). Conotoxin MI. Disulfide bonding and conformational states. J. Biol. Chem., 258, 12247-12251.

Gray, W.R., F.A. Luque, R. Galyean, E. Atherton, R.C. Sheppard, B.L. Stone, A. Reyes, J. Alford, M. McIntosh, B.M. Olivera, L.J. Cruz and R. Rivier (1984). Conotoxin GI: Disulfide bridges, synthesis and preparation of iodinated derivatives. Biochemistry, 23, 2796-2802.

Gray, W.R., D.M. Middlemas, R. Zeikus, B.M. Olivera and L.J. Cruz (1985). Structure-activity relationships in α-conotoxins. In: The Ninth American Peptide Symposium (C.M. Deber, V.J. Hruby and K.D. Kopple, ed.), pp. 823-831. Pierce Chem. Co., Rockford.

Gray, W.R., B.M. Olivera and L.J. Cruz (1988). Peptide toxins from venomous Conus snails. Annu. Rev. Biochem., 57, 665-700.

Hadley, M.E. (1984). Neurohypophysial hormones. In: Endocrinology, pp. 140-159. Prentice Hall, Inc., Englewood Cliffs, NJ.

Hauschka, P.V., S.A. Carr and K. Biemann (1982). Primary structure of monkey osteocalcin. Biochemistry., 21, 638-642.

Hillyard, D.R., B.M. Olivera, S. Woodward, G.P. Corpuz, W.R. Gray, C.A. Ramilo and L.J. Cruz (1988). A molluscivorous Conus toxin; conserved frameworks in conotoxins. Biochemistry, 27, Accepted for publication.

Kerr, L.M. and D. Yoshikami (1984). A venom peptide with a novel presynaptic blocking action. Nature (Lond.), 308, 282-284.

Kerr, L.M., F. Filloux, B.M. Olivera, H. Jackson and J.K. Wamsley (1988). Autoradiographic localization of calcium channels with [^{125}I]ω-conotoxin in rat brain. Eur. J. Pharmacol., 146, 181-183.

Kohn, A.J., P.R. Saunders and S. Wiener (1960). Preliminary studies on the venom of the marine snail Conus. Ann. NY Acad Sci., 90, 706-725.

Lyman, F. (1948). Authentic case of death by poisonous cone shell. Shell Notes, 2, 78-82.

McCleskey, E.W., A.P. Fox, D. Feldman, L.J. Cruz, B.M. Olivera, R.W. Tsien and D. Yoshikami (1987). Multiple types of calcium channels distinguished by a peptide toxin. Proc. Natl. Acad. Sci. USA, 84, 4327-4331.

McIntosh, M., L.J. Cruz, M.W. Hunkapiller, W.R. Gray and B.M. Olivera (1982). Isolation and structure of a peptide toxin from the marine snail Conus magus. Arch. Biochem. Biophys., 218, 329-334.

McIntosh, J.M., B.M. Olivera, L.J. Cruz and W.R. Gray (1984). γ-Carboxyglutamate in a neuroactive toxin. J. Biol. Chem., 259, 14343-14346.

McManus, O.B., J.R. Musick and C. Gonzalez (1981). Peptides isolated from the venom of Conus geographus block neuromuscular transmission. Neurosci. Lett., 24, 57-62.

McManus, O.B. and J.R. Musick (1985). Postsynaptic block of frog neuromuscular transmission by conotoxin GI. J. Neurosci., 5, 110-116.

Moczydlowski, E., B.M. Olivera, W.R. Gray and G.R. Strichartz (1986). Discrimination of muscle and neuronal Na-channel subtypes by binding competition between ^{3}H-saxitoxin and μ-conotoxin. Proc. Natl. Acad. Sci. USA, 83, 5321-5325.

Moczydlowski, E., A. Uehara, K.T. Guo and J. Heiny (1986a). Isochannels and blocking modes of voltage-dependent sodium channels. Ann. NY Acad. Sci., 479, 269-292.

Nishiuchi, Y., K. Kumagaye, Y. Noda, T.X. Watanabe and S. Sakakibara (1986). Synthesis and secondary-structure determination of ω-conotoxin GVIA: A 27-peptide with three intramolecular disulfide bonds. Biopolymers, 25, S61-S68.

Ohizumi, Y., S. Minoshima, M. Takahashi, A. Kajimara, H. Nakamura and J. Kobayashi (1986). Geographutoxin II, a novel peptide inhibitor of Na channels of skeletal muscles and autonomic nerves. J. Pharmacol. Exptl. Therapeutics, 239, 243-248.

Ohizumi, Y., H. Nakamura, J. Kobayashi and W.A. Catteral (1986a). Specific inhibition of [^{3}H] saxitoxin binding to skeletal muscle sodium channels by geographutoxin II, a polypeptide channel blocker. J. Biol. Chem., 261, 6149-6152.

Olivera, B.M., J.M. McIntosh, L.J. Cruz, F.A. Luque and W.R. Gray (1984). Purification and sequence of a presynaptic peptide toxin from Conus geographus venom. Biochemistry, 23, 5087-5090.

Olivera, B.M., W.R. Gray, R. Zeikus, J.M. McIntosh, J. Varga, J. Rivier, V. de Santos and L.J. Cruz (1985). Novel peptide neurotoxins from fish-hunting cone snails. Science, 230, 1338-1343.

Olivera, B.M., L.J. Cruz, V. de Santos, G.W. LeCheminant, D. Griffin, R. Zeikus, J.M. McIntosh, R. Galyean, J. Varga, W.R. Gray and J. Rivier (1987). Neuronal calcium channel antagonists. Discrimination between calcium channel subtypes using ω-conotoxin from Conus magus venom. Biochemistry, 26, 2086-2090.

Olivera, B.M., W.R Gray and L.J. Cruz (1988). Marine snail venoms. In: Handbook of Natural Toxins (A.T. Tu, ed.), Vol. 3, pp. 327-352. Marcel Dekker, Inc., New York and Basel.

Poser, J.W., F.S. Esch, N.C. Ling and P.A. Price (1980). Isolation and sequence of the vitamin K-dependent protein from human bone. J. Biol. Chem., 255, 8685-8691.

Reynolds, I.J., J.A. Wagner, S.H. Snyder, S.A. Thayer, B.M. Olivera and R.J. Miller (1986). Brain voltage-sensitive calcium channel subtypes differentiated by ω-conotoxin fraction GVIA. Proc. Natl. Acad. Sci. USA, 84, 8804-8807.

Rivier, J., R. Galyean, L. Simon, L.J. Cruz, B.M. Olivera and W.R. Gray (1987). Total synthesis and further characterization of the γ-carboxyglutamate-containing "sleeper" peptide from Conus geographus venom. Biochemistry, 26, 8508-8512.

Stenflo, J. and J.W. Suttie (1977). Vitamin K-dependent formation of γ-carboxyglutamic acid. Annu. Rev. Biochem., 46, 157-172.

Yanagawa, Y., T. Abe and M. Satake (1987). μ-Conotoxins share a common binding site with tetrodotoxin/saxitoxin on eel electroplax Na channels. J. Neurosci., 7, 1498-1502.

Yeager, R.E., D. Yoshikami, J. Rivier and L.J. Cruz (1987). Transmitter release from presynaptic terminals of electric organ: Inhibition by the calcium channel antagonist omega *Conus* toxin. *J. Neurosci.*, *7*, 2390-2396.

Zafaralla, G.C., C. Ramilo, W.R. Gray, R. Karlstrom, B.M. Olivera and L.J. Cruz (1988). Phylogenetic specificity of cholinergic ligands: α-Conotoxin SI. *Biochemistry*, *27*, In press.

III. Use of Cloning Techniques in the Study of Toxins

POSTSYNAPTICALLY-ACTING TOXINS AND PROTEINS WITH PHOSPHOLIPASE STRUCTURE FROM SNAKE VENOMS: COMPLETE AMINO ACID SEQUENCES DEDUCED FROM cDNAs and PRODUCTION OF A TOXIN WITH STAPHYLOCOCCAL PROTEIN A GENE FUSION VECTOR.

F. DUCANCEL, G. GUIGNERY-FRELAT, T. TAMIYA*, J-C. BOULAIN and A. MÉNEZ

Service de Biochimie, Département de Biologie, CEN Saclay, 91191 Gif-sur-Yvette, France.
*Present address: Faculty of Science and Technology, Sophia University, Tokyo, Japan

ABSTRACT

We describe the cloning and nucleotide sequences of i) three cDNAs encoding postsynaptically-acting neurotoxins and ii) three cDNAs encoding proteins with phospholipase A_2 structure [PLA_2], present in the venom glands of sea or land snakes. Two of these sequences were already known, but the four others corresponded to hitherto unknown proteins. The signal peptides of the neurotoxins and PLA_2 respectively consisted of 21 and 27 amino acid residues. We also describe the production of a hybrid protein molecule comprising the successive sequences of staphylococcal protein A and a postsynaptically-acting neurotoxin. The amount of hybrid produced per liter of culture was in the milligram range. This hybrid protein had biological properties similar to those of native postsynaptically-acting neurotoxins. Antiserum raised in rabbits against this protein afforded protection both **in vitro** and **in vivo**, from the harmful effects of the toxin.

KEYWORDS

Cloning; cDNA; protein fusion; neurotoxin; phospholipase A2; snake.

INTRODUCTION

Snake venoms are complex mixtures of proteins, some of which are potent toxins. These toxins are capable of killing snake preys by affecting vital processes such as muscle and nerve functions or blood circulation. Snake toxins are usually classified according to their biological activities. However, such classification is rather difficult and even confusing because the biological properties of snake toxins are extremely diverse. In 1979, Karlsson proposed classifying them into two stuctural groups. Although this classification system does not cover all the snake toxins it certainly includes the most common **Elapidae** and **Hydrophiidae** toxins and some **Viperidae** toxins.

The snake toxins in structural group I are single chain proteins of 60 to 74 amino acid residues with four to five disulfide bridges (Karlsson, 1979). Their polypeptide chain is folded into three adjacent loops rich in ß-pleated sheets, emerging from a small globular core containing the disulfides (Low, et al., 1976, Tsernoglou and Petsko, 1977, Walkinshaw et al., 1980, Love and Stroud, 1986, Rees et al., 1987). This group includes [i] the postsynaptically-acting neurotoxins (Endo and Tamiya, 1987) which block the nicotinic acetylcholine receptors, thereby preventing the depolarizing action of acetylcholine (Changeux et al., 1984). These toxins are abundant in the venoms of **Elapidae** and **Hydrophiidae** and constitute minor components of some **Viperidae** venoms (Jiang et al., 1987); [ii] the cardiotoxins, also referred to as cytotoxins or direct lytic factor (Harvey, 1985, Dufton and Hider, 1988). They are capable of various actions including depolarization of excitable cell membranes and cytotoxicity. Cardiotoxins have been found only in **Elapidae** venoms. The acetylcholinesterase-blocking toxins (Karlsson et al., 1985) and muscarinic toxins (Adem et al., 1988) presumably also belong to structural group I; they are both found in mamba (**Dendroaspis** genus) venoms.

The snake toxins in structural group II have a phospholipase A_2 structure [PLA_2]. They are often complexes of 2 to 4 subunits, of which at least one is a PLA_2 with about 120 amino acid residues and 6 to 8 disulfide bridges. As indicated by structural analyses and predictive investigations (Dufton et al., 1983), PLA_2 found in snake venoms are probably folded like PLA_2 from mammalian origin (Dijkstra et al., 1981). Structural group II includes [i] the presynaptically-acting neurotoxins which block acetylcholine release from nerve endings (Harris, 1985). These are the most lethal toxins so far isolated from snake venoms that are found in the venoms of **Elapidae, Hydrophiidae** and **Viperidae**; [ii] the myonecrotic toxins (Harris, 1985) and [iii] the cytolytic toxins (Chwetzoff et al., 1988). It must be stressed that PLA_2-type toxins possess several other kinds of biological properties which have been described in detail in appropriate reviews (Harris, 1985, Chang, 1985, Rosenberg, 1986).

The amino acid sequences and spatial structures of many snake toxins have been reported in the literature. For some of them, our knowledge of their structure-function relationships is progressing (Endo and Tamiya, 1987). However, little is known about snake toxin molecular biology. Clearly, the obtaining of the cDNAs encoding snake toxins is of great importance for at least two reasons: firstly, it would provide information about precursor sequences, which would be most helpful in studying the biosynthesis and evolution of snake toxins. Secondly, the obtaining of cDNAs constitutes the first step towards genetic engineering i.e. towards the possibility of substituting any amino acid residues in snake toxins. However, such procedure obviously requires an expression vector.

In the present paper we report the cloning and sequencing of cDNAs encoding several snake venom gland proteins belonging to structural group I or II. We describe the preparation of a vector allowing the production of a hybrid protein composed of the successive sequences of the protein A from **S. aureus** and erabutoxin a, a postsynaptically-acting neurotoxin. The biological properties of this hybrid protein are also indicated.

MATERIALS and METHODS

Enzymes and chemicals

Restriction enzymes, DNA Polymerase I, DNA ligase, RNase H, terminal deoxynucleotidyl transferase, M-MLV reverse transcriptase, oligo (dT)-cellulose and sequencing kit were purchased from Bethesda Research Laboratories and Appligene. Labeled compounds, $[^{35}S]dCTP\alpha S$ and $[\gamma ^{32}P]dATP$, were provided by Amersham, tritium gas by CEA (Saclay, France). Oligo$(dT)_{12-18}$ and IgG sepharose were from Pharmacia. Chemicals were from Prolabo and Merck.

Bacterial strains, phages and plasmids

E. coli strains MC1061 (Casadaban and Cohen, 1980) and JM 101 (Yannisch-Perron et al., 1985) were used as bacterial hosts. M13 phage vectors were obtained from Amersham and Bethesda Research Laboratories, pBRdG (dG-Tailed Pst I Cleaved pBR322) and pRIT5 plasmids were from Bethesda Research Laboratories and Pharmacia, respectively.

Extraction of mRNA

Extraction of total RNAs from snake venom glands were performed in 5% SDS buffer according to Zitomer and Hall, (1976). The poly$(A)^+$ RNA fraction was isolated by oligo(dT)-cellulose chromatography (Aviv and Leder, 1972).

Synthesis of cDNA

Poly$(A)^+$ RNA was hybridized with oligo$(dT)_{12-18}$ and the cDNA first strand was synthesized using Moloney Murine Leukemia Virus (M-MLV) reverse transcriptase (Gerard and d'Alessio, 1986). The second strand was synthesized according the method of Okayama and Berg (1982) and Gubler and Hoffman (1983).

Cloning and sequencing of cDNA

The double stranded cDNA was inserted into the Pst1 site of the pBR322 plasmid by the dG/dC tailing method (Nelson and Brutlag, 1979) and recombinant plasmids were used to transform **E. coli** strain MC 1061 (Casadaban and Cohen, 1980; Hanahan, 1983). Colonies were transferred to nitrocellulose filters , lysed as described by Thayer (1979) and screened by **in situ** hybridization with ^{32}P labeled oligonucleotide probes. The cDNA fragments were then excised, inserted into the Pst1 site of M13 mp18 vector and sequenced according to Sanger et al. (1977).

Construction of the fusion vector

The commercially available pRIT5 gene fusion vector was used to construct a hybrid structural gene beetwen protein A gene from **Staphylococcus aureus** and erabutoxin a cDNA from **Laticauda semifasciata**. The resulting hybrid protein was expressed in **E.coli**, extracted and purified according to a procedure which will be reported in a subsequent article.

Biological properties of the Protein A-erabutoxin a fusion protein

Radioimmunoassays were carried out as previously described using labeled toxins and Mα2-3 monoclonal antibody (Trémeau et al., 1986). Competition between the radioactive toxin and the protein A-erabutoxin a fusion protein was made according to Faure et al., (1983). Binding inhibition of the radioactive toxin to the nicotinic acetylcholine receptor by an immune rabbit serum raised against the hybrid protein was performed according to Boulain et al., (1982).

Immunization procedure

Male rabbits were injected subcutaneously at multiple sites with 300 μg of IgG purified fusion protein in Freund's complete adjuvant. The animals were boosted at one week intervals with the hybrid protein in Freund's incomplete adjuvant and bled 10 days after the fourth injection.

RESULTS AND DISCUSSION

Nucleotide Sequences of cDNAs encoding postsynaptic neurotoxins

The venoms of **Hydrophiidae** are rich in postsynaptically-acting neurotoxins, especially of the short chain type (60-62 amino acid residues and 4 disulfide bridges). Three years ago, our laboratory reported for the first time the cloning and nucleotide sequence of a cDNA encoding such a toxin (Tamiya et al. 1985). This sequence is illustrated in fig.1. The cDNA has an open reading frame encoding 83 amino acid residues, 62 of which (not underlined) are identical to the corrected amino acid sequence of erabutoxin a (Nishida et al., 1985). Erabutoxin a is one of the two main neurotoxins present in the venom of the sea snake **Laticauda semifasciata**. As many as 10 non polar residues including Val, Leu and Ile, are present amongst the 21 amino acids found in the N-terminal precursor sequence underlined in Fig. 1. This region presumably acts as a signal peptide, thus favorizing the translocation of the 62 residue protein through the **endoplasmic reticulum** membrane.

```
TCCGAAAAAGATCGCAAG ATG AAA ACT CTG CTG CTG ACC TTG GTG GTG GTG
                    M   K   T   L   L   L   T   L   V   V   V
                   -21
ACA ATC GTG TGC CTG GAC TTA GGA TAC ACC AGG ATA TGT TTT AAC CAT
 T   I   V   C   L   D   L   G   Y   T   R   I   C   F   N   H
-10                                 -1   1
CAG TCA TCG CAA CCG CAA ACC ACT AAA ACT TGT TCA CCT GGG GAG AGC
 Q   S   S   Q   P   Q   T   T   K   T   C   S   P   G   E   S
            10                                      20
TCT TGC TAT AAC AAG CAA TGG AGC GAT TTC CGT GGA ACT ATA ATT GAA
 S   C   Y   N   K   Q   W   S   D   F   R   G   T   I   I   E
                            30
AGG GGA TGT GGT TGC CCC ACA GTG AAG CCC GGT ATT AAA CTC AGT TGT
 R   G   C   G   C   P   T   V   K   P   G   I   K   L   S   C
    40                                      50
TGC GAA TCA GAG GTC TGC AAC AAT TAG CTCTACGAGTGGCTAAATTCCTTGAGT
 C   E   S   E   V   C   N   N  end
                    60
TTTACTCTCATTCATCAAGGACCATCCTTCAAAATGTATGCTTCTGGCCTTTACCACCACATG
GTCCATCATCCCCCTCTCCCCTGCTGTCTTTGACACCTCAACATCTTTCCCTTTTCTCTTGAT
CTGTAAGTTTCCTTCTGCTAGTTCTGTAGTTTGAGAATCAAATAAACCTCAGCATTCAAAAAA
AAAAAAAAAAAAAAAAAAAAA
```

Fig.1. Nucleotide sequence of the cDNA encoding **Laticauda semifasciata** erabutoxin a and the protein sequence deduced (Tamiya et al., 1985). The amino acid sequence of the presumed signal peptide is underlined.

The cDNAs encoding two additional short-chain neurotoxins were recently cloned and their nucleotide sequence elucidated (Figs 2 and 3). They were prepared from mRNAs extracted from the venom glands of the olive sea snake **Aipysurus laevis** collected during an expedition on the Great Barrier reef (Australia) in 1987.

The open reading frames of the two cDNAs depicted in figs 2 and 3 code for 81 amino acid residues. The deduced amino acid sequences of the two signal peptides (underlined in the figures) comprise 21 residues. They are identical with that found in the precursor of erabutoxin a (Fig. 1). Previously, Maeda and Tamiya (1976) reported the isolation and amino acid sequence of three toxins, designated as a, b and c, from venom of **A. laevis**. The amino acid sequence of the mature protein (Fig. 2) is identical with that of toxin b. The sequence of the mature protein shown in Fig.3 differs from those of the three toxins a, b and c by two, one and three residues, respectively. It corresponds to a novel protein, designated as toxin d. This toxin may be a minor component of **Aipysurus laevis** venom and/or it may have been absent from the batch of venom investigated by Tamiya and co-workers.

```
        ACACTTTGCAGGCTCCAGAGAAGATTGCAAG ATG AAA ACT CTG CTG CTG ACC
                                         M   K   T   L   L   L   T
                                        -21
TTG GTG GTG GTG ACC ATC GTG TGC CTG GAC TTA GGA TAC ACC TTG ACA
 L   V   V   V   T   I   V   C   L   D   L   G   Y   T   L   T
                -10                                 -1   1
TGT TGC AAC CAA CAG TCA TCG CAA CCT AAA ACC ACT ACA GAT TGT GCA
 C   C   N   Q   Q   S   S   Q   P   K   T   T   T   D   C   A
                            10
GAT AAC TCT TGC TAT AAA ATG ACT TGG AGG GAT CAC CGT GGA ACT AGA
 D   N   S   C   Y   K   M   T   W   R   D   H   R   G   T   R
    20                                      30
ATT GAA AGG GGA TGT GGT TGC CCT CAG GTG AAG CCC GGT ATT AAA CTT
 I   E   R   G   C   G   C   P   Q   V   K   P   G   I   K   L
                    40                                      50
GAA TGT TGC AAA ACA AAC GAA TGC AAC AAT TAG CTCTACGAATGGCTAAATT
 E   C   C   K   T   N   E   C   N   N  end
                                    60
CCTTGAGTTTTGCTCTCATCCATCAAGGACCATCCTTGAAAATTTATGCTTCTGGCCTTTACC
ACCACATGGTCTATCATCCCCCTCTCCCCTGCTGTCTTTGACACCTCAACATCTTTCCCTTTT
CTCTTGTTCTGTAAGTTTCCTTCTGCTAGTTCTGTAGTTTGAGATCAAATAAACCTCAGCATC
CAAAAA
```

Fig.2. Nucleotide sequence of the cDNA encoding **Aipysurus laevis** toxin b and the protein sequence deduced. The amino acid sequence of the presumed signal peptide is underlined.

Postsynaptically-acting neurotoxins bind to nicotinic acetylcholine receptors with specificity and high affinity (Ménez et al.,1984). There is a general agreement that this binding is ensured by multiple residues which have been tentatively identified on the basis of both sequence comparison of homologous neurotoxins and chemical modification experiments (Faure et al., 1983). Twelve positions have been proposed as being involved in neurotoxin binding to nicotinic receptors (Ménez et al., 1984). These are positions 8, 27, 29, 31, 33, 34, 36, 38, 46, 47, 49 and 52. Although they are highly preserved amongst a large set of different neurotoxin sequences, most of these positions are not strictly invariant, suggesting that the actual "toxic" site may differ slightly from one toxin to another.

Examination of the sequences in Figs .1 to 3 reveals that 9 of the above positions are identical in erabutoxin a and **A. laevis** toxins b and d in terms of both codons and amino acids. In contrast, the codons corresponding to the amino acid residues at positions 27, 36 and 52 differ from one toxin to another by one base mutation. The differences are accompanied by a change in the residues at positions 27 (Met-Lys) and 36 (Arg-Ile) whereas the mutation at position 52 remains silent.

```
       ACACTTTGCAGGCTCCAGAGAAGATTGCAAG ATG AAA ACT CTG CTG CTG ACC
                                        M   K   T   L   L   L   T
                                       -21
TTG GTG GTG GTG ACC ATC GTG TGC CTG GAC TTA GGA TAC ACC TTG ACA
 L   V   V   V   T   I   V   C   L   D   L   G   Y   T   L   T
                -10                                 -1   1
TGT TGC AAC CAA CAG TCA TCG CAA CCT AAA ACC ACT ACA GAT TGT GCA
 C   C   N   Q   Q   S   S   Q   P   K   T   T   T   D   C   A
                             10
GAT GAC TCT TGC TAT AAA AAG ACT TGG AAG GAT CAC CGT GGA ACT AGA
 D   D   S   C   Y   K   K   T   W   K   D   H   R   G   T   R
    20                                      30
ATT GAA AGG GGA TGT GGT TGC CCT CAG GTG AAG CCC GGT ATT AAA CTT
 I   E   R   G   C   G   C   P   Q   V   K   P   G   I   K   L
                    40                                      50
GAA TGT TGC AAA ACA AAC GAA TGC AAC AAT TAG CTCTACGAATGGCTAAATT
 E   C   C   K   T   N   E   C   N   N  end
                                    60
CCTTGAGTTTTGCTCTCATCCATCAAGGACCATCCTTGAAAATTTATGCTTCT
```

Fig.3. Nucleotide sequence of the cDNA encoding **Aipysurus laevis** toxin d and the protein sequence deduced. The amino acid sequence of the signal peptide is underlined.

Nucleotide cDNA Sequences Encoding Snake venom PLA_2.

Proteins with phospholipase structure (PLA_2) are found in most snake venoms. Recently, the nucleotide sequence of a cDNA encoding a PLA_2 from the venom gland of the sea snake **Laticauda laticaudata** was reported (Guignery et al., 1987) and is shown in fig.4. The open reading frame is composed of 145 amino acid residues, numbered from -27 to 118. This is a new protein sequence which displays homologies with sequences of snake venom PLA_2, from residue 1 to residue 118 (Tamiya and Yagi, 1985). In particular, the protein possesses 14 cysteine residues at positions 11, 27, 29, 44, 45, 51, 60, 71, 78, 84, 89, 91, 98, 117 like in most other PLA_2. Furthermore, we noted the presence of particularly high homologies in the regions containing residues involved in the catalytic action of PLA_2 (Dijkstra et al., 1981). As a consequence, it is likely that the protein sequence numbered 1-118 in fig. 4 corresponds to that of a new mature PLA_2. The 27 first residues presumably correspond to a signal peptide, as indicated by the large proportion of hydrophobic residues found in this region. There are as many as 12 non-polar residues including Val, Leu or Ile in the N-terminal peptide.

```
      TTCATCTTGCTTGCAGCTTCACCACTGACAAA ATG TAT CCT GCT CAC CTT CTG CTC
                                        M   Y   P   A   H   L   L   L
                                       -27                          -20
CTG TTG GCA GTT TGT GTC TCC CTC TTA GGA GCC TCC GCC ATT CCT CCT CTG
 L   L   A   V   C   V   S   L   L   G   A   S   A   I   P   P   L
                                   -10
CCT CTC AAC CTT GCA CAA TTT GCC CTC GTC ATT AAA TGT GCC GAC AAA GGC
 P   L   N   L   A   Q   F   A   L   V   I   K   C   A   D   K   G
   -1    1                                   10
AAG AGA CCT CGT TGG CAT TAT ATG GAC TAC GGT TGC TAC TGT GGC CCA GGA
 K   R   P   R   W   H   Y   M   D   Y   G   C   Y   C   G   P   G
                 20                                      30
GGT AGC GGG ACA CCG GTA GAC GAG TTG GAT AGG TGC TGC AAA ACA CAT GAT
 G   S   G   T   P   V   D   E   L   D   R   C   C   K   T   H   D
                             40
CAG TGC TAT GCT CAA GCC GAA AAA AAG GGG TGC TAC CCA AAG TTG ACG ATG
 Q   C   Y   A   Q   A   E   K   K   G   C   Y   P   K   L   T   M
 50                                     60
TAT AGT TAC TAC TGT GGC GGA GAT GGA CCC TAC TGC AAT TCA AAA ACG GAA
 Y   S   Y   Y   C   G   G   D   G   P   Y   C   N   S   K   T   E
             70                                      80
TGT CAA CGT TTT GTG TGT GAT TGT GAT GTC AGG GCA GCC GAC TGC TTT GCC
 C   Q   R   F   V   C   D   C   D   V   R   A   A   D   C   F   A
                         90                                     100
AGA TAC CCT TAC AAC AAC AAG AAC TAC AAT ATC AAC ACC AGC AAA CGT TGC
 R   Y   P   Y   N   N   K   N   Y   N   I   N   T   S   K   R   C
                                    110
AAA TGA TATTTGAGAGGCTTCAGCGCAAGGATTGTGGCAGTAACTCACCTGCGCATGGCAATTCT
 K  end
CTGGATGGGCCTCTATTATGTGTATAAAAATAGAAAATTATACATATATGATATTTAAAAAACAAAA
GGAACCGTTTTGTGAACAATAAAGTGAGGTGCCGATAAAAAAAAA
```

Fig.4 . Nucleotide sequence of the cDNA encoding **Laticauda laticaudata** PLA2 and protein sequence deduced (Guignery et al.,1987). The amino acid sequence of the signal peptide is underlined. Ten residues constituting presumably the active site of a PLA_2 (Dijkstra et al., 1981), are emphasized.

More recently, two additional cDNAs encoding new PLA_2 have been cloned and sequenced. They were prepared from mRNAs extracted from the venom glands of the sea snake **Aipysurus laevis** (collected at the Great Barrier Reef, Australia) and the land snake **Notechis scutatus scutatus** (collected near Sydney, Australia). They are presented in figs 5 and 6.

The homology between the protein sequences of the PLA_2 shown in figs. 4, 5 and 6 is obvious. Unlike what was observed for neurotoxins, the sequences of the signal peptides in the three PLA_2 are different. We noted, however, that the C-terminal pentapeptides of these signal sequences contain at least two proline residues. This is clearly different from the consensus pro-sequences found at homologous positions in PLA_2 of mammalian origin (Ohara et al., 1986). These

```
    TCTTGCTTGCAGCTTCACCACTGACAAA ATG TAT CCT GCT CAC CTT CTG GTC CTC
                                  M   Y   P   A   H   L   L   V   L
                                 -27                         -20
TTG GCA GTT TGT GTC TCC CTC TTA GGA GCC TCT GAC ATT CCT CCT CTG CCT
 L   A   V   C   V   S   L   L   G   A   S   D   I   P   P   L   P
                                 -10
CTG AAC CTC TAT CAG TTC GAC AAC ATG ATT CAA TGT GCC AAC AAG GGC AAA
 L   N   L   Y   Q   F   D   N   M   I   Q   C   A   N   K   G   K
-1   1                                   10
AGA GCT ACT TGG CAT TAT ATG GAC TAC GGT TGC TAC TGC GGC TCG GGA GGT
 R   A   T   W   H   Y   M   D   Y   G   C   Y   C   G   S   G   G
            20                                      30
AGC GGG ACA CCG GTA GAT GCG TTG GAT AGG TGC TGC AAA GCA CAT GAT GAC
 S   G   T   P   V   D   A   L   D   R   C   C   K   A   H   D   D
                        40                                      50
TGC TAT GGT GTA GCC GAA GAT AAC GGA TGC TAC CCC AAG TGG ACG TTG TAT
 C   Y   G   V   A   E   D   N   G   C   Y   P   K   W   T   L   Y
                                    60
AGT TGG CAA TGT ACT GAA AAT GTA CCC ACC TGC AAT TCA GAA TCG GGG TGT
 S   W   Q   C   T   E   N   V   P   T   C   N   S   E   S   G   C
        70                                      80
CAA AAA TCT GTG TGT GCT TGT GAC GCC ACA GCA GCC AAG TGC TTT GCC GAA
 Q   K   S   V   C   A   C   D   A   T   A   A   K   C   F   A   E
                    90                                      100
GCC CCT TAC AAC AAC AAG AAC TAC AAT ATC AAC ACC AGT AAT TGC CAA TGA
 A   P   Y   N   N   K   N   Y   N   I   N   T   S   N   C   Q  end
                                110
TATTTGAGAGGCTTCAGCGCAAGGACTGT
```

Fig.5. Nucleotide sequence of the cDNA encoding **Aipysurus laevis** PLA_2 and the protein sequence deduced (Ducancel et al., in press). The amino acid sequence of the signal peptide is underlined.

findings suggest that PLA_2 from **Elapidae** and **Hydrophiidae** are not synthesized as pro-proteins. It is striking that the signal sequences of the three PLA_2 in Figs 4, 5 and 6 and the three neurotoxins in Figs 1, 2 and 3 all possess a cysteine residue. The reason for the presence of this residue is not yet known but it might favor correct folding of the proteins. Examination of the mature sequences revealed that the ten residues presumed to be involved in the active site of mammalian PLA_2 (Dijkstra et al., 1981) are present in the three reptile PLA_2 described here. These are positions 5, 9, 22, 29, 45, 48, 92, 95, 96 and 99. Seven of these preserved residues are coded for by identical codons in all three PLA_2. Silent single base changes were observed at amino acid positions 5, 29 and 92.

```
  TTGCAGCTCACCACTGACAAA ATG TAT CCT GCT CAC CTT CTG GTC CTG TTG ACA
                         M   Y   P   A   H   L   L   V   L   L   T
                        -27                         -20
GTT TGT GTC TCC CTC TTA GAA GCC TCC AGC ATT CCT GCG CGG CCT CTC AAC
 V   C   V   S   L   L   E   A   S   S   I   P   A   R   P   L   N
                        -10                                 -1   1
CTC TAT CAG TTC GGC AAC ATG ATT CAA TGT GCC AAC CAT GGC AGG AGA CCT
 L   Y   Q   F   G   N   M   I   Q   C   A   N   H   G   R   R   P
                                10
ACT TTG GCT TAT GCG GAC TAC GGT TGC TAC TGC GGC GCA GGA GGT AGC GGG
 T   L   A   Y   A   D   Y   G   C   Y   C   G   A   G   G   S   G
    20                                      30
ACA CCG GTG GAT GAG TTG GAT AGG TGC TGC AAA GCA CAT GAT GAC TGC TAT
 T   P   V   D   E   L   D   R   C   C   K   A   H   D   D   C   Y
                40                                      50
GGT GAA GCC GGA AAA AAA GGA TGC TAC CCC ACG TTG ACG TTG TAT AGT TGG
 G   E   A   G   K   K   G   C   Y   P   T   L   T   L   Y   S   W
                            60
CAA TGT ATT GAA AAA ACA CCC ACC TGC AAT TCA AAA ACG GGA TGT GAA CGT
 Q   C   I   E   K   T   P   T   C   N   S   K   T   G   C   E   R
70                                      80
TCT GTG TGT GAT TGT GAT GCC ACA GCA GCC AAG TGC TTT GCC AAA GCC CCT
 S   V   C   D   C   D   A   T   A   A   K   C   F   A   K   A   P
            90                                      100
TAC AAC AAG AAG AAC TAC AAT ATC GAC ACC GAG AAA CGT TGC CAA TGA TAT
 Y   N   K   K   N   Y   N   I   D   T   E   K   R   C   Q  end
                        110
TTGAGAGGCTTCAGCGCAAGGACTGTGGCAGTTACTCACCTGCGCGTGGCAATTCTCTGGACGGGCC
TCTATTATACATATAAAAATAGAAAATTATATATATATAATTATTAAAAAACAAAAGGAACCATTTC
CTGAACAATAAAGTGAGGTGCCGATAAAAAAAAA
```

Fig.6. Nucleotide sequence of the cDNA encoding a PLA_2 from **Notechis scutatus scutatus** and the protein sequence deduced (Ducancel et al., in press). The amino acid sequence of the presumed signal peptide is underlined.

Production of a protein A-neurotoxin fusion protein

We constructed a plasmid containing staphylococcal protein A and erabutoxin a fusion DNAs. Our choice was guided by three factors: firstly, the pRIT5 plasmid contains the protein A cDNA controlled by an efficient protein A promoter and permits the production of large amounts of fusion proteins (Nilsson et al. 1985a). Secondly, fusion proteins are exported to the periplasm where disulfide bonds can form (Nilsson et al. 1985b), and thirdly, it was previously observed that the presence of the protein A moiety in a hybrid molecule enhances the immune response (Lowenadler et al. 1987). The fused cDNAs were therefore constructed by inserting the modified coding region of erabutoxin a cDNA into the multiple cloning site of the pRIT5 gene fusion vector. We called the resulting vector pRIT5-ea. The amino acid sequence deduced for the hybrid protein successively included the signal sequence and IgG binding domain of protein A, a junction peptide comprising 13 amino acid residues, and mature erabutoxin a (see figure

3). Details concerning the construction of the fusion cDNAs will be given in a subsequent report. Two points, however, should be stressed: firstly, a methionine residue was introduced at position -1 of the mature toxin by site-directed mutagenesis, in order to cleave the hybrid protein using cyanogen bromide. In this connection, note that erabutoxin a does not contain any methionine residues. Secondly, we carried out i) partial digestion by Dde1 of a Pst1/EcoR1 fragment containing met-erabutoxin a.; ii) a fill in with dATP and dTTP; iii) insertion into the Sma1 site of the M13 mp18 vector and iv) transfer into pRIT5 expression vector of a EcoR1/BamH1 restriction fragment containing the region coding for erabutoxin a, which was suitably orientated.

The **E.coli** cells were transformed with the pRIT5-ea plasmid and cultured overnight in an appropriate medium. They subsequently underwent a standard osmotic shock procedure at a cold temperature. The periplasmic extract was applied to an IgG Sepharose 6FF column. The eluted molecules containg protein A were analyzed by SDS-gel electrophoresis . As expected, a 38K fusion protein was observed as well as several smaller proteins. These results are similar to those reported by Nilsson et al., (1985b) for the expression of another hybrid protein, using pRIT5 for transformation. The total amount of protein bound to IgG was 5mg per liter, in early stationary phase cultures. The 38K hybrid protein was estimated at 10-20% of this amount.

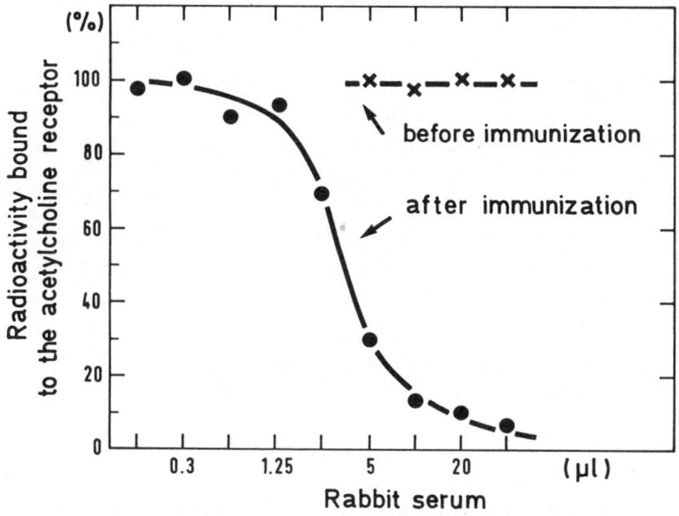

Fig.7. Inhibition of the binding of ^{125}I labeled erabutoxin to the nicotinic acetylcholine receptor by increasing amounts of immune rabbit antiserum raised against protein A-erabutoxin a hybrid protein.

The biological properties of the protein A-erabutoxin a hybrid were investigated. The detailed results will be reported in another paper. They clearly indicated that the hybrid molecule had native neurotoxin-like biological activities. This conclusion was based on the five following observations: firstly, the hybrid protein completely inhibited the binding of a radioactive neurotoxin (Ménez et al. 1971) to Mα2-3, a monoclonal antibody which recognizes all short-chain neurotoxins (Trémeau et al. 1986). Secondly, the hybrid molecule inhibited the binding of the radioactive neurotoxin to its physiological target, i.e. the nicotinic acetylcholine receptor. Thirdly, injection into rabbits of affinity purified fusion protein resulted in the production of neurotoxin-specific polyclonal antibodies, as evidenced by radioimmunoassay procedures. Fourthly, as shown in fig. 7 the antibodies raised against the hybrid molecule inhibited the binding **in vitro** of a radioactive toxin to the nicotinic acetylcholine receptor. Lastly, recent experiments have shown that these anti-hybrid antibodies were also capable of neutralizing the toxic activity of erabutoxin a in mice.

Clearly, the expression vector used in the present study was particularly well-suited for the production of active toxin fused with protein A. Site-directed mutagenesis experiments are in progress in our laboratory with a view to precise delineation of the functional sites of neurotoxins, and subsequently, of snake venom PLA_2.

ACKNOWLEDGMENTS

We are much indebted to Prs H. Cogger (Australian Museum, Sydney, Australia) and H. Heatwole (New South Wales University, Armidale, Australia) as well as to Drs G. Mengden (Australian Museum, Sydney, Australia) and G. Burns (New South Wales University, Armidale, Australia) for their kind and efficient help during field work. Warm thanks are also due to Dr. J. Pusset (CNRS) and to our colleagues from ORSTOM in New Caledonia for their kind assistance in collecting **L. laticaudata** specimens. We are also indebted to P. Legay for his efficient help at developping computing techniques. It should be stressed that biohazards associated with the experiments described in this publication have been examined previously by the French National Control Committee.

REFERENCES

Adem, A., A. Asblom, G. Johansson, P. M. Mbugua and E. Karlsson (1988). Toxins from the venom of the green mamba **Dendroaspis angusticeps** that inhibit the binding of quinuclidinyl benzilate to muscarinic acetylcholine receptors. Biochim. Biophys. Acta, 968, 340-345.

Aviv, H. and P. Leder (1972). Purification of biologically active globin messenger RNA by chromatography on oligothymidylic acid-cellulose . Proc. Natl. Acad. Sci. USA, 69, 1408-1412.

Boulain, J-C., A. Ménez, J. Couderc, G. Faure, P. Liacopoulos and P. Fromageot (1982). Neutralizing monoclonal antibody specific for **Naja nigricollis** toxin α: Preparation, characterization and localization of the antigenic binding site. Biochemistry, 21, 2910-2915.

Casadaban, M.J. and S.N. Cohen (1980). Analysis of gene control signals by DNA fusion and cloning in **Escherichia coli**. J. Mol. Biol., 138, 179-207.

Chang, C.C. (1985). Neurotoxins with phospholipase A_2 activity in snake venoms. Proc. Natl. Sci. Counc. B. ROC., 9, 126-142.

Changeux, J.P., A. Devillers-Thiéry and P. Chemouilli (1984). Acetylcholine receptor: an allosteric protein. Science, 225, 1335-1345.

Chwetzoff, S., M. Takeshi, P. Fromageot and A. Ménez (1988). La phospholipase basique du venin de **Naja nigricollis** est cytotoxique. C.R. Acad. Sci. Paris 306, 31-33.

Dijkstra, B. W., J. Drenth and K.H. Kalk (1981). Active site and catalytic mechanism of phospholipase A_2. Nature, 289, 604-606.

Dufton, M.J., D. Eaker and R.C. Hider (1983). Conformational properties of phospholipases A_2. Eur. J. Biochem., 137, 537-544.

Dufton, M.J. and R.C. Hider (1988). Structure and pharmacology of elapid cytotoxins. Pharmac. Ther., 36, 1-40.

Endo, T. and N. Tamiya (1987). Current view on the structure-function relationships of postsynaptic neurotoxins from snake venoms. Pharmac. Ther., 34, 403-451.

Faure, G., J-C. Boulain, F. Bouet, Th. Montenay-Garestier, P. Fromageot and A. Ménez (1983). Role of indole and amino groups in the structure and function of **Naja nigricollis** toxin α. Biochemistry, 22, 2068-2076.

Gerard, G.F. and D.P. Grandgenett (1975). Purification and characterization of the DNA polymerase and RNase H activities in Moloney murine sarcoma-leukemia virus. J. Virol., 15, 785-797.

Gerard, G.F., J.M. D'Alessio, M.L. Kotewicz and M.C. Noon (1986). Influence on stability in **Escherichia coli** of the carboxy-terminal structure of cloned Moloney murine leukemia virus reverse transcriptase. DNA, 5, 271-279.

Gubler, U. and B.J. Hoffman(1983). A simple and very efficient method for generating cDNA libraries. Gene., 25, 263-269.

Guignery-Frelat G.,F. Ducancel,A. Ménez and J.C. Boulain (1987). Sequence of a cDNA encoding a snake venom phospholipase A_2. Nucleic Acids Research 15, 5892.

Hanahan, D. (1983). Studies on transformation of **Escherichia coli** with plasmids. J. Mol. Biol. 166, 557-580.

Harris, J.B. (1985). Phospholipases in snake venoms and their effects on nerve and muscle. Pharmac. Ther., 31, 79-102.

Harvey, A.L. (1985). Cardiotoxins from cobra venoms: possible mechanisms of actions. J. Toxic.-Toxin Rev., 4, 41-69.

Jiang, M., J. Häggblad and E. Heilbronn (1987). Isolation and pharmacological characterization of a new α-neurotoxin (α-AgTx) from venom of the viper **Agkistrodon Halys** (Pallas). Toxicon, 25, 1019-1022.

Karlsson, E. (1979). Chemistry of protein toxins in snake venoms. In: Snake Venoms, Handbook Exp. Pharm. (C-Y Lee, Ed.), Vol. 52, pp. 159-212.

Karlsson, E., P.M. Mbugua and D. Rodriguez-Ithurralde. (1986). Anticholinesterase toxins. Pharmac. Ther.,30, 259-276.

Love, R.A. and R.M. Stroud (1986). The crystal structure of α-bungarotoxin at 2.5 Å resolution: relation to solution structure and binding to acetylcholine receptor. Protein Engineering, 1, 37-46.

Low, B.W., H.S. Preston, A. Sato, L.S. Rosen, J.E. Searl, A.D. Rudko and J.S. Richardson (1976). Three dimensional structure of erabutoxin b neurotoxic protein: inhibitor of acetylcholine receptor. Proc. Natl. Acad. Sci. USA 73, 2991-2994.

Löwenadler, B., B. Jansson, S. Paleus, E. Holmgren, B. Nilsson, T. Moks, G. Palm, S. Josephson, L. Philipson and M. Uhlen (1987). A gene fusion system for generating antibodies against short peptides. Gene, 58, 87-97.

Maeda, N. and N. Tamiya (1976). Isolation ,properties and amino acid sequences of three neurotoxins from the venom of a sea snake, **Aipysurus laevis**. Biochem. J., 153, 79-87.

Ménez,A., J.L. Morgat, P. Fromageot, A.M. Ronseray, P. Boquet and J.P. Changeux (1971). Tritium labelling of the α-neurotoxin of **Naja nigricollis.** FEBS Lett. ,17, 333-335.

Ménez, A., J-C. Boulain, F. Bouet, J. Couderc, G. Faure, A. Rousselet, O. Trémeau, E. Gatineau and P. Fromageot (1984). On the molecular mechanisms of neutralization of a cobra neurotoxin by specific antibodies. J. Physiol., Paris, 79, 196-206.

Nelson, T. and D. Brutlag (1979). Addition of homopolymers to the 3'-ends of duplex DNA with terminal transferase. Methods Enzymol. ,68, 41-50.

Nilsson, B., L. Abrahamsén and M. Uhlen (1985a). Immobilization and purification of enzymes with staphylococcal protein A gene fusion vectors. The EMBO Journal, 4, 1075-1080.

Nilsson, B., E. Holmgren, S. Josephson, S. Gatenbeck, L. Philipson and M. Uhlen (1985b). Efficient secretion and purification of human insulin-like growth factor I with a gene fusion vector in **Staphylococci**. Nucleic Acids Research , 13, 1151-1162.

Nishida, S., Y. Kokubun and N. Tamiya (1985). Correction of the amino acid sequences of erabutoxins from the venom of the sea snake **Laticauda semifasciata.** Biochem. J., 226, 879-880.

Ohara, O., M. Tamaki, E. Nakamura, Y. Tsuruta, Y. Fujii, M. Shin, H. Teraoka and M. Okamoto (1986). Dog and rat pancreatic phospholipases A_2 : Complete amino acid sequences deduced from complementary DNAs. J. Biochem., 99, 733-739.

Okayama, H. and P. Berg (1982). High-efficiency cloning of full-length cDNA. Mol. Cell. Biol., 2, 161-170.

Rees, B., J.P. Samama, J.C. Thierry, M. Gilibert, J. Fischer, H. Schweitz, M. Lazdunski and D. Moras (1987) Crystal structure of a snake venom cardiotoxin. Proc. Natl. Acad. Sci. USA, 84, 3132-3136.

Rosenberg, P. (1986). The relationship between enzymatic activity and pharmacological properties of phospholipases in natural poisons. In: Natural toxins (J.B. Harris, Ed.) Clarendon Press, Oxford. pp. 129-174.

Sanger, F., S. Nicklen and A.R. Coulson (1977). DNA sequencing with chain-terminating inhibitors. Proc. Natl. Acad. Sci. USA, 74, 5463-5467.

Tamiya, N. and T. Yagi (1985). Non-divergence theory of evolution: sequence comparison of some proteins from snakes and bacteria. J. Biochem., 98, 289-303.

Tamiya,T. A. Lamouroux, J-F. Julien, B. Grima, J. Mallet, P. Fromageot and A. Ménez (1985). Cloning and sequence analysis of the cDNA encoding a snake neurotoxin precursor. Biochimie, 67, 185-189.

Thayer, R.E. (1979). An improved method for detecting foreign DNA in plasmids of **Escherichia coli**. Anal. Biochem., 98, 60-63.

Trémeau, O., J-C. Boulain, J. Couderc, P. Fromageot and A. Ménez (1986). A monoclonal antibody which recognized the functional site of snake neurotoxins and which neutralizes all short-chain variants. FEBS Lett. 208, 236-240.

Tsernoglou, D. and G. A. Petsko (1977). Three-dimensional structure of neurotoxin a from venom of the Philippines sea snake. Proc. Natl. Acad. Sci. USA, 74, 971-974.

Walkinshaw, M.D., W. Saenger and A. Maelicke (1980). Three-dimensional structure of the "long" neurotoxin from cobra venom. Proc. Natl. Acad. Sci. USA, 77, 2400-2404.

Yanisch-Perron, C., J. Vieira and J. Messing (1985). Improved M13 phage cloning vectors and host strains: nucleotide sequences of the M13mp18 and pUC19 vectors. Gene, 33, 103-119.

Zitomer, R.S. and B.D. Hall (1976). Yeast cytochrome c messenger RNA. J. Biol. Chem., 251, 6320-6326.

SCORPION VENOM NEUROTOXINS: cDNA CLONING AND EXPRESSION

By Pierre E. Bougis[1], Hervé Rochat[2], Leonard A. Smith[1]

[1]Toxinology Department, Pathology Division, USAMRIID, Fort Detrick, Frederick, MD 21701, USA

[2]Université d'Aix-Marseille II, Faculté de Médecine Secteur Nord, Biochimie, UDC: CNRS UA 1179 - INSERM U 172, Bd P. Dramard, 13326 Marseille Cedex 15, France

ABSTRACT

As part of our continued interest on the immunochemistry and the structure-activity relationships of scorpion toxins acting on the voltage-sensitive sodium channel, recombinant DNA technology has been used to clone complementary DNA copies of messenger RNAs encoding these toxins. We present the strategy used and the main results obtained concerning the toxin II of the North-African scorpion *Androctonus australis* Hector. The structure determined for the cloned complementary DNA of the toxin II suggest a pretoxin of 85 amino acids in length, having signals for both protein secretion and α-carboxyamidation processes. Upon transfection with the toxin II cDNA, monkey kidney COS cells have transiently expressed a recombinant toxin that possessed both the immunological and biological characteristics of the mature toxin II.

KEYWORDS

Scorpion, Neurotoxin, Cloning, Expression.

INTRODUCTION

About 600 species of scorpions are known and belong to 70 genera and 6 families. Almost all the venomous scorpion species are from the *Buthidae* family. In the last 25 years, over 90 different neurotoxins have been isolated from scorpion venoms. Like many other toxins from animal origin, scorpion toxins are short, single chain, basic proteins of 60 to 65 amino acid residues (Miranda *et al.*, 1970), tightly reticulated by four disulfide bridges (Kopeyan *et al.*, 1974). Information about the three-dimensional structure of these proteins is derived from the crystal structure study of the variant-3 toxin of *Centruroides sculpturatus* Ewing (Fontecilla-Camps *et al.*, 1980). Biologically, most of the scorpion toxins are active either on mammals or on insects (De Dianous *et al.*, 1987). The mammal toxins that have been sequenced thus far fall into four distinctive groups according to both sequence and antigenic homologies (Rochat *et al.*, 1979). The potent toxicity of mammal toxins is related to their ability to bind with high-affinity to the voltage-sensitive sodium channel of excitable cells on sites 3 and 4 for those of the α- or β-type, respectively (Jover *et al.*, 1980; Martin *et al.*, 1987). This specific binding results in the impairing of the initial, rapid depolarization phase of the action potential in nerve and muscle causing the paralytic effect. Herein, scorpion toxins are useful tools to investigate the biochemistry of their ionophore target (Catterall *et al.*, 1986).

The study of structure-activity relationships of this class of neurotoxins is currently under investigation (El Ayeb *et al.*, 1983, 1986). New knowledge may contribute to a definition of the basic structural events responsible for sodium channel gating. In addition, further research may also help to develop a more efficient serotherapy against the worldwide medical problem of scorpionism. Presently, this therapy is limited due to the low abundance and high polymorphism of toxic antigens (El Ayeb and Rochat, 1985). Information on the genetics of the scorpion is limited. However, caryotypes made for different species of scorpion suggest that the number of chromosomes pairs may not be constant. In the case of *Androctonus mauretanicus* 12 pairs of chromosomes (2n=24) have been observed (Goyffon *et al.*, 1971). Using recombinant DNA technology, we are interested in extending our current knowledge on the genetics and the structure-activity relationships of scorpion toxins in order to understand better both their pharmacological activities and their antigenic properties.

CLONING EXPERIMENT

The cloning experiment described here concerns the toxin II of *Androctonus australis* Hector (AaH II). The living area of this scorpion species extend over the north of Algeria and the south of Tunisia. Venoms of animals collected in Chellala (Algeria) and Tozeur (Tunisia) have been already extensively studied. At present, 6 mammal toxins have been characterized using multiple chromatographic steps, as shown in Fig. 1. Except for AaH IV, their amino-acid sequences have been determined. AaH II belongs to the second toxin group and is also representative of toxins of α-type. Some biological properties of AaH toxins are reported in Fig. 2. As many other bio-active peptides scorpion toxin may be α-carboxyamidated. This is the case of AaH II. Scorpion toxins are not usually major components of the venoms. Indeed, using high performance liquid chromatography the AaH venom can be fractionated in numerous components, toxins being minor fractions (Fig. 3). This low abundance in toxins may be of concern for cloning experiments mainly because this may also reflect low level of messenger RNAs (mRNA) encoding toxins.

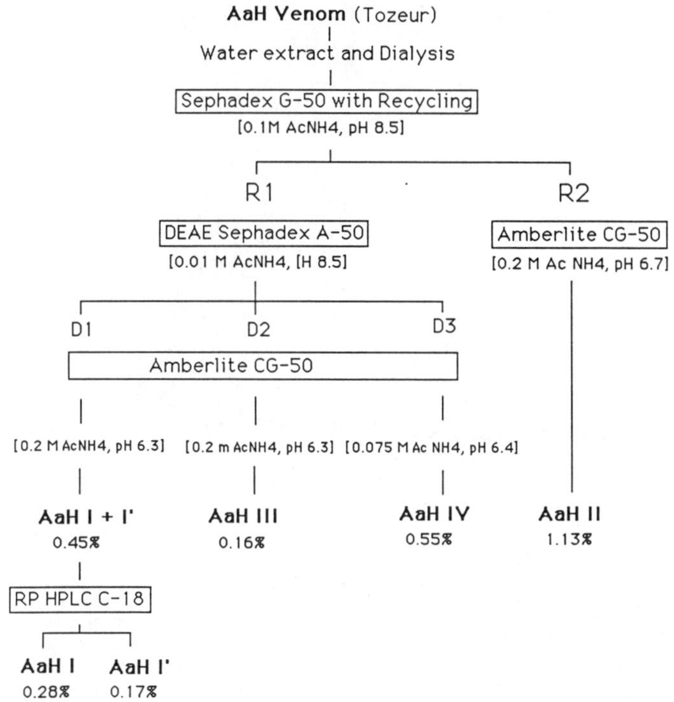

Fig. 1. Purification diagram of *Androctonus australis* Hector toxins lethal to mice, % are of dry venom weight (Martin and Rochat, 1986).

Toxins are synthesized by two specialized exocrine glands that are located in the telson of the scorpion, the last segment of the tail of the animal. The histological profile of these glands has been studied using immunostaining to detect toxins within the cells. Using rabbit AaH II immune serum and peroxidase immuno-developing, AaH II has been located in secretory vacuoles (Fig. 4). Control experiments using rabbit non-immune serum showed no specific

	Mouse LD_{50} (μg/Kg) S.C.	Mouse LD_{50} (μg/Kg) I.C.V.	Fly LD_{50} (μg/100mg)	$K_{0.5}$ / ^{125}I AaH II Rat brain synaptosomes (nM)	$K_{0.5}$ / ^{125}I AaH IT Fly head synaptosomes (nM)
Venom	320				
AaH I/I'/I''	17.5	0.500		4.5	
AaH II	9.4	0.025	not toxic	0.2	>10 000
AaH III	24.0	0.350		3.0	
AaH IV	122.5	0.900		50.0	
AaH IT	not toxic	not toxic	0.002	>10 000	0.3

Fig. 2. Somes biological properties of Androctonus australis Hector toxins, s.c. sucutaneously, i.c.v., intracerebroventricularly (Martin and Rochat, 1984; De Lima et al., 1986; De Dianous et al., 1986).

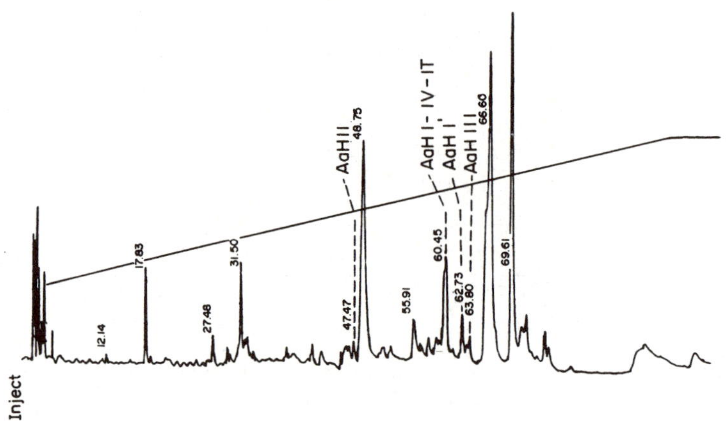

Fig. 3. RP-HPLC diagram of pooled, manual Androctonus australis Hector venom samples, 0.150 mg was injected on the column (Martin et al., 1987).

staining at all. Subsequently, as the first step in cloning a complementary DNA (cDNA) from a mRNA that has been transcribed from the toxin gene, the purification of the population of diverse mRNAs from the telson of the scorpion has been undertaken. The telson may easily obtained but, because of the chitin, the dissection of the two venom glands is not practicable. For this reason, whole homogenized telsons have been used as starting material for the purification of total RNA (Maniatis et al., 1982). The mRNA population was purified from total RNA on oligo d(T) cellulose (Aviv and Leder, 1972). The cloning has been undertaken without any size selection of the mRNA population obtained from scorpion telsons. The cDNA cloning strategy we have used is described in Fig. 5. cDNAs were synthesized from telson mRNAs according to Okayama and Berg (1983) in order to set up the library. This procedure of cloning cDNAs within plasmid vector has the main advantage of generating high number of full-length copies of mRNAs. This specific cloning vector is also an expression vector due to the

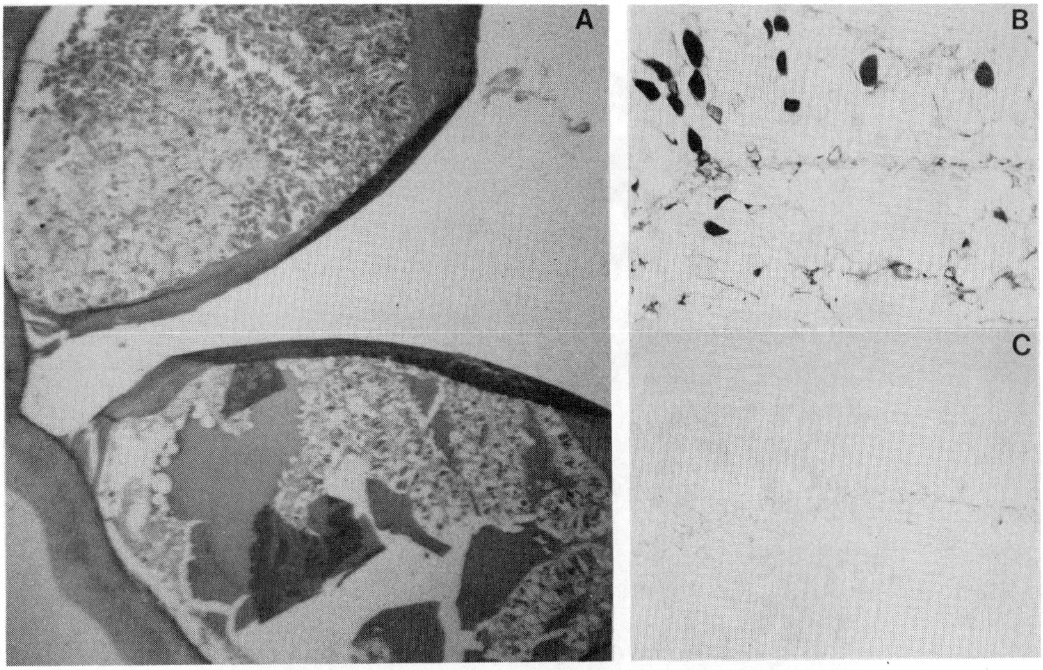

Fig. 4. Some histological aspects of the venom glands of Androctonus australis Hector. The section was transverse to the telson, a) Haemotoxilyn and eosin staining, b) peroxidase immunostaining with AaH II immune rabbit serum, c) control experiment with non immune rabbit serum.

presence of a Simian virus early promoter upstream from the cloned sequence to be expressed and a poly A site downstream from the inserted gene for polyadenylation of the transcribed mRNA.

To screen the library synthetic, oligonucleotide probes (Fig. 6) complementary to the known amino-acid sequence of AaH II (Rochat et al., 1972) were used. A clone (pcD-403) containing the AaH II cDNA has been obtained. Restriction analysis of the clone using Pst I and BamH I enzymes has shown that the insert size was about 500 base pairs, a size in agreement with regard to the 64 amino-acids comprising the toxin. After amplification and subcloning in M13 bacteriophage the nucleotide sequence of the cDNA was determined (Fig. 7). According to this sequence, the AaH II mRNA has the following characteristics. It has a single continuous translational reading frame of 280 nucleotides extending from the first nucleotide sequenced, through two AUG triplets, to a UAA termination codon. The first AUG in the extended reading frame occurs at the 25th nucleotide, followed by a second AUG six codons downstream. We assume that the 5' proximal AUG should be the initiator codon (Kozak, 1984). Additional features of the AaH II mRNA include a 5' nontranslated region of 25 nucleotides and a 3' nontranslated region of 60 nucleotides, followed by a polyadenylation tract. A putative polyadenylation signal (AAUAAA) is found 21 nucleotides upstream from the beginning of the tract (Proudfoot and Brownlee, 1976). The AaH II mRNA predicts a pretoxin consisting of 85 amino-acids (MW, 9537), 21 more than the mature toxin. According to the signal hypothesis for protein secretion, a signal protease cleaves the pretoxin sequence at a serine residue, leading to the removal of a highly hydrophobic signal peptide of 19 amino-acids, the average size usually observed (Austen, 1979). The remaining amino-acid sequence agrees in full with that of AaH II (Rochat et al., 1972), except for the presence of an additional dipeptide (Gly-Arg) at the C-terminal end. Within precursors to secretory peptides, sites for proteolysis and α-amidation are often marked by the sequence -X-Gly-B-B; X is the C-terminal amino-acid in the mature peptide that is α-amidated, and B is either lysine or arginine (Yoo et al., 1982). Among other scorpion neurotoxins, AaH II has been shown to be α-amidated as a C-terminal histidine amide (Rochat et al., 1972). It is not known if the α-carboxyamidation is required for optimal biological activity. The additional dipeptide predicted by the nucleotide sequence agrees with these rules by having only one basic residue.

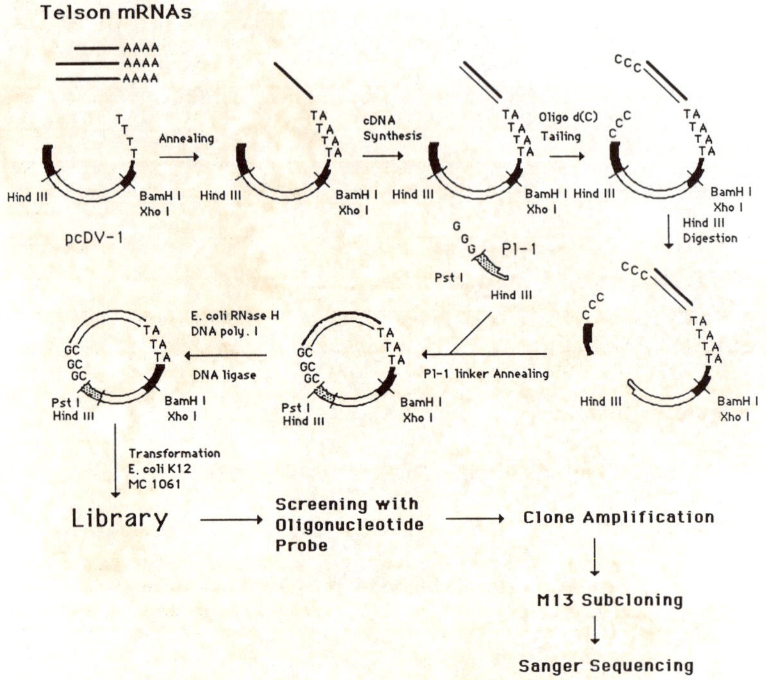

Fig. 5. The cDNA cloning strategy used. According to the Okayama and Berg system (1983), the first step to construct a recombinant plasmid is an annealing step between the poly A tract of the mRNA and the poly T of the plasmid vector (pcDV-1). The next step is the synthesis of the first cDNA strand using the reverse transcriptase primed on the poly T. Subsequently, an oligo d(C) tailing step coupled to an enzymatic digestion using Hind III to generate a sticking end is performed. In order to end with a circular recombinant plasmid the linker PL-1 is used, and later, the mRNA is digested with RNase H in preparation to the second cDNA strand synthesis. E. coli strain K12 MC1061 is then transformed with the total recombinant plasmid population generating the library used to screen for the scorpion toxins.

```
    21                      27                          34                  39
    Tyr Cys Asn Glu Glu Cys Thr Lys Leu Lys Gly Glu Ser Gly Tyr Cys Gln Trp Ala
 5' TAC TGC AAC GAA GAA TGC AC 3'                   5' GGA TAC TGC CAA TGG GC 3'
      T   T   T   G   G   T                               C   T   T   G
                                                          G
                                                          T
```

Fig. 6. Oligonucleotide probes specific to AaH II used for the cloning.

To further prove that the cDNA sequence contained in the clone pcD-403 is sufficient to direct the expression of a biologically active toxin, a transient eukaryotic expression assay system was used (Okayama and Berg, 1983). The rationale for choosing a mammalian expression

```
-25    -20          -10                                 15                  30
TAGAA  AATTCTATAA   AAGCTTCAAA  ATG AAT TAC TTG GTG ATG ATT AGT TTG GCA
                                Met Asn Tyr Leu Val Met Ile Ser Leu Ala

                    45              60                75
CTT CTC TTC GTG ACA GGT GTA GAG AGT GTA AAA GAC GGT TAT ATT GTC GAC GAT
Leu Leu Phe Val Thr Gly Val Glu Ser Val Lys Asp Gly Tyr Ile Val Asp Asp

    90              105                 120                 135
GTA AAC TGC ACA TAC TTT TGT GGT AGA AAT GCA TAC TGC AAC GAG GAA TGT ACC
Val Asn Cys Thr Tyr Phe Cys Gly Arg Asn Ala Tyr Cys Asn Glu Glu Cys Thr

            150                 165                 180
AAG TTG AAA GGT GAG AGT GGT TAT TGC CAA TGG GCA AGT CCA TAT GGA AAC GCC
Lys Leu Lys Gly Glu Ser Gly Tyr Cys Gln Trp Ala Ser Pro Tyr Gly Asn Ala

195                 210                 225                 240
TGC TAT TGC TAT AAA TTG CCC GAT CAT GTA CGT ACT AAA GGA CCA GGA AGA TGC
Cys Tyr Cys Tyr Lys Leu Pro Asp His Val Arg Thr Lys Gly Pro Gly Arg Cys

        255           270          280          290          300
CAT GGC CGA TAA ATTATAAGATGG  AATGTATCCT  AAGTATCAAT  GTTAAATAAA  TATAA
His Gly Arg End

  310      320          330          340          348
TTAAA  AAATTAAAAA  AAAAAAAAAA  AAAAAAAAAA  AAAAAAAA
```

Fig. 7. Nucleotide sequence of pcD-403 cDNA and inferred amino-acid sequence. The pcD-403 cDNA was subcloned into both M13mp18 and M13mp19 within Bam HI and Pst I restriction sites, and DNA sequencing carried out by the dideoxy chain termination method using the 17 bases M13 primer. The 19-amino-acid signal peptide is depicted in the dashed box, the AaH II mature sequence in the solid box, and the α-carboxyamidation signal sequence in the bold solid box. The ATG triplets and the putative poly-adenylation signal are underlined. The dashed lines represent the amino-acid sequences complementary to the oligonucleotide probes used for screening of bacterial colonies.

system is that biological activity of scorpion neurotoxins is, *stricto sensu*, dependent on the correct formation of four disulfide bridges for the proper folding of the protein (Sabatier *et al.*, 1987). Monkey kidney cells (COS-7) were processed for transfection either with pcD-403 or a 5' truncated clone as negative control, or no DNA at all. Supercoiled plasmid DNAs were detected 72 hours after transfection in all the samples except where DNA was omitted. We were not able to detect transcripts of pcD-403 cDNA by specific hybridization, due to their low copy number within cells (data not shown). Toxin expression in cell culture media was analyzed by immunoassay with polyclonal AaH II-specific, rabbit antibodies prepared against the native toxin (El Ayeb *et al.*, 1983). The expression of an immuno-detectable component was maximum by day 6. The highest level of expression detected as AaH II was 0.20 µg *per* 1 x 10^6 cells. We further characterized the expressed component on the basis of its binding properties to both AaH II specific antibodies and rat brain voltage-sensitive sodium channels (Jover *et al.*, 1978). The results established that it had the ability to compete in both immunoassay and receptor assay at an identical level with [^{125}I]-AaH II. This means that the antigenic and toxic sites of this expressed component are closely related or identical to those of AaH II. Upon intracerebroventricular injections, the component was able to promote the death of mice with a symptomatology identical to that of AaH II. As estimated by the preceding immunoassay and receptor assay, its LD_{50} was 0.3 ng *per* mouse, compared to 0.5 ng *per* mouse as we previously determined for native AaH II (De Lima *et al.*, 1986). Accordingly, we assume that the neurotoxic component that COS-7 cells expressed upon their transfection with the clone pcD-403 is the AaH II mature form.

ACKNOWLEDGMENTS

The authors thank Dr. Linda Lee, Dr. Catherine Loridan and Dr. Marie-France Martin for their help. The histological experiments were conducted by the Pathology Division at USAMRIID and we deeply thank Dr. Bill Hall for his involvement in it.

NOTES

The research described in this report was in compliance with the NIH guidelines involving recombinant DNA molecules. The views of the authors do not purport to reflect the positions of the U. S. Department of the Army or the U. S. Department of Defense.

This work was done while P. E. B. held a National Research Council-USAMRIID Research Associateship. Permanent address: Université d'Aix-Marseille II, Faculté de Médecine Secteur Nord, Biochimie, NDC:CNRS UA1179 - INSERM U172, Bd. P. Dramard, 13326 Marseille Cedex 15, France.

REFERENCES

Austen, B. (1979). Predicted secondary structures of amino-terminal extension sequences of secreted proteins. FEBS Lett., 103, 308-313.

Aviv, H. and Leder, P. (1972). Purification of biologically active globin messenger RNA by chromatography on oligothymidine acid-Cellulose. Pro. Natl. Acad. Sci. U.S.A., 69, 1408-1412.

Catterall, W. A. (1986). Molecular properties of voltage-sensitive sodium channels. Annu. Rev. Biochem., 55, 953-985 .

De Dianous, S., Hoarau, F. and Rochat, H. (1987). Re-examination of the specificity of the scorpion Androctonus australis Hector insect toxin towards arthropods. Toxicon, 25, 411-417.

De Lima, M. E., Martin, M. F., Diniz, C. R. and Rochat, H. (1986). Tityus serrulatus toxin VII bears pharmacological properties of both β-toxin and insect toxin from scorpion venoms. Biochem. Biophys. Res. Commun., 139, 296-302.

El Ayeb, M., Delori, P. and Rochat, H. (1983). Immunochemistry of scorpion α-toxins: antigenic homology checked with radioimmunoassays (RIA). Toxicon, 21, 709-716.

El Ayeb, M., Martin, M.F., Delori, P., Bechis, G. and Rochat, H. (1983). Immunochemistry of scorpion α-neurotoxins. Determination of the antigenic site number and isolation of a highly enriched antibody specific to a single antigeneic site of toxin II of Androctonus australis Hector. Mol. Immn., 20, 697-708.

El Ayeb, M. and Rochat, H. (1985). Polymorphism and quantitative variations of toxins in the venom of the scorpion Androctonus australis Hector. Toxicon, 23, 755-760.

El Ayeb, M., Darbon, H., Bahraoui, El M., Vargas, O. and Rochat, H. (1986). Different effects of defined chemical modifications on antigenic and pharmacological activities of scorpion α- and β-toxins. Eur. J. Biochem., 155, 289-294.

Fontecilla-Camps, J. C., Almassy, R. J., Suddath, F. L., Watt, D. D. and Bugg, C. E. (1980). The three dimensional structure of a protein from scorpion venom: a new structural class of neurotoxins. Proc. Nat. Acad. Sci. U.S.A., 77, 6496-6500.

Goyffon, M., Chovet, G. Deloince, R. and Vachon, M. (1971). Etude du caryotypes de quelques scorpions Buthides. Arachnologorum Congressus Internationalis V, 23-27.

Jover, E., Martin-Moutot, N., Couraud, F. and Rochat, H. (1978). Scorpion toxin: specific binding to rat brain synaptosomes. Biochem. Biophys. Res. Commun., 85, 377-382.

Jover, E., Couraud, F. and Rochat, H. (1980). Two types of scorpion neurotoxins characterized by their binding to two separate receptor sites on rat brain synaptosomes. Biochem. Biophys. Res. Commun., 95, 1607-1614.

Kopeyan, C., Martinez, G., Lissitzky, S., Miranda, F. and Rochat, H. (1974). Disulfide bonds of the toxin II of the scorpion Androctonus australis Hector. Eur. J. Biochem., 47, 483-489.

Kozak, M. (1984). Compilation and analysis of sequences upstream from the translational start site in eukaryotic mRNAs. Nucl. A. Res., 12, 857-872.

Maniatis, T., Fritsch, E. F. and Sambroock, J. (1982). Molecular cloning: A laboratory manual, Cold Spring Harbor Laboratory, Cold Spring Harbor, NY.

Martin, M.F. and Rochat, H. (1984). Purification and amino acid sequence of toxin I" from the venom of the North African scropion Androctonus australis Hector. Toxicon, 22, 695-703.

Martin, M.F. and Rochat, H. (1986). Large scale purification of toxins from the venom of the scorpion Androctonus australis Hector. Toxicon, 24, 1131-1135.

Martin, M.F., Garcia y Perez, L.G., El Ayeb, M., Kopeyan, C., Bechis, G., Jover, E. and Rochat, H. (1987). Purification and chemical and biological characterizations of seven toxins from the Mexican scorpion, Centruroides suffusus suffusus. J. Biol. Chem., 262,

4452-4459.

Martin, M. F., Rochat, H., Marchot, P. and Bougis, P. (1987). Use of high performance liquid chromatography to demonstrate quantitative variation in components of venom from the scorpion *Androctonus australis* Hector. *Toxicon*, *25*, 569-573.

Miranda, F., Kopeyan, C., Rochat, H., Rochat, C. and Lissitzky, S. (1970). Purification of animal neurotoxins. Isolation and characterization of eleven neurotoxins from the venoms of the scorpions *Androctonus australis* Hector, *Buthus occitanus tunetanus* and *Leiurus quinquestriatus quinquestriatus*. *Eur. J. Biochem.*, *16*, 514-523.

Okayama, H. and Berg, P. (1983). A cDNA cloning vector that permits expression of cDNA inserts in mammalian cells. *Mol. Cell. Biol.*, *3*, 280-289.

Proudfoot, N. J. and Brownlee, G. G. (1976). 3' non-coding region sequences in eukaryotic messenger RNA. *Nature*, *263*, 211-214.

Rochat, H., Rochat, C., Sampieri, F. and Miranda, F.; Lissitzky, S. (1972). The amino-acid sequence of the neurotoxin II of *Androctonus australis* Hector. *Eur. J. Biochem.*, *28*, 381-388.

Rochat, H. Bernard, P. and Couraud, F. (1979). Scorpion toxins: chemistry and mode of action. In B. Ceccarelli and F. Clementi (Ed.) *Advances in cytopharmacology*. Neurotoxins: tools in neurobiology , Vol. 3, pp. 325-334, Raven Press, New York.

Sabatier, J. M., Darbon, H., Fourquet, P., Rochat, H. and Van Rietschoten (1987). Reduction and reoxidation of the neurotoxin II from the scorpion *Androctonus australis* Hector. *Int. J. Peptide Protein Res.*, *30*, 125-134.

Yoo, O. J., Powell, C. T. and Agarwal, K. L. (1982). Molecular cloning and nucleotide sequence of full-length cDNA coding for porcine gastrin. *Proc. Natl. Acad. Sci. U.S.A.*, *79*, 1049-1053.

STRUCTURE AND FUNCTION OF TETANUS TOXIN. APPROACHES BY DNA AND PROTEIN CHEMISTRY

E. Habermann

Rudolf-Buchheim-Institute of Pharmacology, University of Giessen, 6300 Giessen

ABSTRACT

(1) Tetanus toxin has been sequenced at the DNA level, and found to be highly homologous to botulinum neurotoxins. Its two disulfide bridges have been localized between the light and the heavy chains (cys 438-cys 466) and within the fragment C moiety (cys 1076 - cys 1092). (2) Single-chain toxin has been prepared and subjected to nicking with trypsin, chymotrypsin, elastase, post-arginine cleaving enzyme and clostripain. All nicking sites have been aligned by Edman degradation at different positions within a 1000 Da sequence just preceding cys (466). Single-chain toxin is less potent than its nicked derivatives in terms of general toxicity, neuromuscular blockade, and inhibition of [^{3}H]noradrenaline release from cell cultures and washed brain homogenate. Thus the single-chain toxin may be regarded as a protoxin for different isotoxins. (3) Heavy and light chains of tetanus toxin have been separated by isoelectric focusing on the basis of their very different I.P.'s, and recombined with negligible loss of toxicity. This technique has also been applied to fragments of the toxin. Heavy chain, but not light chain promotes the loss of noradrenaline from brain homogenate and of K^+ from human erythrocytes.

KEYWORDS

Tetanus, botulinum, toxin, sequencing, protoxin, isotoxins, nicking, chains, binding, transmitters.

INTRODUCTION

Clostridia produce many toxins. Cytotoxic agents for instance phospholipases C or oxygen-labile, cholesterol sensitive toxins from Cl.perfringens and Cl.novyi permeabilize cell membranes. Others exert a cytopathic effect by damaging the cytoskeleton. Cl.botulinum C_2 toxin does so by ADP ribosylating G-actin. α-Toxin from Cl.novyi type A and B, and the toxins from Cl. difficile lead to the same changes, however without ADP ribosylation. Cytotoxic and cytopathic toxins damage many types of cells.

Clostridial neurotoxins like tetanus and botulinum toxins (for review see Habermann and Dreyer, 1986; Habermann, 1987) have a comparatively narrow target. They react specifically with presynaptic neuronal structures. They are internalized into the nerve endings, and then transported through the axon and in some cases even through central synapses. The peculiar handling of the toxins by neurons is not unique, but it furnishes the pharmacokinetic background for their specificity and potency. Despite seemingly divergent, even contrary clinical pictures e.g. tetanus vs. botulism, the causative toxins share the ability to inhibit the release of many transmitters. Admittedly the neuromuscular synapse is the main target of botulinum toxins, and the inhibitory spinal synapses of tetanus toxin. However, tetanus toxin blocks also the neuromuscular transmission, and botulinum toxins impede the release of GABA which is an inhibitory transmitter. On the basis of these pharmacological observations, clostridial neurotoxins form one group acting on a process that is generally involved in neurotransmitter release.

This is also true with respect to their chemistry. All toxins are synthesized as single 150 kDa chains and processed into bichainal toxins by limited proteolysis. All toxins contain a ganglioside binding site and, in addition, hydrophobic regions. A non-neutralizing monoclonal antibody recognized the light chains of all neurotoxins except that from Cl. botulinum type A (Tsuzuki et al., 1988). Unfortunately, nothing is known about the molecular mode of action of the neurotoxins.

Notwithstanding the numerous similarities in structure and action, the toxin genes are located and transmitted by different means. The tetanus toxin gene is part of a plasmid; this position has facilitated its cloning and sequencing. In contrast, phages carry the genes for Cl.botulinum C and D toxins and those for Cl.novyi α-toxin which they may transfer to Cl.botulinum type C. The genes for the other toxins appear to be represented by sequences in the bacterial chromosome.

Starting from this background in 1984, and because we were convinced that a better understanding of the toxin actions would require a closer look at their structure, we have initiated a series of new approaches to the biochemistry of tetanus toxin. We have selected this toxin because of its medical importance, and because it can be prepared easily .

NEW APPROACHES

Sequencing of the Tetanus Toxin Gene

Fairweather and Lyness (1986) started with the total bacterial DNA, whereas our group (Eisel et al., 1986) under the guidance of Heiner Niemann analyzed the gene in the 75 kbp plasmid from strain E 88. Shortly, we have isolated the heavy and the light chains of tetanus toxin and also its fragment C (synonymous with BIIb). Among the three N-terminal sequences, that of fragment C turned out to contain a hexapeptide with a moderately degenerated code. A pool of corresponding mixed DNA nucleotides was synthesized and used to screen the restriction fragments from the pE88 plasmid (Fig. 1). A 2.0 kbp EcoRI fragment, designated tet7, was specifically recognized, cloned in E.coli using pUC19 as a vector, and used to screen further libraries obtained from pE88 by digestion with restriction endonucleases. Eight overlapping clones, together spanning > 6000 nucleotides were sequenced on both strands to establish the primary structure of the toxin. A single open reading frame represented 1315 amino acids. It started with a codon for methionine, followed by the known N-terminal proline of the light chain. This proline will be labeled as pos. 1 subsequently. Neither a signal sequence nor prominent hydrophobic sections were found. The upstream sequence contained the Shine-Dalgarno consensus sequence [AGGAGA], and the termination codon for another 21 kDa polypeptide of unknown function. Some stem-loop sequences downstream the toxin gene may constitute transcription termination signals.

Although Fairweather and Lyness (1986) started with total DNA and went on by a way different from ours, their nucleotide sequence was the same. Meanwhile, nearly 30 % of the amino acid alignement has been analyzed by Edman degradation in the course of the work of K. Krieglstein et al. (this meeting). Thus the complete structure appears to be well established.

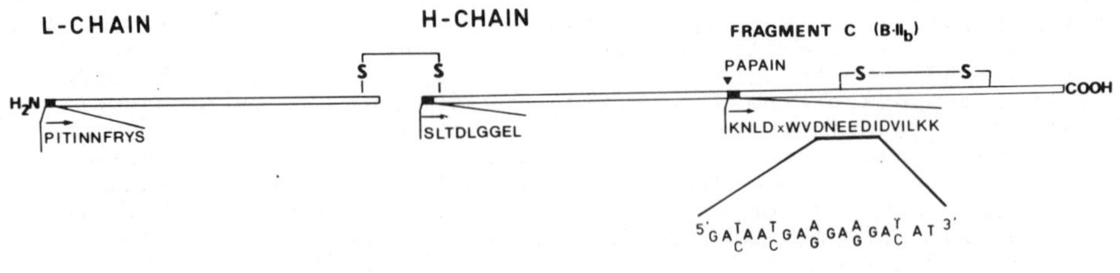

Fig. 1. Structural model of tetanus toxin and partial amino terminal sequences. Partial amino acid sequences of the L- and H-chains as well as of fragments C and BIIb were determined by Edman degradation. A pool of synthetic oligonucleotides corresponding to amino acids 8-13 of fragment C was used to identify the gene encoding tetanus toxin (Eisel et al., 1986).

```
LIGHT CHAINS          1                 10                 20
  TETANUS TOXIN       P I T I N N F R Y S D P V N N D T I I M M E
  BOTULINUM A         P F V N K Q F N Y K D P V N G V D . . . . .
  BOTULINUM B         P V T I N N F N Y N D P I D N N . . . . . .
  BOTULINUM C         X I T I N N F N Y S D P V D N K N I L Y . .
  BOTULINUM E         P - K I N S F N Y N D P V N D R T I L Y I .

HEAVY CHAINS               460                 470                 480
  TETANUS TOXIN     S L T D L G G E L C I K I K N E D L T F I A E K N S
  BOTULINUM A               A L N D L C I K V N N I D L K F . . . . . .
  BOTULINUM A               A L N D L C I K V N N W D L F F S P S E D N
  BOTULINUM B               A - P G I C I D V D N E D L F F I A D . . .
  BOTULINUM E                   K S I C I E I N N G E L - F . . . . . .
```

Fig. 2. Structural homologies between tetanus toxin and botulinum toxins A, B, C and E found in the N-terminal amino acid sequences of the respective L- and H-chains. Amino acids common to tetanus and any botulinum neurotoxin are framed with solid lines (from Habermann 1987, with the data for botulinum C toxin reported by Fujii et al., 1988).

Post-translational modifications and their pharmacological consequences

At the first look the primary structure does not furnish informations on the pharmacokinetics or pharmacodynamics of tetanus toxin. However, it was helpful in two respects. Comparison with known partial sequences of botulinum A, B, C and E toxins disclosed striking homologies (Eisel et al., 1986) between all clostridial neurotoxins, thus adding a structural and phylogenetic argument to the list of their pharmacological and biochemical similarities (Fig. 2). Moreover, the sequence served as a blueprint for our further studies on structure and action. It allowed the localization of the nicking regions between light and heavy chain, and between fragment C and the N-terminal moiety of the heavy chain. The singular Cys (466) of the heavy chain was found close to its N-terminus and to mediate the link with any of the five half-cystines within the light chain. None of the four half-cystines of fragment C is involved in a disulfide bridge with the remainder (called fragment B) of the toxin molecule, because it can be removed in the absence of reducing agents.

On this background we studied the limited proteolysis leading to chain formation, and its pharmacological consequences. First of all single chain toxin had to be prepared free of endogenous protease(s) in larger amounts. We then subjected it to proteolytic cleavage and monitored simultaneously the gel electrophoretic pattern, some physicochemical properties by HPLC, and the pharmacological properties of single-chain toxin and its bichainal derivatives.

Numerous proteases nicked single-chain toxin with surprising specificity, for instance trypsin, chymotrypsin, elastase, post-arginine cleaving enzyme from mouse submaxillary gland, clostripain from Cl. histolyticum and - with lesser specificity - even papain. The resulting light chains differed slightly by their length. Trypsin in higher concentrations led to a light chain that moved electrophoretically with the light chain cut out by the clostridial enzyme(s). After lower trypsin concentrations, a heavier version appeared in SDS gel electrophoresis. The same dose-dependent pattern occurred with clostripain and the post-arginine cleaving enzyme from mouse submaxillary gland. On the other hand, chymotrypsin and elastase produced one light chain of intermediate size. Single-chain toxin did not differ by its molecular weight from any bichainal toxin, so no major sequence was lost by proteolytic attack from the C-terminus of either chain. However, a minor shortening at the C-terminus of the heavy chain would have escaped our detection.

Nicking rendered the toxin more hydrophilic in hydrophobic interaction chromatography, and more acidic as revealed by HPLC with DEAE or QAE ion exchanger. Binding to brain membranes in high or low ionic strength buffer was not changed by nicking.

Limited proteolysis of the single-chain toxin by all enzymes mentioned increased the pharmacological potency, whose degree was independent of the nicking proteases but differed with the test system. The activation factor was only two to three upon subcutaneous injection in mice, but about five to ten when inhibition of $[^3H]$noradrenaline release was measured on washed brain homogenate. The paralytic power on the indirectly stimulated mouse hemidiaphragm was increased about 20 fold by nicking. The activation factors should be regarded as minimum values, since the intrinsic proteases of the test system may substitute for the extrinsic nicking enzymes. Thus the single-chain toxin is a protoxin, and is processed posttranslationally to different isotoxins. The term "tetanus toxin" is the common name for the primary gene product and its various derivatives. The list of nicking proteases contains not only the endogenous enzyme(s) from Cl.tetani, but also enzymes from at least one other bacterium as well as enzymes from the host. All of them might contribute to the activation of single-chain toxin in clinical tetanus (Weller et al., 1988).

As judged from the gel electrophoretic behaviour of the light chains, the

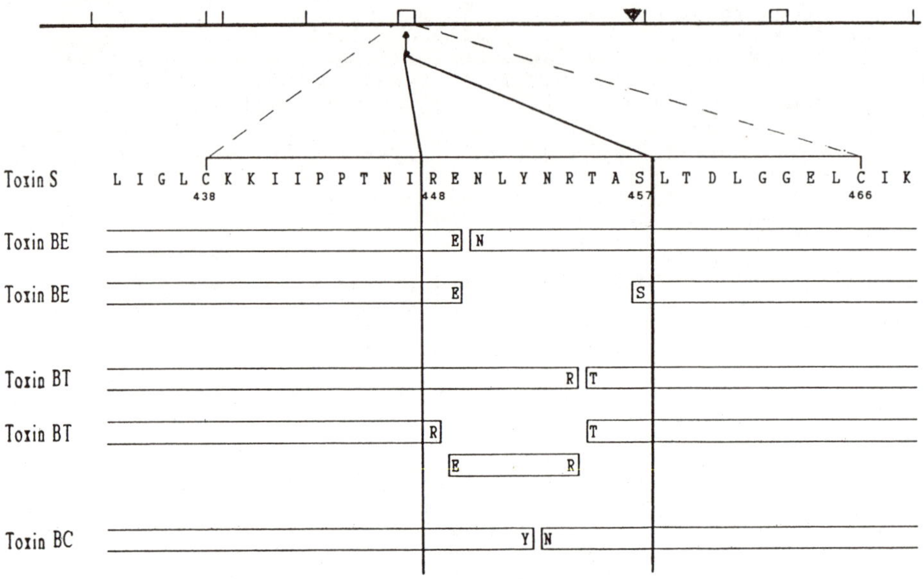

Fig. 3. Disulfides and nicking of tetanus toxin. The horizontol upper line symbolizes the alignement of the half-cystines of tetanus toxin (Eisel <u>et al.</u>, 1986). The position of the disulfide bridge between the chains (left) and within fragment C (right) has been taken from Krieglstein <u>et al</u>. (this meeting). The release of fragment C by papain is indicated by ▼ . An exploded view is given for the extremely narrow nicking region between pos. 448 and 457, showing the loci of limited proteolysis as analyzed by Krieglstein <u>et al</u>. Toxin S is single-chain toxin. BE marks the two bichainal extracellular toxins differing by the length of their respective heavy chains. BT shows the results of exposure to lower (upper bars) and higher (lower bars) trypsin concentrations. BC indicates the precise nicking by chymotrypsin.

protease-sensitive sequence was predicted to span maximally 10 - 15 amino acids and to end with the N-terminus of the heavy chain. Complete structural analysis of the nicking region was obtained by Edman degradation of the unnicked protoxin in comparison with the differently nicked toxins. Chain separation was not necessary because the N-terminus of the protoxin was homogeneous, and its first ten amino acids exactly corresponded with the sequence derived from DNA analysis. Limited proteolysis by trypsin and chymotrypsin turned out to be very specific. Since our sequencing experiments will be presented by K. Krieglstein et al in this meeting, they are mentioned here only as far as necessary for considerations on structure-action relationships. Chymotrypsin cleaved the bond following tyr (452). Trypsin in small concentrations split behind arg (454), with higher concentrations also behind arg (448). The connecting peptide was also sequenced. On reassessment of the bichainal toxin from clostridial cultures, it was found that its heavy chain started not only with ser (457) as previously reported. Three fourth of the heavy chain present possessed asn (450) as its N-terminus. To identify the C-terminus of the light chain from this toxin, we prepared the respective cyanogen bromide fragment, split it with post-lysine cleaving enzyme and subjected the resulting peptide to complete Edman degradation. It ended with glu (449) neighbouring the N-terminus found for the larger version of the heavy chain (Krieglstein et al, 1988).

It is concluded that the nicking region comprises less than 1 % of the length of single-chain toxin. Nicking is relevant for activation, although the freshly exposed amino acids may vary. As mentioned, nicking renders the toxin more hydrophilic and acidic, which may promote the internalization or the interaction with its targets. Nicking does not change the binding properties.

Separation, Properties and Recombination of the Chains.

Tetanus toxin contains ten half-cystines. As mentioned, one disulfide bridge connects cys 466 with one of the five half-cystines of the light chain. It will be dealt with by K. Krieglstein et al. (1988) that the interchain link is between cys (438) and cys (466). Moreover we have positioned the second disulfide bridge as part of a short loop between cys (1076) and cys (1092) within the C-fragment. All other half-cystines are free. The data are important in some respects. Firstly, they show a tendency towards forming the smallest disulfide loops possible. Secondly, they map out the nicking region since separation of the chains always requires reduction. Thirdly, they are helpful for a better understanding of the separation, modification and reassembly of the chains of the toxin. This will be dealt with now.

Matsuda and Yoneda (1976) have reported the separation and reassociation of the chains of tetanus toxin. Like others, we found it difficult to reproduce their work. Since we intended to study the properties of the two chains and to derivatize them separately, we developed a new preparative technique based on isoelectric focusing in 2 M urea under reducing conditions. The light chain has its isoelectric point at pH 4.8, the heavy chain at 7.2. There is also an - albeit slight - difference between bichainal extracellular (I.P. at pH 5.9) and single-chain (I.P. at pH 6.2) toxin, as expected from our data with ion exchange chromatography. Moreover isoelectric focusing separates fragment B into light chain and the N-terminal moiety of the heavy chain. The technique opened the way for a separate study of the heavy and the light chain. It also gave evidence for three different forces holding the chains together: covalent linkage by the disulfide, ionic attractions and hydrogen bonds.

The light chain did neither compete with radiolabeled tetanus toxin for binding, nor did it so far act on any pharmacological system. However, the chain has not yet been injected intracellularly. A - still hypothetical - target must be excluded by that way, since fragment B inhibited exocytosis from bovine adrenal medullary cells (Penner et al., 1986).

Like fragment C, the heavy chain competes with ^{125}I-toxin for binding in low molarity buffer. With respect to binding in high molarity buffer, heavy chain is much less affine than toxin, again like fragment C. Heavy chain exerts some membranal effects which indicate the formation of small pores. For instance. it decreases the content of radioactivity in washed rat brain homogenate which had been preloaded with ^{3}H-noradrenaline.Moreover, it promotes K^+ loss from human erythrocytes. Thus it is tempting to assume that the heavy chain is involved in the internalization of the toxin. Curiously enough, tetanus toxin does not share the direct membranal effects exerted by heavy chain.

Recombination of the heavy and light chain can be achieved by dialysis of their mixture against a slightly alkaline buffer. The resulting material behaves like genuine toxin in all tests used. Recent experiments have shown that toxin fragments and separately modified chains can be also recombined (Weller et al, to be published).

CONCLUSIONS AND FUTURE ASPECTS.

Sequencing of the tetanus toxin gene has furnished crucial data to define the clostridial neurotoxins as members of one family of proteins. It has paved the way to an understanding of its posttranslational modification. In connection with approaches by preparative biochemistry, classical sequencing and pharmacology the single-chain protoxin has been discriminated from different bichainal isotoxins. The disulfide bridges have been localized. The chains have been separated, characterized according to their binding and actions, and recombined.

More questions can now be asked. Gene technology should furnish toxin derivates which have been altered by way of site-directed mutagenesis. Chains prepared by that way could then be recombined with chains derived from native toxin, and the resulting materials subjected to the battery of binding and pharmacological assays now available. The minimal structural requirements for binding, action and axonal transport could be assessed. Hybrid toxins could be attempted through pairing the individual chains with alien partners.

Since all of these approaches could also be extended to botulinum toxins, a rich field is open for future work.

REFERENCES

Eisel, U., W. Jarausch, K. Goretzki, A. Henschen, J. Engels, U. Weller, M. Hudel, E. Habermann and H. Niemann (1986). Tetanus toxin: Primary structure, expression in E.coli, and homology with botulinum toxins. EMBO J., 5, 2495-2502.

Fairweather, N.F. and V.A. Lyness (1986). The complete nucleotide sequence of tetanus toxin. Nuc. Acid. Res., 14, 7809-7812.

Fujii, N., K. Oguma, N. Yokosawa, K. Kimura and K. Tsuzuki (1988). Characterization of bacteriophage nucleic acids obtained from Clostridium botulinum types C and D. Appl. Envir. Microbiol., 54, 69-73.

Habermann, E. (1987). Clostridial neurotoxins. - The search for a common mode of action. Proc. 38th Colloq. Mosbach. Springer Verlag, Berlin, Heidelberg. pp 160-175.

Habermann, E. and F. Dreyer (1986). Clostridial neurotoxins. Handling and action at the cellular and molecular level. Current Topics Microbiol. Immunol., 129, 93-179.

Krieglstein, K., A. Henschen, U. Weller and E. Habermann (1988). Tetanus toxin: Primary structure, disulfide bridges and proteolytic modifications of the extracellular form. This meeting.

Matsuda, M. and M. Yoneda (1976). Reconstitution of tetanus neurotoxin from two antigenically active polypeptide fragments. Biochem. Biophys. Res. Comm., 68, 668-674.

Penner, R., E. Neher and F. Dreyer (1986). Intracellularly injected tetanus toxin inhibits exocytosis in bovine adrenal chromaffin cells. Nature, 324, 76-78.

Tsuzuki, K., N. Yokosawa, B. Syuto, I.Ohishi, N. Fujii, K. Kimura and K. Oguma (1988). Establishment of a monoclonal antibody recognizing an antigenic site common to Clostridium botulinum type B, C_1, D and E toxins and tetanus toxin. Infect. Immun., 56, 898-902.

Weller, U., M. Dauzenroth, D. Meyer zu Heringdorf and E. Habermann (1988). The chains of tetanus toxin. Separation, recombination and biological properties. Europ. J. Biochem., submitted.

Weller, U., F. Mauler and E. Habermann (1988). Tetanus toxin: Biochemical and pharmacological comparison between its protoxin and some isotoxins obtained by limited proteolysis. Naunyn-Schmiedeberg's Arch. Pharmacol., in press.

THE CLONING OF TOXIN AND OTHER CLOSTRIDIAL GENES

T. RUBIDGE, R.W. TITBALL, AND K.L. MARTIN

Chemical Defence Establishment, Porton Down,
Salisbury, Wiltshire, U.K.

ABSTRACT

Clostridial toxins are important in a wide variety of disease conditions. This paper reviews progress in cloning Clostridial toxin and other genes and discusses their structure and function with respect to promoter regions, signal sequences, termination regions and nucleotide and codon usage.

KEYWORDS

Clostridium; toxin; gene; promoters; signal sequence; codon.

INTRODUCTION

The ubiquity of species of Clostridia in the environment can be related to their ability to form desiccation resistant spores and their pathogenic potential can often be related to their ability to produce toxins. *C. perfringens*, for example, secretes toxins implicated in disease in birds (Al-Shiekly and Truscott, 1977), pigs, calves, lambs (Kennedy *et al*., 1977), man (Lawrence and Walker, 1976) and other animals (Niilo, 1965). Clostridial toxins may be of extreme potency; *C. botulinum* produces one of the most potent toxins known and is one cause of fatal poisoning. Infection of wounds by soil-borne *C. tetani* can lead rapidly to death through the action of the toxin upon the central nervous system (Bizzini, 1979).

The genus has, however, been relatively neglected compared to the more generally studied organisms of molecular microbiology - *Escherichia coli, Bacillus subtilis* and *Saccharomyces cerevisiae*. This paper seeks to review current data on the cloning of the genes for Clostridial toxins and the structure of the genes revealed by analysis of the nucleotide sequences. By further extending the analysis to other cloned Clostridial genes it is possible to begin the assembly of a picture of gene structure in the genus.

CLONING OF TOXIN GENES FROM *CLOSTRIDIUM* SPP.

Tetanus toxin, produced by *C. tetani* and responsible for the spastic paralytic symptoms associated with the organism's pathological effects, is amongst the better studied toxins of the Clostridia. The heavy chain of the toxin may be cleaved with papain to give two fragments, B and C (Matsuda and Yoneda, 1975). In 1986, Fairweather and his colleagues reported cloning the entire fragment C and part of the fragment B coding regions using plasmid pAT153 in *E. coli* (Fairweather *et al*., 1976). They were able to confirm the identity of the fragment C coding region by translating its nucleotide sequence into a putative amino acid sequence and comparing this with the known amino acid sequence of the fragment's amino terminal sequence. Additionally the affinity of antibody raised against native fragment C with fusion proteins produced by the fragment C coding region cloned in the expression vector pWRL507 was demonstrated. Fragment C contains epitopes which react with neutralising antibody.

C. difficile secretes two toxins, A and B, implicated in diarrhoeal disease. Muldrow et al., (1987) constructed a genomic library using the phage vector lambda gt11 and recombinant clones expressing toxin epitopes were detected using anti-toxin A antibody. Despite the instability of the 22 plaques initially identified (35,000 were screened) 1 was found sufficiently stable to permit further study but restriction analysis revealed the cloned insert to be only 0.3 kbp in length. It was not cytotoxic for mammalian tissue cells.

Possibly the Clostridial species to receive most attention for its extrachromosomal genetics has been C. perfringens. For example, plasmids conferring resistance to tetracycline and chloramphenicol on naturally occurring strains have been isolated, characterized (Rood et al., 1978; Abraham et al., 1985) and cloned in pBR322 to form chimeric plasmids (Abraham and Rood, 1985). Such chimeric plasmids may be useful as shuttle plasmids for E. coli and C. perfringens (Squires et al., 1984). In addition, chloramphenicol resistance transposons have been described (Abraham and Rood, 1987).

Amongst the spectrum of toxins produced and secreted by C. perfringens the genes for both the alpha toxin, which is a phospholipase C activity, and the bacteriocin, BCN5, have been cloned. The alpha toxin was cloned and sequenced independantly by two groups (Titball et al., 1988a, 1988b, Kehoe, 1988; Leslie et al., 1988) using plasmid vectors - pUC18 and pACYC184 respectively. The toxin clones possessed a promoter recognized by the E. coli host cells and the signal sequence was cleaved. The mature cloned toxin was experimentally indistinguishable from native toxin but was found to be associated predominantly with the periplasmic compartment. It was presumed that cell lysis was adequate to allow the detection of toxin on agar medium supplemented with sheep red blood cells or egg yolk emulsion. The extraction procedure used to prepare DNA from the entire genome for the cloning C. perfringens alpha toxin did not allow any observations to be made regarding the location of the toxin gene. The tetanus toxin gene is plasmid-borne (Fairweather et al., 1986) and the same may be true of the alpha toxin gene.

The bacteriocin, BCN5, has activity against C. perfringens and is borne on the plasmid pIP404. Garnier and Cole (1986) located within a 3.8 kbp fragment of the plasmid an open reading frame of appropriate length to encode a protein of 96,591 daltons similar to the molecular weight of the bacteriocin. The complete identity of the protein with BCN5 could not be confirmed since no activity could be detected when the fragment was cloned into E. coli. Although authors considered that a biased codon usage prevented E. coli from expressing an active product the bias is similar to that established for the active cloned alpha toxin (Clostridial codon usage is discussed more fully below). Since bcn5-related proteins could not be detected in association with the E. coli lacZ gene product in fusion proteins it is, perhaps, more likely that there was a marked instability of the product of the cloned gene product.

A DNA fragment encoding part of the enterotoxin of C. perfringens has been cloned by Wernars (1988) using the plasmids pUC18 and pUC19. Two different strains showed minor differences in nucleotide sequence but the amino acid sequences were identical. The same vectors were used successfully to clone portions of the type B toxin of C. botulinum. The cloning of botulinum toxins continues to attract the attention of several independant groups.

Other toxin genes might not be easy to clone and express in E. coli; workers have looked without success for the expression of C. perfringens theta, nu and kappa toxins in E. coli using plasmid genomic libraries. Other groups have met with similar lack of success with theta toxin in both plasmid and phage libraries. Whether this represents the inability of E. coli to express the genes of whether the toxins are lethal to the host cell remains to be established.

THE CLONING OF OTHER GENES FROM CLOSTRIDIUM SPP.

The cloning of the structural genes encoding the enzymes of the cellulosome in C. thermocellum and C. acetobutylicum attracted the early attention of groups seeking to elucidate more clearly the genetic control of cellulolysis.

Cornet *et al.* (1983a; 1983b), working with *C. thermocellum*, established a library of DNA fragments in the size range 25 to 40 kbp using the cosmid pHC79. Apart from demonstrating complementation of auxotrophic mutations they reported two clones with carboxymethylcellulase (CMCase) activity. When the DNA fragments within these clones were subcloned using plasmid pBR322 the genes were localized on fragments approximately 2.6 kbp in length. In both cases the expression of the genes (*celA* and *celB*) was unaffected by their orientation within the recombinant plasmids, suggesting that functional promoters recognized by *E. coli* had been cloned with the DNA encoding the active polypeptides.

Despite being secreted by *C. thermocellum* the activities expressed by cloned genes were not released from the cells. In *E. coli* both beta glucosidase and CMCase activities were present in the cytoplasm with a proportion of the latter reaching the periplasmic space. When the *celA* gene was further cloned into *Saccharomyces cerevisiae* the activity was located only in the cytoplasm (Sacco *et al.*, 1984).

Further genes concerned in cellulose hydrolysis have been cloned (Piruzyan *et al.*, 1985; Romaniec *et al.*, 1987). Ten clones expressing activities involved in cellulolysis by *C. thermocellum* have been identified (Millet *et al.*, 1985). The cloned promoter regions were recognized by the host *E. coli* cells. Characterization of the activities was performed on cell-free extracts but no data were reported concerning the sub-cellular localization of the activities. Using a lambda phage to clone large DNA fragments, Schwarz *et al.* (1985) reported clones expressing four glucanase and two glucosidase activities.

The nucleotide sequences of the *C. thermocellum celA* and *celD* genes encoding the extracellular endoglucanases A and D have been published (Beguin *et al.*, 1985; Joliff *et al.*, 1986). The initiation codon of the former was identified as GTG which is very inefficiently utilised by *S. cerevisiae*. Fortuitously, an ATG codon was located downstream of the start of the putative bacterial signal sequence suggesting that the functional *celA* gene cloned in *S. cerevisiae* (Sacc *et al.*, 1984) was deficient in the first 21 amino acid residues of the signal sequence. The role of signal sequences in the expression of cloned Clostridial genes is discussed below.

The products of cloned genes from *C. acetobutylicum* are not efficiently transported from the host cells. Zappe *et al.* (1986) concluded that the small amounts of activity necessary for detection of activity on agar medium were released only through cell lysis. Genes complementing mutations *E. coli* (*proA2* and *leuB6*) have been cloned and *Bacillus subtilis* has been used to clone and express the gene for alpha-isopropyl malate dehydrogenase activity from *C. acetobutylicum* (Efstathiou and Truffaut, 1986).

Nitrogenase in *C. pasteurianum* comprises an iron protein and the iron-sulphur protein ferredoxin. Graves *et al.* (1985) reported the cloning of the structural gene for ferredoxin and the elucidation of its nucleotide sequence. An open reading frame coding for a polypeptide containing 56 amino acid residues was identified. Further sequence data, for the *nifH1* and *nifH2* genes, are available (Chen *et al.*, 1986). A partial nucleotide sequence was reported at the same time for the *nifD* gene whilst the *nifH3* was also cloned. The *mop* gene encoding the molybdenum-pterin binding protein and the galactokinase gene have been cloned (Daldal and Applebaum, 1985; Hinton and Freyer, 1986). The nucleotide sequence of the former was also reported.

When the gene encoding 10-formyltetrahydrofolate synthetase in *C. acidiurici* was cloned the promoter region was functional in *E. coli* (Whitehead and Rabinowitz, 1986). The propyl beta-isomalate dehydrongenase (Ishii *et al.*, 1983) and the hydrogenase (Karube *et al.*, 1983) genes of *C. butyricum* have been cloned.

NUCLEOTIDE SEQUENCE DATA FOR CLONED CLOSTRIDIAL GENES

Thirteen sequences, either complete or partial, of cloned Clostridial genes have been published (TABLE 1). Five are toxins and two are extracellular enzymes. Caution must be exercised in drawing conclusions concerning the structure and function of Clostridial genes from such sparse data. Nevertheless, it is possible to begin to establish where Clostridial genetic organization differs from that of other bacteria and where structures and functions are conserved.

TABLE 1. CLONED CLOSTRIDIAL GENES

Organism / gene	cloned into	sequence	ref
Clostridium acetobutylicum			
endoglucanase	pEcoR251	no	1
cellobiase	pEcoR251	no	1
arg / *his*	pEcoR251	no	1
pro / *leu*	pHV33	no	2
Clostridium acidiurici			
10-formyltetra-hydrofolate synthetase	pUC8	no	3
Clostridium butyricum			
hydrogenase	pBR322	no	4
isopropylmalate dehydrogenase	pBR322	no	5
Clostridium difficile			
toxfragA	lambda gt11	no	6
Clostridium pasteurianum			
nifH1	pBR322	yes	7
nifH2	pBR322	yes	7
nifH3	pBR322	no	7
nifD	pBR322	partial	7
gal	pBR322	partial	8
fd	pBR322	yes	9
mop	pBR322	yes	10
Clostridium perfringens			
Tn4451 Cm r	pUC18	no	11
Tn4452 Cm r	pUC18	no	11
pJU121 (tet r)	pBR322	no	12
pJU122 (tet r)	pBR322	no	12
pJU281 (tet r)	pBR322	no	12
pCW3 (tet r)	pBR322	no	13
alpha tox	pUC18	yes	14
alpha tox	pACYC184	yes	15
bcn5	pUC8/pHV33	yes	16
Clostridium tetani			
toxfragB	pWRL507	partial	17
toxfragC	pWRL507	yes	17
Clostridium thermocellum			
endoglucanase	pBR322	no	18
>2 x *cel*	pBR322	no	19
celA	pBR322	yes	20
celA	pG63-11	no	21
celA	pCT182/pBR322	no	22
celB	pCT182/pBR322	no	22
celD	pACYC184/pUC8	yes	23
4 x glucanase	lambda 1059	no	24
2 x glucosidase	lambda 1059	no	24

References: 1- Zappe *et al.* (1986), 2- Efstathiou and Truffaut (1986), 3- Whitehead and Rabinowitz (1986), 4- Karube *et al.* (1983), 5- Ishii *et al.* (1983), 6- Muldrow *et al.* (1987), 7- Chen *et al.* (1986), 8- Daldal and Applebaum (1985), 9- Graves *et al.* (1985), 10- Hinton and Freyer (1986), 11- Abraham and Rood (1987), 12- Squires *et al.* (1984), 13- Abraham and Rood (1985), 14- Titball *et al.* (1988b), 15- Leslie *et al.* (1988), 16- Garnier and Cole (1986), 17- Fairweather *et al.* (1986), 18- Piruzyan *et al.* (1985), 19- Romaniec *et al.* (1987), 20- Beguin *et al.* (1985), 21- Sacco *et al.* (1984), 22- Cornet *et al.* (1983), 23- Joliff *et al.* (1986), 24- Schwarz *et al.* (1985).

STRUCTURE OF CLONED CLOSTRIDIAL PROMOTER SEQUENCES

Where a cloned Clostridial gene has been expressed it has been under the control of the native promoter. Each putative promoter sequence can be compared with the E. coli (Rosenburg and Court, 1979) and Bacillus (Moran et al., 1982) RNA polymerase binding region consensus sequences. Graves and Rabinowitz (1986) have suggested that there might be "extended" promoter recognition sites outside of the Pribnow (-10) and -35 sequences but the data presently available do not permit this suggestion to be further investigated. A further comparison can be made between putative promoter regions in Clostridia and the Shine-Dalgarno ribosome binding region established for other bacteria (Shine and Dalgarno, 1975).

There is considerable agreement between the -10 and -35 consensus sequences established for E. coli and B. subtilis and those identified for Clostridia (TABLE 2). The -10

TABLE 2. PUTATIVE PROMOTER SEQUENCES FOR CLOSTRIDIAL GENES

GENE		-35	N	-10	N	SD	N	init	ref
C. pasteurianum:									
nif H1		ni	-	TATAAT	222	AGGAGGA	7	ATG	1
nif H2		TTGACA	17	TATAAT	73	AGGAGGA	7	ATG	1
nif D		ni	-	ni	-	ATGAGGG	9	GTG	1
ORF		TTGTAG	17	TATAAT	129	GGAAGGA	10	GTG	1
galactokinase		AAGACA	18	TATTAT	-	ni	-	ATG	2
ferredoxin		TTTAAA	17	TATGGT	21	AGGAGGT	9	ATG	3
ORF		ni	-	ni	-	AGGGGGA	7	ATG	3
mop		TTGTAT	16	TATAAT	42	AGGAGGA	7	ATG	4
C. perfringens:									
alpha toxin		GTGAGC	17	TATAAT	58	CGGGGGA	8	ATG	5,6
bcn5		TTGAAG	13	TATATT	77	GAGAGGT	7	ATG	7
C. thermocellum:									
celA	a.	TTGGGT	19	TATAAT	32	AGGAGGA	7	GTG	8
	b.	TTGTAT	22	TATAAT	126	AGGAGGA	7	GTG	8
celD		CTGTAT	13	TATAAT	95	AGGGGGA	12	ATG	9
ORF		TTGTTT	16	TAATAT	8	TGGAGGT	5	ATG	8
C. tetani:									
tetanus toxin		ni	-	ni	-	ni	-	ni	10
Consensi:									
E. coli		TTGACA	15-18	TATAAT	-	AGGAGGT	-	ATG	11,12
B. subtilis		TTGACA	17	TATAAT	-	AGGAGGG	9	-	13

Notes: The Pribnow sequence is denoted by "-10" and the ribosome binding sequence (Shine-Dalgarno) by "SD". Nucleotides intervening between the -35, -10 and SD sequences are shown in the columns headed "N". Initiation codons are shown in the column "init". Where a functional sequence has not been identified "ni" has been inserted in the table. "ORF" signifies an open reading frame.

References: 1- Chen et al. (1986), 2- Daldal and Applebaum (1985), 3- Graves et al. (1985), 4- Hinton and Freyer (1986), 5- Titball et al. (1988b), 6- Kehoe (1988), 7- Garnier and Cole (1986), 8- Beguin et al. (1985), 9- Joliff et al. (1986), 10- Fairweather et al. (1986), 11- Rosenburg and Court (1979), 12- Shine and Dalgarno (1975) 13- Squires et al. (1984)

sequence is the more highly conserved and, like that sequence in E. coli, all published Clostridial sequences are of the form TANNNT (N represents the bases adenine or thymine). Of the thirteen Clostridial sequences only four diverge from TATAAT. In the case of the open reading frame identified adjacent to the glucanase gene in C. thermocellum the second and third bases are inverted (TAATAT) (Beguin et al., 1985) whereas in the galactokinase gene of C. pasteurianum there is a centrally reiterated T (TATTAT) (Daldal and Applebaum, 1985). This same organism shows the only instance of bases other than adenine and thymine (TATGGT) being present. The nine B. subtilis -10 sequences reported by Moran et al. (1982) show more variation than do the twelve sequences identified in Clostridia. All the Clostridial genes which have been cloned are expressed during the vegetative growth phase. There may be separate RNA polymerases active during sporulation similar to those identified in B. subtilis (Losick and Pero, 1981).

Within the -35 region of the Clostridial genes there is, again, a high degree of conservation but less than within the B. subtilis genes. The ferredoxin gene of C. pasteurianum shows greatest divergence from the wider consensi. It would be premature to consider that this constitutes evidence for a pair of -10 and -35 sequences with affinity for a sigma factor other than sig55. Nevertheless, the B. subtilis gp28 -35 sequences also show the triplet adenine residues and the presence of a guanine residue within the Pribnow sequence (Losick and Pero, 1981). Although multiple sigma factors are implicated in the temporal control of events related to sporulation sig37 and sig28 can be identified in growing cells of B. subtilis.

The constancy of the distance between the two polymerase binding regions (never less than 13 nor more than 19 except in one case where it is 22) probably reflects the function of the regions in binding sequentially two sites separated on the same sigma factor protein. The difference between the distance in Clostridia and the 15 to 18 established for E. coli (Rosenburg and Court, 1979) might indicate a slight difference in protein factor structures. Upstream of this sequence, however, we have identified a sequence - TTGAAG - N13 - TATATT - which conforms well with other proposed Clostridial promoters. If this constitutes the polymerase binding region for the gene then the spacing between the -35 and the Pribnow sequences is one of the shortest for a Clostridium sp. and less than that of the E. coli consensus distance. Joliff et al. (1986) also felt there was insufficient homology between the sequence of the celD gene and consensi for E. coli and B. subtilis to identify -35 and Pribnow sequences. We have identified a Pribnow-like sequence (TATAAT) 95 nucelotides upstream of the putative Shine-Dalgarno sequence. Upstream 13 nucleotides from the putative Pribnow sequence there is a sequence (CTGTAT) which shows homology with other such regions within the promoters of other genes in C. thermocellum.

The GGAGG sequence associated with ribosome binding sites is well-conserved in Clostridia. Of the three sequences which do not conform to the pattern two show a quintuplet of guanine residues and the third has a reiterated adenine residue. The free energies of binding of the Clostridial sequences are slightly less (ranging from -7.6 to -18.8 kcalorie) than the twelve putative binding sites reported by Moran et al. (1982) for B. subtilis (which ranged from -16 to -23 kcalorie).

The spacing of the ribosome binding site with respect to the -10 box shows a wide variation, ranging from 8 to 222 bases. The open reading frame identified downstream of the nifH2 gene in C. pasteurianum shows a spacing of 129 bases. There are, however, two additional -10-like sequences downstream of that identified in TABLE 2. The complete structure of the proposed promoter complex is:

TTGTAG-N17-TATAAT-N22-TATAAT-N3-TATAAT-N89-GGAAGGA-N10-ATG

A second promoter showing repeated polymerase binding regions is present upstream of the glucanase gene of C. thermocellum (Beguin et al., 1982). Here there are further -10 and -35 sequences upstream of the sequences nearest the ribosome binding site. The structure of the complete complex is:

TTGTAT-N19-TATAAT-N63-TTGGGT-N19-TATAAT-N32-AGGAGGA-N6-GTG

The functions of these multiple promoter elements are unclear.

A preliminary consensus has been established to describe the -10, the -35 and the ribosome binding sequences in Clostridia (TABLE 3). Within the -35 sequence greatest conservation can be seen at the first, second and third bases (TTG---). The final three positions are less well-conserved but, with each position considered separately, the consensus appears to be TTGTAT. This differs from the TTGACA established for E. coli and B. subtilis. The -10 and -35 sequences for the ferredoxin gene of C. pasteurianum might be recognised by a second sigma factor.

The -10 consensus sequences for Clostridia, E. coli and B. subtilis are identical and there is close identity with the ribosome binding site. The second pair of guanine residues in the sequence GGAGG is almost entirely conserved - the first pair is less so. The only divergences from the highly conserved second pair of guanine residues are the AGGAGA sequences established for C. perfringens enterotoxin and the C. botulinum B toxins (Wernars, 1988). The ribosome binding sites were 19 and 12 nucleotides respectively upstream of the initiation codon ATG - further than most. These data have not been shown

TABLE 3. CONSENSUS SEQUENCES FOR PUTATIVE CLOSTRIDIAL PROMOTERS

a. -35 sequence from 10 promoters:

position	1	2	3	4	5	6
	T7	**T9**	T-	**T5**	T1	**T5**
	A1	A1	A-	A4	**A5**	A2
	G1	G-	**G10**	G1	G2	G2
	C1	C-	C-	C-	C2	C1

b. Pribnow sequence from 11 promoters:

position	1	2	3	4	5	6
	T11	T-	**T10**	T2	T1	**T11**
	A-	**A11**	A1	**A9**	**A10**	A-
	G-	G-	G-	G-	G-	G-
	C-	C-	C-	C-	C-	C-

c. Shine-Dalgarno sequence from 13 promoters:

position	1	2	3	4	5	6	7
	T1	T1	T-	T-	T-	T-	T3
	A9	A1	A1	**A10**	A-	A-	**A9**
	G2	**G11**	**G12**	G3	**G13**	**G13**	G1
	C1	C-	C-	C-	C-	C-	C-

Notes: For each position within the sequences the frequency with which each base occurs follows the base. The bases of the consensus are emboldened.

in the Tables pending the elucidation of the full promoter sequence. Since expression of *C. perfringens* enterotoxin is an event related to sporulation the description of the -10 and -35 sequences will be valuable in revealing the possible existence in the species of multiple sigma factors.

STRUCTURE OF CLONED CLOSTRIDIAL SIGNAL SEQUENCES

Secreted proteins possess a structured N-terminal amino acid signal sequence to facilitate their export from the cell. The signal sequence is cleaved during the export process to release the mature protein. Only with the alpha toxin gene of *C. perfringens* and the *celA* and *celD* genes of *C. thermocellum* have the full nucleotide sequences of the signal polypeptide segments been elucidated. In each case there is good agreement with the structure of such sequences in Bacilli (Neugebauer *et al.*, 1981; Murphy *et al.*, 1984).

Approximately a quarter to one third of each signal sequence, the leading portion, shows a preponderance of hydrophilic amino acid residues with lysine being well-represented among these. Signal sequences in Gram positive organisms are longer than those found in Gram negative bacteria possibly reflecting the greater thickness of the peptidoglycan component of the Gram positive cell wall. In addition, the C-terminal, comprising much of the sequence recognized by the signal cleavage peptidase, is consistent with the pattern described by Heijne (1985) (although the examples of procaryotic signal sequences he uses are essentially those of Gram negative microbes).

Despite showing only a small amino sequence homology plots of the hydrophobic moment and the hydrophobicity (using both the Kyte and the Hopp and Woods algorithms utilised by the DNAstar program) of the *celA* and alpha toxin gene products show a high degree of coincidence. After the first 15 residues the coincidence becomes poor but can be reformed by aligning the sequences upon the C-terminal residue - reflecting the additional four amino acids found within the *celA* signal sequence and which can be visualized as an extension of the hydrophobic region at the 5'-end. Between the plots for the *celA* and the *celD* gene products homology is particularly close when the two are aligned at the C-terminal. In this case, there is more agreement between the amino acid sequences and the functions of the active mature proteins encoded by the genes are closely related. It is probably within the structure of the signal sequence that the mechanism resides which accounts for the distribution between cell fractions of the *celA* gene product when expressed in *C. thermocellum*, *E. coli* and *S. cerevisiae*. In *C. thermocellum* he structure reflects the extracellular function of the cellulolytic complex of enzymes - the metabolism of insoluble cellulosic substrates. In *E. coli* the entire open reading frame encoding the amino acid signal sequence and the amino acid sequence of the structural protein is translated but the complexity of the Gram negative cell wall and membrane complex prevents secretion of the active protein which remains confined to the periplasm and cytoplasm. In *S. cerevisiae*, which begins transcription only at the in-frame ATG codon, the signal sequence is deficient in 21 amino acid residues at the 5'-terminus and the resulting protein is unable to penetrate the cytoplasmic membrane.

Like the celA gene product, the C. perfringens alpha toxin, when cloned into E. coli, failed to reach the culture medium other than through cell lysis (Titball et al., 1988a, 1988b). In no reported case has a gene encoding a normally extracellular Clostridial product been successfully cloned into E. coli in such a way as to permit the continued active secretion of the gene product. This probably reflects the fact that proteins which are truly exported from E. coli require specialised cell wall transport systems. The amino acid sequence revealed by the nucleotide sequence of bcn5 (Garnier and Cole, 1985) shows no similarity with the structures of the signal sequences in the genes of Clostridium and Bacillus spp.. If the regulation of BCN5 production is similar to that in other colicins then export will be shown to be mediated through the action of a second gene product (Pugsley, 1984).

CODON USAGE OF CLOSTRIDIA

We have compared the nucleotide usage shown in all sequenced Clostridial genes with randomly selected genes of B. subtilis and E. coli (15198 and 15444 nucleotides respectively) (TABLE 4a). The bias in the Clostridial nucleotide usage is not restricted merely to the low level of utilisation of the bases G and C. There is a pronounced asymmetry in the usage of A and T between the coding and non-coding strands; A represents 36.5% of the nucleotides of the latter whereas T represents only 28.4%. The asymmetry of nucleotide distribution along the DNA strand reveals a structure whose purpose is unclear but which might be implicated in a further control function. Plots of the frequency of G+C within 50 base windows along the coding regions and flanking sequences for the genes celA, bcn5, nifH2, nifH1 and the structural gene for alpha toxin reveal areas of particularly low G+C frequency associated with the sequences upstream of the promoters.

Garnier and Cole (1986), in order to account for the lack of expression of the cloned bcn5 gene, suggested that there was an inadequate concentration of rarely used tRNAs in the E. coli host that were required by the biased codon usage of the Clostridial gene. This is unlikely to be the cause of the effect since the codon usage in the other fully sequenced, cloned Clostridial toxin - alpha toxin - is substantially similar to that of bcn5. For the cloned nifH1 and nifH2 genes a rule was established (Chen et al., 1986) where codons of the type (C/G)(C/G)(N) always showed A or U at the third position. We have compiled a codon usage chart for all the published Clostridial sequences (TABLE 4b) which confirms only a strong bias toward A or U at the third position. The codon usage for arginine is particularly biased and the codon CGG may be forbidden. Although there is no evidence to support the thesis, the presence of an inosine residue at the third position of the anticodon of the arginyl-tRNA would preclude the recognition of a G as the thirdbase in the CGG codon (Watson et al., 1987). Such a mechanism will clearly restrict the utility of Clostridia for the expression of cloned heteorologous genes containing the CGG codon for arginine.

TERMINATION SIGNALS IN CLONED CLOSTRIDIAL GENES

Both termination codons, TAA and TAG, are represented within the cloned genes of Clostridia but the latter has been observed only in the case of the celA gene of C. thermocellum (Beguin et al., 1985). All the termination codons exist singly with the exception in the case of the alpha toxin gene of C. perfringens which shows a rarer tandem termination codon of structure TAA.TAA.---.TAA (Titball et al., 1988b; Kehoe, 1988). Sequences conforming to the pattern of rho-independant terminators have been found in the nifH2, ferredoxin and mop genes of C. pasteurianum but not in that species' other sequenced genes and in the celA gene of C. thermocellum.

ACKNOWLEDGEMENTS

During the writing of this review the comments of Lynne Wall and David Kelly were most helpful. We wish to thank also Mrs June Hodge for preparing the manuscript for publication.

TABLE 4. NUCLEOTIDE USAGE IN E. COLI, B. SUBTILIS AND IN CLOSTRIDIUM SPP. AND CODON USAGE IN CLOSTRIDIUM

a. Nucleotide usage

	Bases	Nucleotide frequency %				
		G+C	A	T	G	C
Clostridium spp.	12504	35.1	36.5	28.4	21.0	14.1
B. subtilis	15198	45.5	29.9	24.6	24.8	20.7
E. coli	15444	52.7	24.2	23.2	28.1	24.6

b. Codon usage

1.	2.	3.	1.	2.	3.	1.	2.	3.	1.	2.	3.
ala	GCA	142	glu	GAA	179	lys	AAA	214	thr	ACA	103
	GCC	21		GAG	52		AAG	74		ACC	30
	GCG	20								ACG	7
	GCU	87	gly	GGA	185	met	AUG	88		ACU	92
				GGC	32						
arg	AGA	110		GGG	19	phe	UUC	44	trp	UGG	66
	AGG	13		GGU	124		UUU	97			
	CGA	5							tyr	UAC	46
	CGC	3	his	CAC	15	pro	CCA	65		UAU	173
	CGG	0		CAU	47		CCC	9			
	CGU	9					CCG	30	val	GUA	109
			ilu	AUA	195		CCU	50		GUC	9
asn	AAC	86		AUC	31					GUG	27
	AAU	200		AUU	94	ser	AGC	34		GUU	134
							AGU	70			
asp	GAC	69	leu	CUA	30		UCA	92			
	GAU	195		CUC	10		UCC	22			
				CUG	17		UCG	10			
cys	UGC	10		CUU	63		UCU	60			
	UGU	44		UUA	145						
				UUG	51	ter	UAA	7			
gln	CAA	77					UAG	1			
	CAG	25					UGA	0			

1. - amino acid encoded; 2. - codon; 3. - frequency of use

REFERENCES

Abraham, L.J. and J.I. Rood (1987). Identification of Tn4451 and Tn4452, chloramphenicol resistance transposons from *Clostridium perfringens*. *Journal of Bacteriology 169*, 1579-1584.

Abraham, L.J. and J.I. Rood (1985). Cloning and analysis of the *Clostridium perfringens* tetracycline resistance plasmid, pCW3. *Plasmid 13*, 155-162.

Abraham, L.J., A.J. Wales and J.I. Rood (1985). Worldwide distribution of the conjugative *Clostridium perfringens* tetracycline resistance plasmid, pCW3. *Plasmid 14*, 37-46.

Al-Shiekly, F. and R. Truscott (1977). The interaction of *Clostridium perfringens* and its toxins in the production of necrotic enteritis of chickens. *Avian Disease 21*, 256-263.

Beguin, P., P. Cornet and J.-P. Aubert (1985). Sequence of a cellulase gene of the thermophilic bacterium *Clostridium thermocellum*. *Journal of Bacteriology 162*, 102-105.

Bizzini, B. (1979). Tetanus toxin. *Microbiological Reviews 43*, 596-620.

Chen, K.C.-K., J.-S. Chen and J.L. Johnson (1986). Structural features of multiple *nifH*-like sequences and very biased codon usage in nitrogenase genes of *Clostridium pasteurianum*. *Journal of Bacteriology 166*, 162-172.

Cornet, P., J. Millet, P. Beguin and J.-P. Aubert (1983a). Characterization of two cel (cellulose degradation) genes of *Clostridium thermocellum* coding for endoglucanses. *Bio/Technology* 589-593.

Cornet, P., D. Tronik, J. Millet and J.-P. Aubert (1983b). Cloning and expression in *Escherichia coli* of *Clostridium thermocellum* genes coding for amino acid synthesis and cellulose hydrolysis. *FEMS Microbiology Letters 16*, 137-141.

Daldal, F. and J. Applebaum (1985). Cloning and expression of *Clostridium pasteurianum* galactokinase gene in *Escherichia coli* K-12 and nucleotide sequence analysis of a region affecting the amount of the enzyme. *Journal of Molecular Biology 186*, 533-545.

Efstathiou, I. and N. Truffaut (1986). Cloning of *Clostridium acetobutylicum* genes and their expression in *Escherichia coli* and *Bacillus subtilis*. *Molecular and General Genetics 204*, 317-321.

Fairweather, N.F., V.A. Lyness, D.J. Pickard, G. Allen and R.O. Thomson (1986). Cloning, nucleotide sequencing, and expression of tetanus toxin fragment C in *Escherichia coli*. *Journal of Bacteriology* *165*, 21-27.

Garnier, T. and S.T. Cole (1986). Characterization of a bacteriocin plasmid from *Clostridium perfringens* and molecular genetic analysis of the bacteriocin-encoding gene. *Journal of Bacteriology* *168*, 1189-1196.

Graves, M.C. and J.C. Rabinowitz (1986). *In vivo* and *in vitro* transcription of the *Clostridium pasteurianum* ferredoxin gene. *Journal of Biological Chemistry* *261*, 11409-11415.

Graves, M.C., G.T. Mullenbach and J.C. Rabinowitz (1985). Cloning and nucleotide sequence determination of the *Clostridium pasteurianum* ferredoxin gene. *Proceedings of the National Academy of Sciences USA* *82*, 1653-1657.

von Heijne, G. (1985). Signal sequences: the limits of variation. *Journal of Molecular Biology* *184*, 99-105.

Hinton, S.M. and G. Freyer (1986). Cloning, expression and sequencing the molybdenum-pterin binding protein (*mop*) gene of *Clostridium pasteurianum* in *Escherichia coli*. *Nucleic Acids Research* *14*, 9371-9380.

Ishii, K., T. Kudo, H. Honda, and K. Horikoshi (1983). Molecular cloning of beta-isopropylmalate dehydrogenase gene from *Clostridium butyricum* M588. *Agricultural and Biological Chemistry* *47*, 2313-2317.

Joliff, G., P. Beguin, and J.-P. Aubert (1986). Nucleotide sequence of the cellulase gene *celD* encoding endoglucanase D of *Clostridium thermocellum*. *Nucleic Acids Research* *14*, 8605-8613.

Karube, I., N. Urano, T. Yamada, H. Hirochika and K. Sakaguchi (1983). Cloning and expression of the hydrogenase gene from *Clostridium butyricum* in *Escherichia coli*. *FEBS Letters* *158*, 119-122.

Kehoe, M. (1988). Department of Microbiology, University of Newcastle upon Tyne. U.K. Personal communication.

Kennedy, K.K., S.J. Norris, W.H. Beckenbauer, and R.G. White (1977). *Clostridium perfringens* type C and type D toxoid. *American Journal of Veterinerary Research* *38*, 1515-1518

Lawrence, G. and P.D. Walker (1976). Pathogenesis of enteritis necroticans in Papua New guinea. *Lancet* *1*, 125-126.

Leslie, D., N. Fairweather, C. Dougan and M. Kehoe (1988). Cloning and expression in *Escherichia coli* of the -toxin determinant from *Clostridium perfringens*. In: *Bacterial Protein Toxins* (Fehrenbach *et al*. eds.) pp 235. Gustav Fischer, New York.

Losick, R. and J. Pero (1981). Cascades of sigma factors. *Cell* *25*, 582-584.

Matsuda, M. and M. Yoneda (1975). Isolation and purification of two antigenically active, "complementary" polypeptide fragments of tetanus neurotoxin. *Infection and Immunity* *12*, 1147-1153.

Millet, J., D. Petre, P. Beguin, O. Raynaud and J.-P. Aubert (1985). Cloning ten distinct DNA fragments of *Clostridium thermocellum* coding for cellulases. *FEMS Microbiology Letters* *29*,145-149.

Moran, C., S. LeGrice, G. Lee, M. Stephens, A.L. Sonenshein, J. Pero and R. Losick (1982). Nucleotide sequences that signal the initiation of transcription and translation in *Bacillus subtilis*. *Molecular and General Genetics* *186*, 339-346.

Muldrow, L.L., G.C. Ibeanu, N.I. Lee, N.K. Bose and J. Johnson (1987). Molecular cloning of *Clostridium difficile* toxin A gene fragment in lambda gt11. *FEBS Letters* *213*, 249-253.

Murphy, N., D.J. McConnell and B.A. Cantwell (1984). The DNA sequence of the gene and genetic control sites for the excreted *Bacillus subtilis* enzyme beta-glucanase. *Nucleic Acids Research* *12*, 5355-5367.

Neugebauer, K., R. Sprengel and H. Schaller (1981). Penicillinase from *Bacillus licheniformis*: nucleotide sequence of the gene and implcations for the biosynthesis of a secretory protein in a Gram positive bacterium. *Nucleic Acid Research* *9*, 2577-2588.

Niilo, L. (1965). Bovine enterotoxaemia. III. Factors affecting the stability of the toxins of *Clostridium perfringens* types A, C and D. *Canadian Veterinerary Journal* *6*, 38-42.

Piruzyan, E.A., M.A. Mogutov, G.A. Velikodvorskaya and V.K. Akimenko (1985). Cloning and expression of the structural gene for endoglucanase from the cellulolytic complex of *Clostridium thermocellum* F7 in cells of *Escherichia coli* K12. *Doklady Akademii Nauk SSSR* 63-965.

Pugsley, A.P. (1984). The ins and outs of colicins. 1. Production and translocation across membranes. *Microbiological Science* *1*, 168-175.

Romaniec, M.P.M., N.G. Clarke and G.P. Hazlewood (1987). Molecular cloning of Clostridium thermocellum DNA and the expression of further novel endo- -1,4-glucanase genes in Escherichia coli. Journal of General Microbiology 133, 1297-1307.

Rood, J.I., V.N. Scott and C.L. Duncan (1978). Identification of a transferable tetracycline resistance plasmid (pCW3) from Clostridium perfringens. Plasmid 1, 563-570.

Rosenberg, M. and C. Court (1979). Regulatory sequences involved in the promotion and termination of RNA transcription. Annual Reviews of Genetics 13, 319-353.

Sacco, M., J. Millet and J.-P. Aubert (1984). Cloning and expression in Saccharomyces cerevisiae of a cellulase gene from Clostridium thermocellum. Ann. Microbiol. (Inst. Pasteur) 135A, 485-488.

Schwarz, W., K. Bronnenmeier and W.L. Staudenbauer (1985). Molecular cloning of Clostridium thermocellum genes involved in beta-glucan degradation in bacteriophage lambda. Biotechnology Letters 7, 859-864.

Shine, J. and L. Dalgarno (1975). Determinant of cistron specificity in bacterial ribosomes. Nature 254, 34-38.

Squires, C.H., D.L. Heefner, R.J. Evans, B.J. Kopp and M.J. Yarus (1984). Shuttle plasmids for Escherichia coli and Clostridium perfringens. Journal of Bacteriology 159, 465-471.

Titball, R.W., S.E.C. Hunter, B.C. Morris, A.D. Shuttleworth and T. Rubidge (1988a). Molecular cloning of Clostridium perfringens alpha toxin. In: Bacterial Protein Toxins (Fehrenbach et al. eds.) pp 255-256. Gustav Fischer, New York.

Titball, R.W., S.E.C. Hunter, K.L. Martin, B.C. Morris, A.D. Shuttleworth, D.W. Anderson, T. Rubidge and D.C. Kelly (1988b). Molecular cloning and nucleotide sequence of the alpha toxin (phospholipase C) of Costridium perfringens. Infection and Immunity. in press

Watson, J.D., N.H. Hopkins, J.W. Roberts, J.A. Steitz and A.M. Weiner (1987). Molecular Biology of the Gene. Vol. 1. General principles. pp 438-440. Menlo Park, Calif.: The Benjamin/Cummings Publishing Company, Inc.

Wernars, K. (1988). Laboratory of Water and Food Microbiology, National Institute of Public Health and Environmental Protection, Bilthoven, Netherlands. Personal communication.

Whitehead, T.R. and J.C. Rabinowitz (1986). Cloning and expression in Escherichia coli of the gene for 10-formyl tetrahydrofolate synthetase from Clostridium acidiurici ("Clostridium acidi-urici"). Journal of Bacteriology 167, 205-209.

Zappe. H., D.T. Jones and D.R. Woods (1986). Cloning and expression of Clostridium acetobultylicum endoglucanase, cellobiase and amino acid biosynthesis genes in Escherichia coli Journal of General Microbiology 132, 1367-1372.

Note added in proof:

Since the preparation of this paper a structure for the putative tetanus toxin gene promoter has been published. The identified sequence was of the structure:

TTTACA-N14-TATGTT-N121-AGGAGAT-N7-ATG

This structure is similar to those of other Clostridial genes but the only other Clostridial promoter shown to possess a triplet T within the -35 region and a G within the -10 region is that for the ferredoxin gene (TABLE 2).

Reference: Niemann, H., B. Anderson Beckh, T. Binz, U. Eisel, S. Demotz, T. Mayer and C. Widman (1988). Tetanus toxin: Evaluation of the primary sequence and potential applications. In: Bacterial Protein Toxins (Fehrenbach et al. eds.) pp 29-38. Gustav Fischer, New York.

IV. Three-Dimensional Structures of Toxins

THREE-DIMENSIONAL STRUCTURES AND STRUCTURE-FUNCTION RELATIONSHIPS OF SCORPION NEUROTOXINS

J.C. Fontecilla-Camps*, J.C. Genovesio-Taverne* and C. Habersetzer-Rochat%

* Laboratoire de Cristallographie et de Cristallisation de Macromolécules Biologiques - CNRS. Faculté de Médecine, Secteur Nord. Bd. Pierre Dramard 13326 Marseille Cedex 15, FRANCE

% CRMC²-CNRS, Campus Luminy, Case 913, 13288 Marseille Cedex 9, FRANCE

ABSTRACT

The comparison of the available three-dimensional structures of mammal -directed α- and ß-scorpion toxins shows that both types of molecules share most of their secondary structural features. The modulation of their different modes of action seems to depend on changes in the length and orientation of loops near the "conserved" surface of scorpion toxins. Computer modelling of a insect-directed scorpion toxin confirms this notion and suggests a pattern in the way the various specific activities have been generated.

KEYWORDS

X-Ray Crystallography; Scorpion Toxins; Molecular Modelling; Structure- Function Relationships; Protein Evolution

INTRODUCTION

Scorpion toxins constitute a group of small basic neurotoxic proteins (Rochat et al. 1979) generally composed of 60 to 70 amino acids and cross-linked by four disulfide bridges (Kopeyan et al. 1974; Darbon et al. 1982). They display high binding affinities for the Na^+ channels of excitable cells thereby affecting the gating properties of the channels (Feller et al. 1985). Although they have significantly homologous amino acid sequences, the different toxins display various degrees of toxicity toward different animal classes : venoms from the _Buthinae_ family of scorpions contain toxins which are preferentially directed against mammals, insects or crustaceans (Zlotkin et al. 1971, Babin et al. 1974; Zlotkin et al. 1975; Lester et al. 1982). Mammal-directed toxins have been divided into two groups α and ß (Jover et al. 1980a; Couraud et al. 1982), depending on mode of action, cooperative binding with other toxins, and dependence of membrane potential for binding. Not surprisingly, a series of studies have shown that α-toxins and ß-toxins do not bind to the same site on the Na channel (Jover et al. 1980b; Wang and Strichartz, 1983; Darbon et al. 1983; Angelides and Nutter, 1984)

Crystallographic Studies of Scorpion Toxins

To date, four crystal structures involving three different toxins have been determined by X-Ray methods. The first study reported the structure of variant 3 from _Centruroides sculpturatus_ Ewing (CsE v3) (Fontecilla-Camps et al. 1980) later refined to 1.8 Å resolution (Almassy et al. 1983). Subsequently, the CsE v3 model was used to solve the structure of variant 2 (CsE v2) (Zell et al. 1985), a protein closely related to CsE v3 (Babin et al. 1974). CsE v3 and CsE v2 are weakly toxic proteins (Babin et al. 1974) that display extensive amino acid sequence similarities with the very potent ß-toxins such as _Centruroides_ suffussus suffussus toxin II. Because of this and given the fact that no potent ß-toxin X-Ray structure has yet been established, CsE v3 has been used as a model for this class of toxins. The comparison of the available scorpion toxin amino acid sequences allowed Fontecilla-Camps et al (1980) to define three highly conserved stretches among scorpion toxins comprising residues 1-6, 45-48 and 51-53 of CsE v3. Subsequently, it was established that these regions were brought to close proximity by the folding of the CsE v3 polypeptide chain; their exposed residues then define a "conserved" patch on the molecular surface. On the same side of this conserved patch, and partially overlapping it, CsE v3 has the great majority of the hydrophobic residues exposed to the solvent medium. The region containing the combination of conserved and hydrophobic residues was given the name of "conserved- hydrophobic" surface.

In the case of toxin II from Androctonus australis Hector (AaH II) two crystal forms were obtained : a monoclinic one, space-group C2 (Sampieri et al. 1979), grown at pH 8.5, and a better diffracting orthorhombic form, space-group $P2_1 2_1 2_1$ grown at pH 7.0. The orthorhombic crystal form has been solved and refined to 1.8 Å resolution (Fontecilla-Camps et al. 1988). and the AaH II model obtained was used to solve the monoclinic form of the same toxin to 2.5 Å resolution (Genovesio-Taverne et al. manuscript in preparation). AaH II corresponds to the most potent scorpion α-toxin isolated to date and it represents a whole group of molecules with a wide range of toxicity (Rochat et al. 1979). Our discussion will be mostly based on the orthorhombic model since it is known in greater detail than the monoclinic one.

Comparison of α- and ß-toxins

Both α- and ß-toxins present a compact region composed of three of the four disulfide bridges, about two and a half turns of α-helix, and three strands of antiparallel ß-sheet structure. These equivalent regions of AaH II and CsE v3 can be superimposed to a close fit (Figure 1).

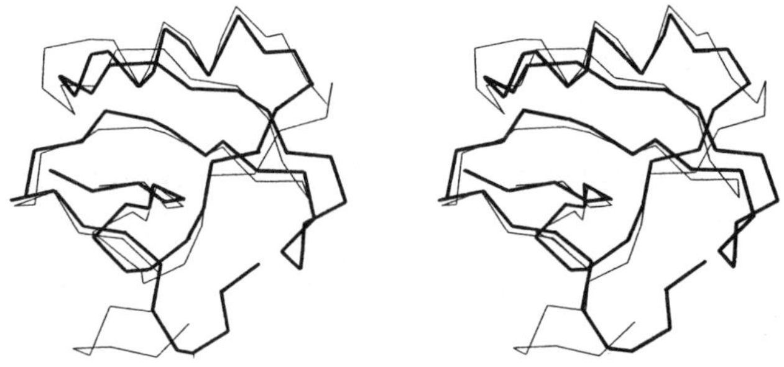

Fig. 1 Superposition of the C- carbon backbones of CsE v3 (thin lines) and AaH II (thick lines)

It is outside this highly organized region that most of the amino acid insertions and deletions are found. Thus, most of the loops protruding from it have different lengths in α- and ß-toxins. The most important differences correspond to the 5-residue insertion of α-toxins and the orientation of the C-terminal region. A direct consequence of the presence of the 5-residue insertion loop is the formation of a cavity which is filled by a series of water molecules and where Lys 58 establishes several hydrogen bonds both with water molecules and carbonyl oxygens from the toxin polypeptide chain. This arrangement that stabilizes several loops of the AaH II molecule is unique to α-toxins (Figure 2)

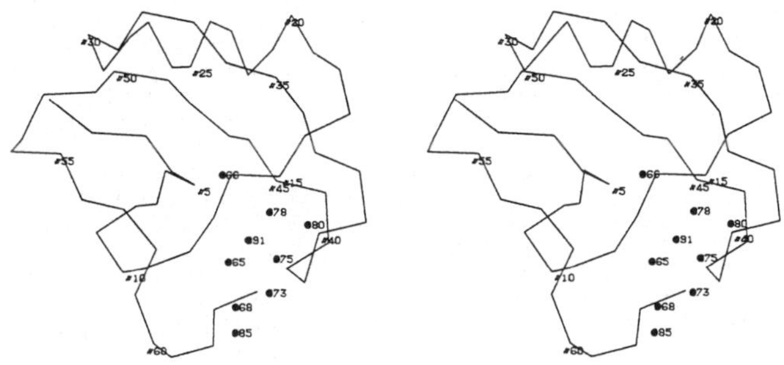

Fig. 2. C- backbone of AaH II. The dark dots represent the position of highly ordered water molecules. The ascending numbering of these solvent molecules reflects their increasing degrees of thermal and/or static disorder.

The comparison of the "conserved-hydrophobic" surface in CsE v3 with the equivalent region of AaH II allows for the following observations: a) at the molecular surface the conserved aromatic residues in positions 4 and 47 of CsE v3, the lysine residue in position 1, and Pro 52 occupy very similar positions in both toxins; b) the acidic sidechains in positions 2 and 53 are oriented rather differently in the two molecules. In AaH II the side chain of Asp 3 forms a hydrogen bond with the NH group of residue 50 and that of Asp 53 is involved in a salt-bridge with the ε-NH2 group. In CsE v3 the equivalent acidic functions do not seem to be involved in intramolecular interactions; c) the internal residues Leu 5, Val 6, Ala 45 and Leu 51 of CsE v3 occupy positions that are similar to those of Ile 6, Val 7, Ala 45 and Leu 51 of AaH II.

AaH II shows a less asymmetric distribution of aromatic residues than CsE v3. This is partially due to the presence of one additional tyrosine and one phenylalanine on the side opposite to the "conserved-hydrophobic" surface. Nevertheless, the α-toxin contains five tyrosines and one tryptophane on or close to the conserved patch. Four of the five tyrosine residues (Tyr 42, 5, 47 and 49) form an arrangement which is reminiscent of that found in the crystal of L-Tyrosine·HCl (Frey et al. 1973), the aromatic cycles being oriented perpendicular to each other in a "herring bone" fashion (Figure 3). This peculiar arrangement minimizes the exposure to the solvent medium of these big, hydrophobic sidechains. In fact, the mean calculated solvent accessible surface for these residues is 67.3 Å². As a comparison, His 64, which is quite exposed to the solvent, has a calculated accessible area of 193 Å². CsE v3, on the other hand, does not show such extensive interaction of aromatic residues. Only Tyr 4 and Trp 47 seem to interact with each other. The other tyrosine sidechains, which are not equivalent to those of AaH II, are either oriented towards the exterior or form hydrophobic interactions with other residues.

AaH II and CsE v3 have amino acid sequences that are identical at 21 positions (29.6%) (Table I). If conservative changes are included, then the two molecules are equivalent at 28 positions (39.4%). On the other hand, from a structural view point, 55% of all C-a positions in the two toxins fall within 0.5 Å. If other topologically-related C-alpha positions are considered, one may conclude that 25 % of all C-a positions are not equivalent when the two molecules are compared.

<u>The superreactive Lysine 58</u>

Of the different chemical modification experiments carried out on AaH II the most revealing are the various modifications of the superreactive Lys 58 which, depending on the reagent, can result in total loss of activity (Habersetzer-Rochat and Sampieri, 1976, Darbon et al. 1983). Interestingly, the naturally-occurring toxin Bot IX which has a valine residue in position 58 is about 100 times less active that AaH II (Sampieri et al. 1987). Figure 4 shows the environment of Lys 58 as found in the orthorhombic crystal structure of AaH II. Lys 58 is quite buried and seems to stabilize a series of loops of the toxin molecule through hydrophobic interactions and hydrogen bond formation. Chemical modification reactions affecting the interactions of this lysine residue would be expected to perturb the overall conformation of the active surface thus inducing a loss of pharmacological activity. Darbon et al (1983) have shown that selective biotinylation of this lysine residue results in complete loss of activity. However, results obtained with amidinyl and iminobiotinyl derivatives of lysine 58 indicate that the presence of a ionizable group close to the position originally occupied by the e-amino group seems to preserve most of the toxic action (Darbon, 1987). This suggests that at least some of the interactions of Lys 58 with other parts of the molecule are conserved when this residue is amidinylated. On the other hand, since reactions that introduce small modifying groups (e.g. acetylation) are as effective as biotinylation in abolishing the biological effects of AaH II (Habersetzer-Rochat and Sampieri, 1976) the bulkiness of the modifying group does not appear to determine the degree of loss of pharmacological activity. Based on these results alone, it is tempting to postulate that the role of Lys 58 is more structural than functional; the position occupied by this residue (Fig. 1) would seem to rule out its involvement in a direct interaction with the toxin receptor site unless some substantial molecular movements take place upon binding. In order to shed some light on this problem we started the X-Ray analysis of the monoclinic form of AaH II which, as mentioned above, crystallizes at pH 8.5 i.e. the pH used in most of the chemical modification reactions. Our preliminary results on the refinement of this structure at 2.5 Å show that its C-terminal region (residues 55 to 64) displays a great deal of thermal motion and/or static disorder. Of the 8 highly ordered water molecules found in this region in the orthorhombic form, only 4 are detected in the monoclinic one (Genovesio-Taverne et al. in preparation). This seems to indicate that the molecule is more flexible than would be expected based on the orthorhombic structure alone. It is difficult at this point to dissociate the effects due to the pH of crystallization from those of the different crystal packing.

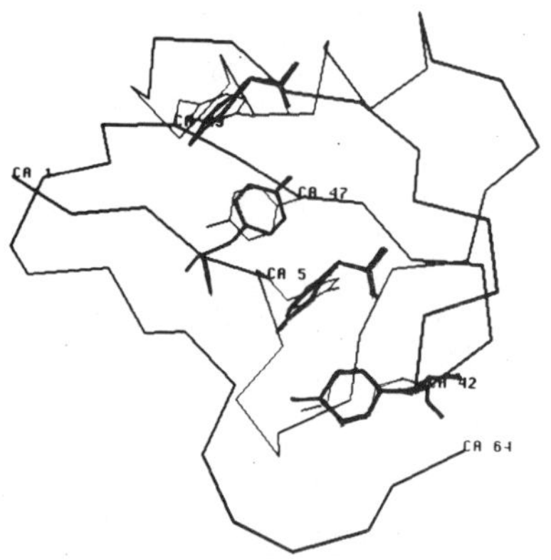

Fig. 3. Superposition of tyr 5, 42, 47, and 49 of AaH II with similarly-oriented tyr molecules (thick lines) of tyrosine·HCl (Frey et al. 1973)

TABLE I

AMINO ACID SEQUENCES OF AaH II, VARIANT 3 AND AaH IT

Each sequence (reviewed in Fontecilla-Camps et al., 1981) has been numbered independently.

					5						10				
AaH II	Val	Lys	Asp	Gly	Tyr	Ile	Val	Asp	Asp	---	Val	Asn	CYS	Thr	Tyr
						5					10				
var 3	---	Lys	Glu	Gly	Tyr	Leu	Val	Lys	Lys	Ser	Asp	Gly	CYS	Lys	Tyr
					5						10				
AaH IT	Lys	Lys	Asn	Gly	Tyr	Ala	Val	Asp	---	Ser	Ser	Gly	Lys	Ala	Pro
	15								20					25	
AaH II	Phe	CYS	Gly	Arg	---	---	---	Asn	Ala	Tyr	CYS	Asn	Glu	Glu	CYS
	15					20					25				
var 3	Gly	CYS	Leu	Lys	Leu	Gly	Glu	Asn	Glu	Gly	CYS	Asp	Thr	Glu	CYS
	15								20					25	
AaH IT	Glu	CYS	Leu	Leu	---	---	---	Ser	Asn	Tyr	CYS	Asn	Asn	Gln	CYS
						30					35				
AaH II	Thr	Lys	---	---	Leu	Lys	Gly	Glu	Ser	Gly	Tyr	CYS	Gln	Trp	Ala
	30					35					40				
var 3	Lys	Ala	Lys	Asn	Gln	Gly	Gly	Ser	Tyr	Gly	Tyr	CYS	Tyr	Ala	---
					30					35					
AaH IT	Thr	Lys	Val	---	His	Tyr	Ala	Asp	Lys	Gly	Tyr	CYS	CYS	Leu	---
	40					45					50				
AaH II	Ser	Pro	Tyr	Gly	Asn	Ala	CYS	Tyr	CYS	Tyr	Lys	Leu	Pro	Asp	His
						45					50				
var 3	---	---	---	---	Phe	Ala	CYS	Trp	CYS	Glu	Gly	Leu	Pro	Glu	Ser
					40					45					50
AaH IT	---	---	---	---	Leu	Ser	CYS	Tyr	CYS	Phe	Gly	Leu	Asn	Asp	Asp
	55						60					64			
AaH II	Val	Arg	Thr	Lys	Gly	---	Pro	---	Gly	Arg	CYS	His	---	---	---
						60					65				
var 3	Thr	Pro	Thr	Tyr	Pro	Leu	Pro	Asn	Lys	Ser	CYS	---	---	---	---
					55						60				
AaH IT	Lys	Lys	Val	Leu	Glu	Ile	Ser	---	Asp	Thr	Arg	Lys	Ser	Tyr	CYS
AaH II	---	---	---	---	---	---									
var 3	---	---	---	---	---	---									
	65					70									
AaH IT	Asp	Thr	Thr	Ile	Ile	Asn									

In both structures Lys 58 establishes a series of intramolecular interactions that make it the least exposed of the 5 lysine residues of AaH II. Buried lysine side chains may have local pK's which are lower than normal (Booshard et al. 1979)) resulting in an increase in the proportion of unprotonated ε-amino groups, the reactive form in the nucleophilic reaction.

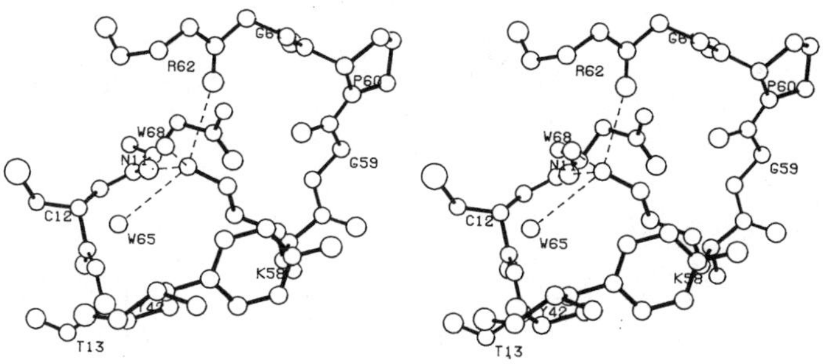

Fig. 4. The environment of Lys 58 in the orthorhombic crystal structure of AaH. Water molecules are indicated by * and hydrogen bonds by dotted lines.

Modelling of the insect-directed scorpion toxin and evolutionary considerations

A general difference is found between the α- and ß- toxins and the toxins specifically active on insects. Alpha- and ß-toxins which are preferentially active on mammals, have the same disulfide bridge pattern (Kopeyan et al. , 1974; Fontecilla-Camps et al, 1980; Gregoire et Rochat, 1983). The insect-directed toxin ,purified from A. australis Hector (AaH IT) has been shown to possess a differently located disulfide bridge resulting from a change in the position of the first half-cystine relative to - and ß-toxins (Darbon et al, 1982). This altered disulfide bridge pattern has also been found in insect toxins from the scorpions Leirus quinquestratus quinquestratus and Buthus martensis (Kopeyan, Ji, personal communications). Thus, this feature may be characteristic of a class of insect-directed toxins and important in determining their specificity. The conservancy of the secondary structure elements observed in the mammal-directed α and ß-scorpion toxins suggested that although one of its 4 disulfide bridges is found in an atypical position, the AaH IT molecule should also have a series of structural elements common to the other toxin types. In order to test this hypothesis, we decided to model AaH IT using the known scorpion toxin structures as guides.

Fisrt, AaH IT was aligned relative to the other two toxins by maximizing amino acid sequence homologies. Subsequently, the starting model of AaH IT was generated from the three-dimensional structures of var 3 and AaH II by using computer graphics (program FRODO, Jones, 1978). FRODO was also useful in keeping a reasonable stereochemistry during the modelling. One required restraint in the model-building procedure was the formation of the atypical disulfide bridge between Cys 37 and Cys 64. A series of energy-minimization cycles using the program EREF (Jack and Levitt, 1978) was performed. During this procedure most of the unfavorable atomic contacts were removed generating a physically plausible model.

The model of AaH IT is shown in figure 5. The conformation of the last 6 C-terminal residues is tentative. This stretch was modelled as an extra strand of ß-sheet structure based only on topological considerations and secondary structure predictions carried out using the method of Dufton and Hider (1977).

The modelling suggests that as opossed to mammal-directed toxins, in AaH IT the four disulfide bridges are found at the same end of the molecule. In this respect, AaH IT shows a superficial resemblance to snake neurotoxins.

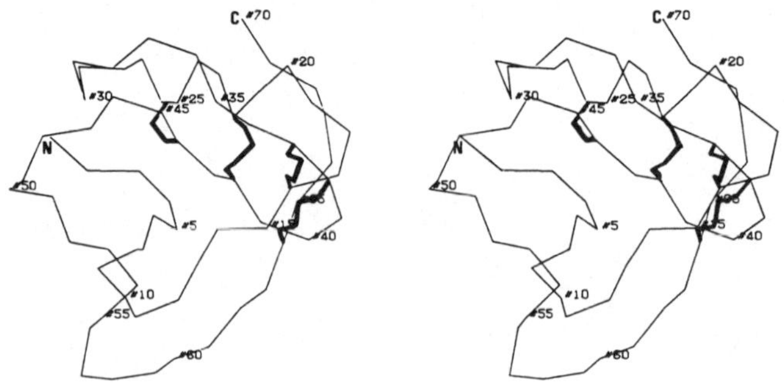

Fig. 5. Stereo drawing showing the theoretical model of AaH IT. Disulfide bridges are indicated by thick lines.

CONCLUSIONS

It seems clear that although α and ß-toxins have different binding sites, they present the same side to the receptor.This surface contains the conserved-hydrophobic surface plus a number of residues located nearby essential for activity. The most interesting case is that of Lys 58, the buried superreactive Lys residue of α-toxins which is also essential for the toxic activity.

The functional diversity found among scorpion toxins should be the consequence of their structural differences. Thus, as α-toxin activity may be at least partially modulated by the 5-amino acid insertion characteristic of these toxins and the ß-toxin activity by the presence of lysine residues in positions 13 and 63 (Darbon and Angelides, 1984), it may be that a topologically equivalent zone is responsible for the insect-specific toxicity of AaH IT. This zone is represented by the C-terminal portion of the molecule.

References

Almassy, R.J., Fontecilla-Camps, J. C., Suddath, F. L. and Bugg, C. E. (1983). Structure of Variant-3 scorpion neurotoxin from Centruroides sculpturatus Ewing, refined at 1.8 Å resolution. J. Mol. Biol. 170, 497-527

Angelides K.J. and Darbon, H. (1984). Molecular and cellular mapping of the voltage-dependant Na channel. Biophys. J., 45 35-37

Babin, D.R., Watt, D.D., Goos, S.M., and Meejneck, R.V. (1974). Amino acid sequences of neurotoxic protein variants from the venom of Centruroides sculpturatus Ewing. Arch. Biochem. Biophys. 164,694-706

Couraud F.,Jover, E., Dubois, J.M. and Rochat, H. (1982). Two types of scorpion toxin receptor sites, one related to activation, the other to inactivation of the action potential sodium channel. Toxicon, 20 9-16

Darbon, H., Zlotkin, E., Kopeyan, C., Van Rietschoten J. and Rochat H. (1982). Covalent structure of an insect toxin from the North African scorpion Androctonus australis Hector. Int. J. Peptide Protein Res. 22,320-330

Darbon, H. and Angelides, K.J. (1984). Structural mapping of the voltage-dependent Na channel. J. Biol. Chem., 259, 6074-6084

Feller, D.J., Talvenheino, J.A., Catterall, W. A. (1985). The sodium channel from rat brain: reconstitution of voltage dependent scorpion toxin binding in vesicles of defined lipid composition. J. Biol. Chem. 260, 11542-11547

Fontecilla-Camps, J.C., Almassy, R.J., Suddath, F. L., Watt, D.D.and Bugg, C. E. (1980). Three-dimensional structure of a protein from scorpion venom: a new structural class of neurotoxins. Proc. Natl. Acad. Sci. USA 77, 6496-6500

Fontecilla-Camps, J.C., Almassy, R. J., Ealick, S. E., Suddath, F. L., Watt, D.D., Feldmann, R. J. and Bugg, C. E. (1981). Architecture of scorpion neurotoxins : a class of membrane-binding proteins. Trends Biochem. Sci., 6, 291-296

Fontecilla-Camps J.C., Habersetzer-Rochat C. and Rochat H. (1988). Orthorhombic crystals and three-dimensional structure of the potent toxin II from the scorpion Androctonus australis Hector. Proc. Natl. Acad. Sci. USA (in the press).

Frey, M., Koetzle, T.F., Lehmann, M.S. and Hamilton W.C. (1973). Precision neutron diffraction determination of protein and nucleic acid components. X. A comparison between the crystal and molecular structures of L-tyrosine and L-tyrosine hydrochloride. J. Chem. Phys., 58, 2547-2556

Genovesio-Taverne, J.C., Habersetzer-Rochat, C., Sampieri, F. and Fontecilla-Camps, J.C. (manuscript in preparation).

Gregoire, J. and Rochat, H. (1983). Covalent structure of toxins I and II from the scorpion Buthus occitanus tunetanus. Toxicon, 21, 153-162.

Habersetzer-Rochat, C. and Sampieri, F. (1976). Structure-function relationships of scorpion neurotoxins. Biochemistry, 15, 2254-2261

Jack, A. and Levitt, M. (1978). Refinement of large structures by simultaneous minimization of energy and R-factor. Acta Crystallogr. A34, 931-935

Jones, T.A. (1978). A graphics model building and refinement system for macromolecules. J. Appl. Crystallogr. 11, 268-272

Jover, E., Martin-Moutot, N., Couraud, F. and Rochat, H. (1980a). Binding of scorpion toxins to rat brain synaptosomal fractions. Effects on membrane potential, ions and other neurotoxins. Biochemistry, 19, 463-469

Jover, E., Couraud, F. and Rochat, H. (1980b). Two types of scorpion neurotoxins characterized by their binding to two separate receptor sites on rat brain synaptosomes. Biochem. Biophys. Res. Commun. 95, 1607-1614

Kopeyan, C., Martinez, G., Lissitzky, S., Miranda, F. and Rochat, H. (1974). Disulfide bonds of Toxin II of the scorpion Androctonus australis Hector. Eur. J. Biochem., 47, 483-489

Lester, D., Lazarovici, P., Pelhate, M. and Zlotkin E. (1982). Purification, characterization and action of two insect toxins from the venom of the scorpion Buthacus judaicus. Biochem. Biophys. Acta, 701, 370-381

Meves, H., Rubly, N. and Watt, D.D. (1982). Effects of toxins isolated from the venom of the scorpion Centruroides sculpturatus on the Na currents of the node of Ranvier. Pflugers Arch. 393, 56-62

Rochat C., Sampieri, F., Rochat, H., Miranda, F. and Lissitsky, S. (1972). Iodination of neurotoxins I and II of the scorpion Androctonus australis Hector. Biochimie 54, 445-449

Rochat, H., Bernard, P. and Couraud, F. (1979). Scorpion Toxins : chemistry and mode of action. Adv. Cytopharmacol. 3, 325-334

Sampieri, F. and Habersetzer-Rochat C. (1978). Structure-function relationships in scorpion neurotoxins : identification of the superactive lysine residue in toxin I of Androctonus australis Hector. Biochem. Biophys. Acta, 535, 100-109

Sampieri,F., Habersetzer-Rochat C., Martin, M.F., Kopeyan, C. and Rochat, H. (1987). Amino acid sequence of toxin XI of the scorpion Buthus occitanus tunetanus Int J Peptide Protein Res, 29, 231-237

Wang, G. K. and Strichartz, G. (1983) Purification and physiological characterization of neurotoxins from venoms of the scorpions Centruroides sculpturatus and Leirus quinquestriatus. Molecular Pharmacology, 23, 519-533

Zell, A., Ealick, S.E. and Bugg, C.E. (1985). Three-dimensional structures of scorpion neurotoxins. In Molecular Architecture of Proteins and Enzymes. Academic Press, New York. pp. 65-97

Zlotkin, E., Rochat, H., Kopeyan C., Miranda, F and Lissizky, S. (1971). Purification and properties of the insect toxin from the venom of the scorpion Androctonus australis Hector. Biochimie, 53, 1073-1078

Zlotkin, E., Martinez, G., Rochat, H. and Miranda, F. (1975). A protein toxic to crustacea from the venom of the scorpion Androctonus australis Hector. Insect Biochem., 5, 243-250

THE THREE DIMENSIONAL STRUCTURE OF THE ENZYMATIC PLANT TOXIN RICIN

JON ROBERTUS

Department of Chemistry, University of Texas,
Austin, Texas, 78712, U. S. A.

ABSTRACT

Ricin is the most thoroughly studied example of a class of enzymatic toxins isolated from higher plants. The intact toxin has a 30,000 dalton cell surface recognition protein (B chain) linked by a disulfide bond to a 30,000 dalton enzyme (A chain) which attacks eucaryotic ribosomes, inactivating them by removing a single adenine base. The X-ray crystal structure has been solved to 2.8Å resolution. It reveals that B chain is a dumbbell shaped structure in which each domain binds cell surface galactosides. In each domain, galactose binds by lying roughly parallel to an aromatic side chain of the protein, while specific hydrogen bonds are formed between the protein and the hydroxyl groups of the sugar. The A chain is more globular in shape and sits between the two domains of B chain. A chain has a pronounced cleft which binds the adenine product of its catalytic reaction. The cleft also contain many residues conserved in a variety of related proteins, which helps confirm that the binding and catalytic site for the N-deglycosidation reaction has been identified.

KEYWORDS

Ricin; plant toxin; N-glycosidase; x-ray structure; lectin.

BACKGROUND

Many bacteria, fungi and higher plants contain powerful protein toxins. The exact role of these toxins is uncertain or may vary from species to species. For example, the toxins may serve to deter predators or they may kill neighboring cells, providing a rich breeding ground for the toxin producing cells. It seems likely that plant toxins are defensive in nature.

Plant toxins fall into two broad groups - heterodimers and monomers. The heterodimers are true cytotoxins, like ricin (Olsnes and Pihl, 1982), abrin (Olsnes and Pihl, 1973), and modeccin (Refsnes et al., 1977). They have an A or active chain which enzymatically attacks ribosomes, and a B or binding chain which binds cell surfaces, usually via galactoside recognition. This binding triggers endocytosis, leading to toxin uptake (Nicolson et al., 1975). In addition, there is a group of single chain plant toxins which are evolutionarily related to the A chains of heterodimers (Ready et al., 1984) but which lack a B chain. As a result, they are not true cytotoxins; if they can be delivered into a cell, however, they are as toxic as the true cytotoxins. Examples of this latter class are PAP (Irvin, 1975), PAP-II (Irvin et al., 1980), dodecandrin (Ready et al., 1984), gelonin (Stirpe et al., 1980), and tritin (Roberts et al., 1979). This class of proteins is referred to as ribosome inhibiting proteins or RIP's. Probably the most thoroughly studied plant toxin is ricin. It is a member of the heterodimer class and consists of a 32,000 dalton A chain linked by a disulfide bond to a 32,000 dalton B chain. Both chains are glycosylated, possessing high mannose carbohydrate groups. The amino acid sequence of ricin has been determined chemically (Funatsu et al., 1978, 1979), as well as from the nucleotide sequences of both the cDNA (Lamb et al., 1985)

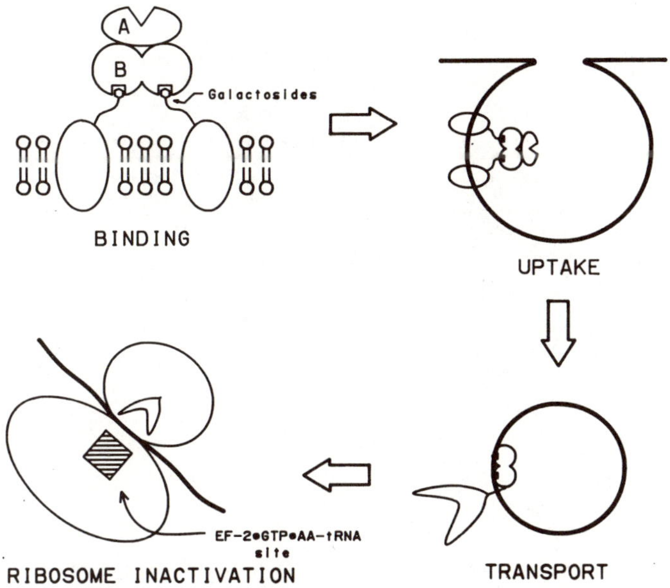

Fig. 1. Schematic of eucaryotic cell intoxication by ricin. Ricin B chain binds to galactoside containing cell surface reaptors, triggering endocytosis. The A chain is released from the B chain, probably accompanied by a conformational change, and crosses the vesicle membrane. In the cytoplasm, it attacks ribosomes, removing a single adenine base from 28S rRNA.

and the genomic DNA (Halling et al., 1985). A and B chain have a strong affinity for one another, mediated by hydrophobic forces, and their association is necessary for toxicity (Lewis and Youle, 1986). The role of the disulfide bond in cytotoxicity is unclear. Some data has been interpreted to mean that the linkage is not critical for toxicity except in maintaining protein-protein interactions at very low toxin concentration (Lewis and Youle, 1986). On the other hand, alkylation of the interchain cysteine appears to retard cellular uptake although surface binding and ribosome inactivation are not effected (Wright and Robertus, 1987).

The overall mechanism of cellular intoxication by ricin is shown in Fig 1. The process begins when ricin B chain attaches to cell surface receptors, thought to be glycoproteins, triggering endocytosis (Nicolson et al., 1975). The B chain is known to bind two galactosides in a non-cooperative manner (Zentz et al., 1978; Houston and Dooley, 1982). Chemical modification studies have implicated Tyr 248 in a 'strong' galactose binding site (Mise et al., 1986), and tryptophan in the 'weak' site (Hatakeyama et al., 1986). It is clear however, that B chain has a higher affinity for natural cell surface receptor groups than for simple sugars (Baenziger and Fiete, 1979).

After cell surface binding, ricin is taken into a membrane bound vesicle. This vesicle may carry ricin to other organelles, such as the golgi, so it is unclear at what point ricin crosses the membrane and reaches the cytoplasm. It is likely, however, that the conditions in the endosome or other organelle are reducing and allow the A and B chains to separate. The A chain then crosses the membrane, probably as a result of some conformational change. There is conflicting evidence as to whether the B chain plays a major role in membrane transport, although there is no doubt that intact ricin is taken into vesicles far more efficiently than is A chain alone.

Once the A chain of ricin reaches the cytoplasm of a typical eukaryotic cell, it enzymatically attacks the 60S ribosomal subunit and disrupts protein synthesis. Ricin has a $K_m = 0.1\ \mu M$ for ribosomes and shows a $k_{cat} = 1500\ min^{-1}$ (Olsnes et al., 1975). Bacterial ribosomes are not susceptible to ricin intoxication (Olsnes et al., 1973). It has recently been shown that ricin acts as an N-glycosidase, specific removing a single adenine base from the 28S rRNA. (Endo et al., 1987; Endo and Tsurugi, 1987).

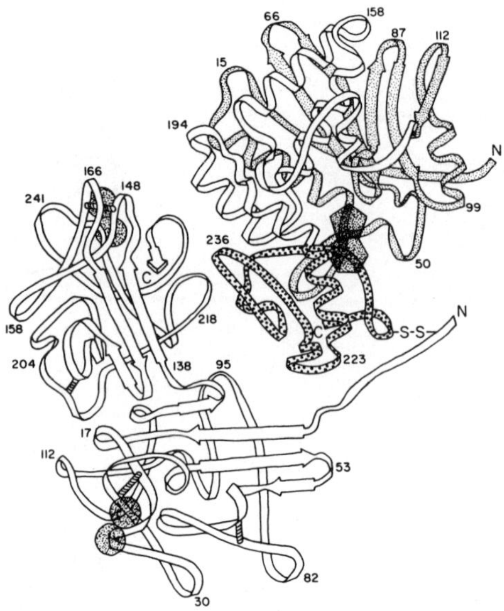

Fig. 2. A ribbon model of ricin. The A chain in the upper right is shown to be divided into three folding domains. The binding site for adenine is shown as a stippled purine. A disulfide bond, lower right, holds the A chain to the B chain (lower left). The B chain lectin is a two domain structure, each of which binds a galactoside (stippled disks).

Ricin has been used extensively in the creation of immunotoxins, molecules in which whole ricin or the A chain is crosslinked to antibodies raised against tumor cells. In essence, the antibody is used to guide the plant toxin to the tumor cells for selective killing. In practice the conjugates have had mixed success, depending largely on the choice of antibody and the cell line to be killed. Even so, immunotoxins are in clinical trials and hold considerable promise for cancer therapy. The entire field, from toxin action to clinical work, has recently been reviewed (Frankel, 1988).

CRYSTAL STRUCTURE OF RICIN

An electron density map was computed from 2.8Å data collected from native ricin and two isomorphous heavy atom derivatives (Montfort _et al_., 1987). The map was fairly easy to interpret and an atomic model of the protein was constructed. Figure 2 is a schematic drawing of the model in which the path of the backbone atoms is shown. The A chain is a globular molecule in the upper right. The B chain has two roughly spherical domains, with the A chain nestling into the gap between the B chain domains.

Contacts between Chains

It has been known for some time that hydrophobic forces hold the chains together and that their association does not depend on the interchain disulfide bond (Houston, 1980). It has also been shown that release of the A chain from the B chain apparently exposes hydrophobic residues which enhance protein association with membranes and may also be important for toxin transport (Uchida _et al_., 1980). Lewis and Youle showed that the association constant for the A and B chains was of the order of 5×10^6 and was entropically driven; that is, hydrophobic forces drive the association interactions (Lewis and Youle, 1986).

In considering the structure of the A-B interface, one should bear in mind that the change in free energy for association of the chains is on the order of -9 to -10 Kcal/mole (Lewis and Youle, 1986). It has been shown that the change in free energy of moving a methyl group from water to octanol is - 0.1 Kcal/mole and that of moving a benzene ring is - 3.6 Kcal/mole (Hansch and Coats, 1970). This suggests that the number of residues making apolar contacts across the A-B interface, which would otherwise be exposed to solvent when dissociated, may be quite small.

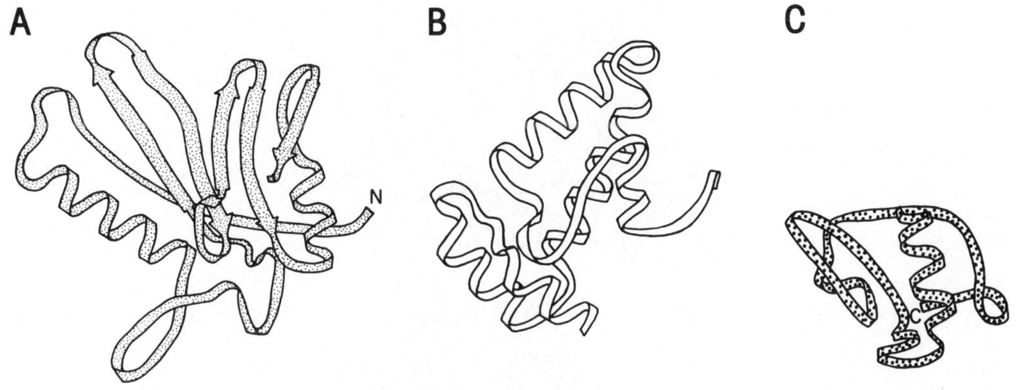

Fig. 3. The three domains of A chain. A) Domain 1, residues 1-114, is dominated by parallel sheet structure. B) Domain 2, residues 115-120, is almost exclusively helices. C) Domain 3, residues 211-267, is a cylindical structure which makes most of the hydropholis contacts with B chain.

Although the A and B chains show substantial contact (Fig. 2) most of the nonpolar interactions occur over a localized region in which five A chain groups and six B groups form an "oily patch". A total of five phenylalanines, two leucines, two prolines, a tyrosine and an isoleucine are involved.

A Chain Structure

We have broken the A chain fold into three domains, shown in Fig. 3. Domain 1 (Fig. 3a) is formed by the amino terminal 114 residues and shows the only extended B sheet in ricin. In addition to this six stranded sheet, domain 1 has two α helices. Domain 2 (Fig. 3b) is composed of residues 115-210 and has five helices. This domain lays over domain 1 and makes a few weak contacts with B chain. Domain 3 (Fig. 3c) consists of residues 211-267 and has a rather cylindrical shape. It interacts with domains 2 and 3 and also with B chain. In fact, five of the six nonpolar A chain groups in the interface are from domain 3.

Ricin A chain is known to act as a specific glycosidase (Endo et al., 1987; Endo and Tsurugi, 1987), removing an adenine from 28S rRNA. Our x-ray structure shows a prominent cleft which is shown in Fig. 4 and which we assume contains the active site. Two lines of evidence support this. First, we have diffused adenine, the reaction product, into our crystals and see that it binds in this cleft. Secondly, conservation of sequence among various RIPS suggests the importance of residues in this cleft.

It was recently shown, however, that there are strong amino acid sequence similarities among three plant toxins -- ricin, trichosanthin (Xuejun and Jiahuai, 1986)), and the barley translation inhibitor (Asano et al., 1986). Furthermore, domains two and three of these toxins appear homologous to E. coli RNase H and to a major peptide from Rous sarcoma virus reverse transcriptase (Ready et al., 1988). This analysis reveals only five absolutely conserved residues across this wide range of proteins, three of which are clustered in the active site cleft. They correspond to ricin positions Glu 177, Asn 209, and Trp 211. In addition, a basic residue, Arg 180, is conserved in four of the five proteins. It seems very likely that these residues are involved in substrate binding or catalysis by ricin. Trp 211 may intercalate RNA bases, while Arg 180 likely forms salt links to the phosphate backbone. Asn 209 can make hydrogen bonds to the bases, and Glu 177 may also perform that role or act as a general base in the adenine base hydrolysis. In addition to these residues conserved in many different proteins, it is likely that each specific protein class makes use of other residues depending on the task to be performed. For example, the analogs of two tyrosine residues, 80 and 123, are conserved in all the plant toxins. Our x-ray studies show they are both in the active site area and indeed Tyr 123 hydrogen bonds to the conserved Glu 177.

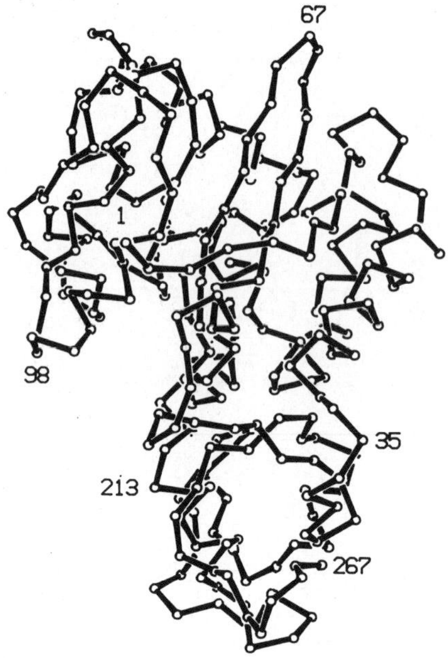

Fig. 4. The active site cleft of A chain. The α carbon skeleton is shown turned roughly 60° to the common view of ricin (Fig. 2). A distinct cavity is seen, which binds adenine, the product of the enzymatic reaction.

The details of the enzyme mechanism remain to be worked out but it seems reasonable that it must involve an acid to protonate the leaving adenine, and a carboxylate to stabilize the likely carboxonium ion formed when the C-N bond is broken.

B Chain Structure

We had shown some time ago that the ricin B chain is a gene duplication product, exhibiting about 32% amino acid identity between its two halves (Villafranca and Robertus, 1981). Each half is built around a pair of disulfide loops, and we expected the protein to form two domains, each binding one lactose. Our crystal contained the disaccharide lactose and we expected one sugar bound to each B domain. In each domain, the galactose moiety lies in a shallow binding cleft, formed by the aromatic ring of a side chain and by a slight kink in a locally straight section of polypeptide backbone. In domain 1, the aromatic ring is that of Trp 37. The sugar binding is stabilized by hydrogen bonds to Asn 46, Lys 40, and Gln 35. Asn 46 and Lys 40 form bonds to OH 3 and OH 4 of the galactose, respectively, and help determine the epimeric specificity of the binding site. The key residue, Asn 46, is held in position by a hydrogen bond to Asp 22. A hydrogen bond also appears to be formed between Gln 35 and OH 6 of the galactose. This arrangement is shown in Figure 5a.

In domain 2 the galactose rings lie over and roughly parallel to the aromatic ring of Tyr 248. Asn 255 is crucial to epimeric binding specificity, forming a hydrogen bond to the galactose OH 4. The position of Asn 255 is stabilized by a hydrogen bond to Asp 234. A water molecule, bound to Asn 255, forms a hydrogen bond with OH 3 of the galactose and is in a position analogous to Lys 40 of domain 1. There is no analog of Gln 35 in the domain 2 galactose binding site (Figure 5b).

An investigation of the B chain structure, together with amino acid sequence comparisons (Robertus and Ready, 1984) convinced us that each domain of the lectin protein arose from the triplication of an ancient gene which coded for a 40 amino acid galactose binding protein (Rutenber *et al.*, 1987). This simple peptide domain is also seen in discoidin I, a galactose binding protein from the slime mold *Dictyostelium discoideum*. Since the mold is not even in the same phylogenetic kingdom with higher plants, we concluded that this galactose binding unit is very ancient, and may be one of the primitive building blocks from which modern protein are assembled.

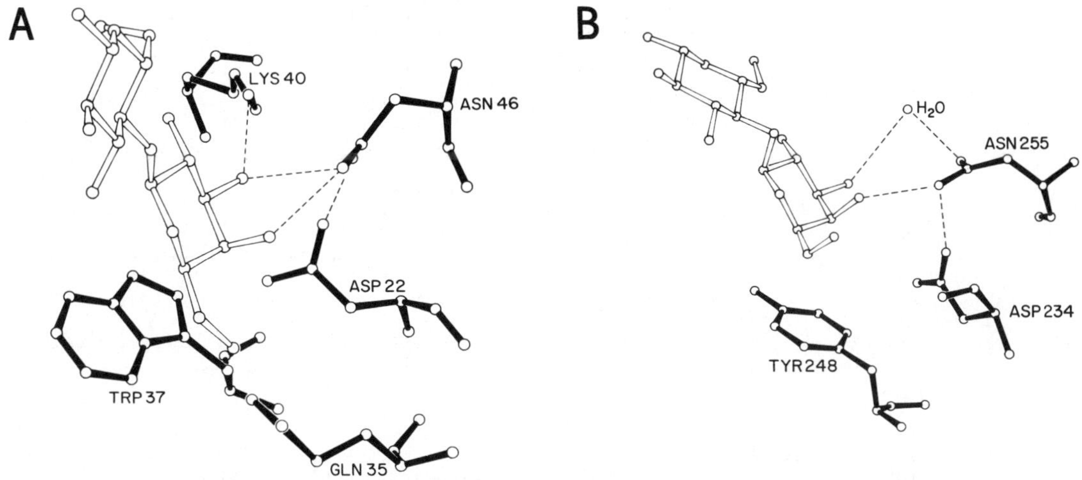

Fig. 5. Lactose binding by ricin B chain. Part A shows lactose as seen binding to domain 1. The same motif is seen in domain 2 (part B) although Tyr replaces Trp as the base of binding. In each case, only the galactose moiety of lactose makes specific interaction with the protein.

FUTURE WORK

We have recently crystallized ricin A chain expressed from a gene cloned into E. coli (Robertus et. al., 1987). That structure, and a comparison with the A chain of intact ricin should allow us to define conformational changes which may occur when A and B chain separate. These changes may be involved in 'activation' of the active site cleft and may also rearrange the surface which interacts with B chain in such a way as to facilitate membrane transport.

As mentioned, we have been able to bind adenine to ricin. We plan to extend these studies to larger, more substrate-like ribonucleotides. Hopefully these studies will allow us to accurately define the mechanism of ricin action. Finally, we have crystallized several other toxins, including PAP. We hope to compare this representative of the single chain RIP's with the ricin A chain to elucidate constant features of their common mechanisms of ribosome intoxication.

REFERENCES

Asano, K., Svensson, B., Svendsen, I., Poulsen, F. M., Roepstorff, P. (1986). The Complete Primary Structure of Protein Synthesis Inhibitor II From barley Seeds," Carlsberg Res. Commun. 51, 129-141.

Baenziger, J.U. and Fiete, D. (1979). "Structural Determinants of Ricin communis Agglutinin and Toxin Specificity for Oligosaccharides," J. Biol. Chem. 254, 9795-9799.

Endo, Y., Mitsui, K., Motizuki, M. and Tsurugi, K. (1987). "Mechanism of Action of Ricin and Related Toxic Lectins on Eukaryotic Ribosomes: The site and the characteristics of the modification in 28S rRNA caused by the toxins," J. Biol. Chem. 262, 5908-5912.

Endo, Y. and Tsurugi, K. (1987). "RNA N-glycosidase Activity of Ricin A-chain: Mechanism of action of the toxin lectin ricin on eukaryotic ribosomes," J. Biol. Chem. 262, 8128-8130.

Frankel, A. E., editor (1988). Immunotoxins. Kluwer Academic Publishers, Boston, MA.

Funatsu, G., Kimura, M. and Funatsu, M. (1979). "Primary Structure of Ala Chain of Ricin D," Agric. Biol. Chem. 43, 2221-2224.

Funatsu, G., Yoshitake, S. and Funatsu, M. (1978). "Primary Structure of Ile Chain of Ricin D," Agric. Biol. Chem. 42 , 501-503.

Halling, K.C., Halling, A.C., Murray, E.E., Ladin, B.F., Houston, L.L. and Weaver, R.F. (1985). "Genomic Cloning and Characterization of a Ricin Gene from Ricinus communis," Nucl. Acids Res. 13, 8019-8033.

Hansch, C. and Coats, E. (1970). "α-Chymotrypsin: A Case Study of Substituent Constants and Repression Analysis in Enzymic Structure-Activity Relationships," J. Phar. Sci. 59, 731-743.

Hatakeyama, T., Yamasaki, N. and Funatsu, G. (1986). "Evidence for Involvement of Tryptophan Residue in the Low-Affinity Saccharide Binding Site of Ricin D," J. Biochem. 99, 1049-1056.

Houston, L.L. (1980). "Differential Fluorescence Enhancement of 8-Anilino-1-Naphthalene Sulfonic Acid by Ricin A and B Chains," Biochem. Biophys. Res. Comm. 92, 319-326.

Houston, L.L. and Dooley, T.P. (1982). "Binding of Two Molecules of 4-Methylumbelliferyl Galactose or 4-Methylumbelliferyl N-Acetylgalactosamine to the B Chains of Ricin and Ricinus communis Agglutinin and to Purfied Ricin B Chain," J. Biol. Chem. 257, 4147-4151.

Irvin, J.D. (1975). "Purification and Partial Characterization of the Antiviral Protein from Phytolacca americana which Inhibits Eukaryotic Protein Synthesis," Arch. Biochem. Biophys. 169, 522-528.

Irvin, J.D., Kelly, T. and Robertus, J.D. (1980). "Purification and Properties of a Second Antiviral Protein from Phytolacca americana which Inactivates Eukaryotic Ribosomes," Arch. Biochem. Biophys 200, 418-425.

Lamb, F.I., Roberts, L.M. and Lord, J.M. (1985). "Nucleotide Sequence of Cloned cRNA Coding for Preproricin," Eur. J. Biochem. 148, 265-270.

Lewis, M.S. and Youle, R.J. (1986). "Ricin Subunit Association: Thermodynamics and the Role of the Disulfide Bond in Toxicity," J. Biol. Chem. 261, 11571-11577.

Mise, T., Shimoda, T. and Funatsu, G. (1986). "Identification of Tyrosyl Residue in the Gigh Affinity Saccharide-Binding Site of Ricin D," Agric. Biol. Che. 50, 151-155.

Montfort, W., Villafranca, J.E., Monzingo, A.F., Ernst, S., Katzin, B., Rutenber, E., Xuong, N.H., Hamlin, R. and Robertus, J.D. (1987). "The three-dimensional Structure of Ricin at 2.8Å," J. Biol. Chem. 262, 5398-5403.

Nicolson, G.L., Lacorbiere, M. and Hunter, T.R. (1975). "Mechanism of Cell Entry and Toxicit of an Affinity-purified Lectin from Ricinus communis and Its Differential Effects on Normal and Virus-transformed Fibroblasts," Cancer Res. 35, 144-155.

Olsnes, S., Fernandez-Puentes, C., Carrasco, L. and Vasquez, D. (1975). "Ribosome Inactivation by the Toxic Lectins Abrin and Ricin: Kinetics of the Enzymic Activity of the Toxin A-Chains," Eur. J. Biochem. 60, 281-288.

Olsnes, S., Heiberg, R. and Pihl, A. (1973). "Inactivation of Eucaryotic Ribosomes by the Toxic Plant Proteins Abrin and Ricin," Mol. Biol. Rep. 1, 15-20.

Olsnes, S. and Pihl, A. (1982). "Toxic Lectins and Related Proteins, in The Molecular Action of Toxins and Viruses (Cohen, P. and Van Heynigen, S. eds) pp 52-105, Elsevier Biomedical Press, New York.

Olsnes, S. and Pihl, A. (1973). "Isolation and Properties of Abrin: A Toxic Protein Inhibiting Protein Synthesis: Evidence for Different Biological Functions of Its Two Constituent-Peptide Chains," Eur. J. Biochem. 35, 179-185.

Ready, M. P., Adams, R. P. and Robertus, J. D. (1984). "Dodecandrin, A New Ribosome-Inhibiting
Protein From Phytolacca Dodecandra," Biochem. Biophys. Acta 791, 314-319.

Ready, M. P., Katzin, B. J. and Robertus, J. D. (1988). "Ribosome Inhibiting Proteins, Retroviral Reverse Transcriptases, and RNase h Share Common Structural Elements," Proteins: Structure, Function, and Genetics 3, 53-59.

Ready, M., Wilson, K., Piatak, M. and Robertus, J.D. (1984). "Ricin-like Plant Toxins are Evolutionarily Related to Single-chain Ribosome-inhibiting Proteins from Phytolacca," J. Biol. Chem. 259, 15252-15256.

Refsnes, K., Haylett, T., Sandvig, K. and Olsnes, S. (1977). "Modeccin-A Plant Toxin Inhibiting Protein Synthesis," Biochem. Biophys. Res. Commun. 79, 1176-1183.

Roberts, W. and Stewart, T. (1979). " Purification and Properties of a Translation Inhibitor from Wheat Germ," Biochemistry 18, 2615-2621.

Robertus, J.D., Piatak, M., Ferrie, R. and Houston, L.L. (1987). "Crystallization of Ricin A Chain Obtained from a Cloned Gene Expressed in Escherichia coli," J. Biol. Chem. 262 19-20.

Robertus, J. D. and Ready, M. P. (1984). "Ricin B Chain and Discoidin I Share a Common Primitive Protein Fold," J. Biol. Chem. 259, 13593-13956.

Rutenber, E., Ready, M., Robertus, J. D. (1987). "Structure and Evolution of Ricin B Chain," Nature 326, 624-626.

Stirpe, F., Olsnes, S. and Pihl, A. (1980). "Gelonin A New Inhibitor of Protein Synthesis, Nontoxic to Intact Cells: Isolation characterization and Preparation of cytotoxic complexes with concanavalin A," J. Biol. Chem. 255, 6947-6953.

Uchida, T., Mekada, E. and Okada, Y. (1980). "Hybrid Toxin of the A Chain of Ricin Toxin and a Subunit of Wistaria floribunda Lectin: Possible importance of the Hydrophobic Region For Entry of Toxin Into the Cell,"J. Biol. Chem. 255, 6687-6693.

Villafranca, J.E. and Robertus, J.D. (1981). "Ricin B Chain Is a Product of Gene Duplication," J. Biol. Chem. 256, 554-556.

Wright, H. T. and Robertus, J. D. (1987). "The Intersubunit Disulfide Bridge of Ricin Is Essential For Cytotoxity," Archives of Biochemistry and Biophysics 256, 280-284.

Xuejun, Z. and Jiahuai, W. (1986). "Homology of Trichosanthin and Ricin A Chain," Nature 321, 477-478.

Zentz, C., Frenoy, J.P. and Bourrillon, R. (1978). "Binding of Galactose and Lactose to Ricin: Equilibrium Studies," Biochem. Biophys. Acta 536, 18-26.

V. Clinical Aspects and Therapies

PATHOPHYSIOLOGY AND TREATMENT OF SCORPION POISONING

L. FREIRE-MAIA and J.A. CAMPOS*

Departamento de Farmacologia, Instituto de Ciências Biológicas, Universidade Federal de Minas Gerais and *Departamento de Pediatria, Faculdade de Medicina da UFMG and Hospital João XXIII, Belo Horizonte, Brasil.

ABSTRACT

The authors describe the pathophysiology of scorpion poisoning in animals, and the clinical findings and treatment in children. They conclude that the scorpion venom acts at the peripheral nervous system, with release of chemical mediators (e.g., acetylcholine and catecholamines) and that part of the effects are reflex in nature and secondary to stimulation of vagal afferent fibers. The treatment of 168 children severely poisoned by *Tityus serrulatus* scorpion venom in an Intensive Care Unit consisted of symptomatic measures, support of vital functions and neutralization of circulating venom. From 1972 to 1987 3860 adults and children were poisoned by scorpions, with a mortality rate of 0.28%.

KEYWORDS

Pathophysiology; scorpion poisoning; scorpion toxins; mechanism of action; clinical findings; treatment.

INTRODUCTION

Scientists all over the world have been interested in scorpion venoms because of the high incidence of fatal cases of scorpion poisoning (Magalhães, 1946; Efrati, 1949; Silva, 1950; Waterman, 1957; Mazzoti and Bravo Becherelle, 1961; Russell, 1967; Bücherl, 1978; Habermehl; 1981; Goyffon *et al.*, 1982; Gueron and Ovsyshcher, 1987). Treatment of severe cases of poisoning in Intensive Care Units has decreased the mortality rate in the last years (Campos *et al.*, 1979, 1980; Rimsza *et al.*, 1980; Herskovich *et al.*, 1985). On the other hand, many investigators have shown that crude scorpion venoms or toxins purified from the venoms evoke complex effects on sodium channels, with release of chemical mediators. Purification procedures have revealed that the active components of venoms from several scorpion species are polypeptides (see reviews in Rochat *et al.*, 1979; Possani *et al.*, 1984). On the other hand, the toxicity of venoms from scorpions of several species shows great variations. The most toxic scorpion species in the world are *Leiurus quinquestriatus*, *Androctonus crassicanda*, *Centruroides noxius* and *Tityus serrulatus* (Hassan, 1984).

Neurotoxins are present in the majority of scorpion venoms and some of them have also in their composition autacoids such as serotonin in *Leiurus quinquestriatus* (Adam and Weiss, 1958) and histamine in *Palamneus gravimanus* (Ismail *et al.*, 1975).

For these reasons the pathophysiology of scorpion poisoning may vary, according to the scorpion species. We will describe the pathophysiology of poisoning induced by the South American scorpion *Tityus serrulatus*, comparing it with reports on different scorpion species.

PATHOPHYSIOLOGY

A. Cardiovascular effects

1. Hypertension

Intravenous injections of *Tityus serrulatus* or *Centruroides suffusus* scorpion venoms in anesthetized dogs or cats induced arterial hypertension which was explained by actions of the venoms either on medulla (Magalhães, 1938) or spinal cord (Del Pozo, 1968). However, the hypertension elicited by *T. serrulatus* venom was not prevented by ganglionic blockade, but was abolished by an alpha adrenergic blocking agent; these results indicated, therefore, that hypertension was not due to a central but rather to a peripheral effect of the venom, through stimulation of alpha adrenergic receptors (Ramos and Corrado, 1954; Freire-Maia and Ferreira, 1961).

Experiments performed with a purified scorpion toxin showed that the hypertension induced in anesthetized intact rats was not prevented by hexamethonium but was decreased by reserpine, guanethidine or phenoxybenzamine, and prevented by guanethidine in adrenalectomized animals. These data indicated that the hypertension was caused by the release of catecholamines from adrenal glands and postganglionic nerve endings (Freire-Maia and Diniz, 1970; Freire-Maia *et al.*, 1974). On the other hand, the hypertension induced by crude venom of *T. serrulatus* in dogs was explained by actions at the sympathetic post-ganglionic fibers (Corrado *et al.*,1974). Based on these experiments in rats and dogs we can postulate that the hypertensive effect induced by scorpion toxin is due to the release of catecholamines from both adrenal glands and postganglionic nerve endings. The hypothesis that part of the hypertensive effect was due to the release of catecholamines from adrenal glands was supported by experiments which showed that *T. serrulatus* scorpion venom produced a depletion of adrenal catecholamines (Celeste - Henriques, 1968) and that *Leiurus quinquestriatus* and *Androctonus australis* scorpion venoms induced discharge of catecholamines into the blood accompanied by hypertension (Beauvallet *et al.*, 1972; Moss *et al.*, 1973).

The venom from the scorpion *Buthus minax* also induced hypertensive effect in cats and rats, which was prevented by alpha adrenergic blockade with phenoxybenzamine or tolazoline (Ismail *et al.*, 1973). On the other hand, the hypertensive effect evoked by *Leiurus quinquestriatus* scorpion venom in dogs was, only, transiently reduced by phentolamine (Gueron *et al.*, 1980).

Venoms from scorpions *Centruroides sculpturatus* and *Leiurus quinquestriatus* were able to release renin, even in phenoxybenzamine-treated rats (La Grange, 1977). This effect could be mediated by catecholamines released by venoms acting on beta adrenergic receptors in the kidney, since it is known that renin secretion is associated, in part, with stimulation of beta adrenergic receptors.

Arterial hypertension could, also, be due in part to an increased myocardial contractility, since it was shown that venom obtained from *Leiurus quinquestriatus* increased in dogs the dp/dt of the left ventricle (Braun *et al.*, 1970; Gueron *et al.*, 1980).

In conclusion, the arterial hypertension induced by scorpion toxin is due to:

1. Release of catecholamines from adrenal glands and postganglionic nerve endings;
2. The catecholamines action on alpha adrenergic receptors, increasing the peripheral resistance;
3. The catecholamines action, also, on beta adrenergic receptors, either increasing the cardiac contractility or releasing renin from the kidneys.

2. Cardiac arrhythmias

Several investigators have described complex cardiac arrhythmias induced by scorpion venoms (Magalhães, 1938; Poon-King, 1963; Gueron *et al.*, 1967; Gueron and Yarom, 1970; Campos *et al.*, 1980).

We have shown in our laboratory, that injection of small doses of a purified scorpion toxin (*Tityus serrulatus*) in anesthetized rats evoked sinus tachycardia, whereas larger doses produced sinus bradycardia, sinoatrial (SA) and atrioventricular(AV) block,ventricular ectopic beats and idioventricular rhythm (Freire-Maia and Diniz, 1970; Freire-Maia *et al.*, 1974). We have also shown that bilateral vagotomy did not prevent the arrhythmias;in vagotomized animals physostigmine enhanced, hexamethonium decreased and atropine abolished the bradycardia . Moreover, propranolol prevented or abolished the sinus tachycardia and changed the ventricular into a sinus rhythm. Based on these results we concluded that the sinus bradycardia, SA and AV block were due to release of acetylcholine by actions of the toxin on vagal ganglia and postganglionic nerve endings in the heart and that the sinus tachycardia, the ventricular ectopic beats and the idioventricular rhythm were caused by activation of beta adrenergic receptors in the heart by catecholamines released by the toxin (Freire-Maia and Diniz, 1970; Freire-Maia et al., 1974).

Injections of a toxin, isolated from Androctonus australis scorpion venom, evoked electrocardiographic changes such as descrease of T wave amplitude,AV dissociation and ectopic beats in anesthetized rats. Blockade of sodium channels with tetrodotoxin prevented the cardiotoxic action of the venom in these animals (Tazieff-Depierre, 1971).

Injection of Buthus minax scorpion venom into rabbits caused either bradycardia or tachycardia (Ismail et al., 1976). According to the authors, the tachycardia was explained by sympathetic stimulation, which is in accordance with our previous data (Freire-Maia and Diniz, 1970; Freire-Maia et al., 1974). As far as the bradycardia is concerned, Ismail et al. (1976) assumed that it was due to a "central vagal stimulation", since it was blocked by atropine. We had previously showed that bilateral vagotomy did not prevent the bradycardia, while atropine abolished it, indicating a peripheral action of scorpion toxin. The authors have also reported an "anterior wall infarction", induced by scorpion venom in the rabbit heart. "Myocardial infarcts" induced by scorpion venom have also been reported by other investigators (Gueron et al., 1967; Gueron and Yarom, 1970; Tazieffe-Depiere, 1971; Yarom et al., 1974). We believe that the effects on ST segment and T wave described by those authors could be better explained by a relative and temporary myocardial hypoxia due to a decrease in coronary blood flow, during tachycardia and positive inotropic effect (Campos et al., 1980; Almeida et al., 1982). An increase in oxygen consumption induced by catecholamines released by scorpion toxin could also play a role in the relative myocardial hypoxia. Finally, a direct effect of catecholamines on the ventricular action potential could contribute to the changes observed in ST segment and T wave.

3. Effects of scorpion venom on the isolated heart

Corrado et al. (1968) showed that the crude venom of the scorpion Tityus serrulatus produced in isolated guinea pig heart a short-lasting bradycardia followed by a conspicuous increase in the force and the rate of cardiac contractions. The authors concluded that both effects were indirect and due to a local release of acetylcholine and noradrenaline.

The crude venom of Buthus minax also produced a positive inotropic effect on isolated rabbit and guinea pig hearts (due to release of catecholamines), but an alteration in rate was not observed (Ismail et al., 1973). However, in reserpine-treated animals the venom induced bradycardia, blocked by atropine. These data indicated that the parasympathetic effects were masked by sympathetic stimulation.

The venoms of scorpions Androctonus australis, Leiurus quinquestriatus and Buthus occitanus induced a positive inotropic effect and bradycardia in the isolated guinea pig heart (Cheymol et al., 1974). According to the authors, atropine abolished the positive inotropic effect. It is unlikely that a blockade of muscarinic receptors could abolish a positive inotropic effect, which is due to release of catecholamines. On the other hand, the authors also reported a "fibrillation" induced by those venoms. We think that a diagnosis of fibrillation should be more accurate when established by electrical activity recordings of the heart rather than by observing the contractile force recordings.

It has been shown that a toxin purified from the venom of the scorpion Leiurus quinquestriatus released noradrenaline (NA) from isolated rat atrial strips. The release of NA resembled that induced by nerve stimulation, because it was calcium-dependent (Moss et al., 1974).

Yarom et al. (1974) recorded the electrical activity of isolated rat heart and showed that the venom of the scorpion Leiurus quinquestriatus evoked ectopic beats,widening of the QRS complex, atrioventricular block, idioventricular rhythm, atrial fibrillation and myocardial infarct patterns. The heart rate response was variable. The authors also reported temporary ultrastructural changes of the heart, similar to those induced by large doses of noradrenaline.

A direct demonstration of the release of noradrenaline (NA) in isolated guinea pig atria by a toxin extracted from the venom of Tityus serrulatus was made by Langer et al.(1975). In atria previously labeled with ^{3}H-noradrenaline, scorpion toxin enhanced the spontaneous outflow of radioactivity. ^{3}H-noradrenaline accounted for 60% of the total increase in outflow of radioactivity elicited by the scorpion toxin and the ^{3}H-deaminated glycol (^{3}H - DOPEG) represented the main metabolite formed (35% of the total release). As ^{3}H-DOPEG is formed preferentially in adrenergic nerve endings, these data indicate that a significant fraction of the labelled transmitter released by the scorpion toxin is metabolized presynaptically. The authors also showed that the scorpion toxin enhanced the NA release elicited by nerve stimulation, through a prejunctional effect, which was unrelated to the factors known to influence NA release.

Grupp *et al*. (1980) have described a direct effect of the venom from scorpion *Leiurus quinquestriatus* on contractile force of isolated guinea pig atria and papillary muscles. As venom from this species contains 5-HT (Adam and Weiss, 1958), it would be of interest to repeat the experiments using a 5-HT antagonist, since it is known that this autacoid induces an increase in contractile force of isolated heart.

The results so far discussed have shown that scorpion venoms of several species produce contradictory results when applied to isolated heart preparations. Because of these differences our group performed experiments in isolated guinea pig hearts using a purified toxin extracted from the venom of *Tityus serrulatus* (Almeida *et al*., 1982). We showed that the scorpion toxin-induced increase in contractile force was dose-dependent, whereas the positive chronotropic effect was not. The absence of a direct relation between dose and positive chronotropic effect might be due to the bradycardia evoked by a larger dose of scorpion toxin, in some experiments. Therefore, a similar dose of toxin could induce a positive chronotropic effect in one guinea pig and a negative chronotropic effect in another. The increase in rate was due to a sinus tachycardia, whereas the decrease was due to sinus bradycardia, sinus arrest or atrioventricular block.

We have also shown that after the initial events evoked by scorpion toxin, periodic changes in heart rate, contractile force and coronary flow were observed during a period of 5-15 min. The periodic increase in heart rate was associated with an increase in contractile force, whereas the coronary flow varied inversely with the rate and the contractile force.

Recording of the electrical activity of the heart showed that the periodic changes of cardiac rate were due to wandering pacemakers; as atropine prevents the appearance of such pacemakers, it seems likely that they are related to release of acetylcholine by toxin (Almeida *et al*., 1982; Freire-Maia, 1983).

On the other hand, a toxin purified from *Androctonus australis* scorpion venom induced a positive chronotropic effect and arrhythmias in nerve-free cultured chick embryo heart cells, explained by an increase in Na^{+} and Ca^{++} uptakes (Fayet *et al*., 1974; Couraud and Jover, 1984). These data seem to indicate that there is an essential difference in the response to scorpion toxin between the embryonic and adult heart cells, since the effects on the latter depend on the presence of nerve fibers (Zlotkin *et al*., 1978).

4. Hypotension

We have shown that scorpion toxin (*Tityus serrulatus*) induced hypotensive effects before or after the hypertension in anesthetized rats (Freire-Maia and Diniz, 1970; Freire-Maia *et al*., 1974, 1976a). The small hypotensive effect recorded in some animals, before the pressor effect, occured simultaneously with bradycardia and could be due to a reduction of the cardiac output. Injections of large doses of the toxin induced hypertension followed by bradycardia, periodic respiration, hypotension, apnea, and death. Previous injection of atropine potentiated the pressor response and prevented the bradycardia, but did not prevent the periodic respiration, hypotension, apnea and death. In the artificially ventilated animals, the toxin also produced hypertension, bradycardia, hypotension and death. Atropinization of animals, under artificial ventilation, has shown that scorpion toxin still produced hypertension followed by hypotension, but no bradycardia. The hypotensive effect was of smaller magnitude and death did not occur during the time of the experiment, that was 2 h 30 min. It seems likely, therefore, that apnea and bradycardia are responsible, at least in part, for hypotension and death in these anesthetized animals (Freire-Maia *et al*. 1976a).

Crude venom from the scorpion *Buthus minax* produced a small hypotensive effect (Ismail *et al*., 1973) and venoms from scorpion *Androctonus australis*, *Leiurus quinquestriatus* and *Buthus occitanus* also induced hypotensive effects (Cheymol *et al*., 1974). However, quantitative data on the subject were not published.

5. Pulmonary edema

Many patients stung by scorpions of several species died with pulmonary edema (Waterman, 1938; Magalhães, 1946; Stahnke, 1950; Gueron et al., 1967; Gueron and Yarom, 1970; Reddy et al.,1972; Campos et al., 1979, 1980).

Gueron and Yarom (1970) reported the cardiovascular manifestations of severe scorpion sting in Israel, from 1960 to 1968. Eighty-two patients were hospitalized in this period stung by B. quinquestriatus scorpions, with 9 deaths. The authors reported the autopsies performed in these patients. The lungs showed different degrees of pulmonary edema, accompanied by diffuse areas of alveolar hemorrhage. Similar results were also observed in dogs following injection of the venom (Yarom and Braun, 1970). Intravenous injection of Tityus serrulatus scorpion venom induced pulmonary edema in rats. Microscopical examination of the lungs showed pulmonary edema and hemorrhage, alveolar wall thickening and increased cellularity (Rossi et al., 1974).

To study the mechanism of pulmonary edema we injected a purified scorpion toxin (Tityus serrulatus) intravenously in unanesthetized rats. Ganglionic blockade with hexamethonium or beta adrenergic blockade with propranolol did not change significantly the magnitude of the lung edema induced by the toxin, but alpha adrenergic blockade with phenoxybenzamine prevented the production of the edema. Moreover, atropine increased the severity of the lung edema elicited by the toxin (Freire-Maia et al., 1978). We have also shown that scorpion toxin induced a dramatic systolic and diastolic arterial hypertension in unanesthetized rats, before the appearance of signs of pulmonary edema (e.g., froth in the mouth and dyspnea).Our data also showed that the severity of pulmonary edema was directly related to the dose of toxin and duration of intoxication (Azevedo et al., 1983). The velocity of rise of systemic arterial pressure following injection of scorpion toxin in unanesthetized rats seemed to be another factor in the genesis and severity of pulmonary edema. Therefore, the experiments of our group showed that the hemodynamic effect, characterized by an abrupt and dramatic rise of systemic arterial pressure (afterload), due to release of catecholamines and stimulation of alpha adrenergic receptors, plays an important role in the pathogenesis of acute pulmonary edema. The acute arterial hypertension would evoke a left ventricular failure and pulmonary edema.It seems likely that bradycardia protects the animals, since injection of atropine increased the severity of the lung edema (Freire-Maia et al., 1978).

In the presence of severe sinus tachycardia due to beta adrenergic stimulation (Corrado et al., 1968; Freire-Maia et al., 1974; Almeida et al., 1982), the filling of the left ventricle should be impaired, with a consequent decrease in the cardiac output. A decrease of left ventricular compliance induced by catecholamines released by scorpion venom could also result in an impairment of ventricular filling and heart failure (Gueron et al., 1980). Myocardial damage, attributable to a sympathomimetic overstimulation, induced by venoms from scorpions of several species, could also play a role in the genesis of heart failure and pulmonary edema (Poon-King, 1963; Gueron et al., 1967; Gueron and Yarom, 1970; Yarom and Braun, 1970; Efrati, 1978; Gueron and Ovsyshcher, 1987).

Therefore, the heart failure induced by scorpion venom might be due to some of several mechanisms, such as an increase in afterload, a decrease of left ventricular compliance, the presence of a severe sinus tachycardia and myocardial damage.

Another factor contributing to the genesis of pulmonary edema would be an increase in venous return. As we have said previously, scorpion toxin increase the level of catecholamines present in the blood (Beauvallet et al., 1972; Moss et al., 1973), that would contract the smooth muscle of peripheral veins, increasing the venous return. Moreover, the toxin could contract the veins by a direct effect (Savino and Catanzaro, 1979) contributing to an increase of the venous return. This would induce to an increase in preload leading to pulmonary congestion. This hypothesis is supported by previous experiments which showed an increase in pulmonary arterial pressure following the injection of Leiurus quinquestriatus scorpion venom in dogs (Braun et al., 1970).

The pulmonary edema induced by catecholamines in unanesthetized rats is due to the joint action of vasopressor effects and kinin release in the lungs (Rotschild and Castania, 1976; Azevedo et al., 1979). As the lung edema elicited by scorpion toxin in unanesthetized rats is similar to that evoked by catecholamines (Freire-Maia et al., 1978; Azevedo et al.,1983), it seems likely that the edema induced by toxin could be explained, at least in part, by kinin release. Histamine is also released from the lungs after injection of Tityus serrulatus scorpion venom or adrenaline (Beraldo and Dias da Silva, 1966; Oliveira Antônio et al., 1973) and could also play a role in the genesis of pulmonary edema. Other chemical mediators are possibly released by scorpion toxin, since indomethacin decreased the severity of the pulmonary edema induced by toxin in the rat (Freire-Maia _et al_., 1978).

These data indicate, therefore, that the pulmonary edema evoked by scorpion toxin is caused, at least in part,by release of substances which increase vascular permeability. On the other hand, venom of the scorpion _Tityus serrulatus_ or one of its toxic fractions (tityustoxin), kept in contact with the peripheral cut end of sensory nerves,induce the release of a permeability increasing factor, responsible for edema formation (Garcia Leme _et al_.,1978). According to the authors the action of the toxin is not attributable to acetylcholine, histamine, serotonin, prostaglandins and bradykinin. It seems likely that this novel permeability factor originating in sensory fibers could contribute for the formation of pulmonary edema, following injection of scorpion toxin.

All these data indicate that the pathogenesis of acute pulmonary edema induced by scorpion toxin is very complex. It is important to keep this in mind during the treatment of patients stung by scorpions (Freire-Maia and Campos, 1987).

B. Respiratory arrhythmias

Injections of crude venoms from several scorpion species in dogs,cats and rats produce complex respiratory arrhythmias, such as tachypnea, hyperpnea, periodic respiration and respiratory paralysis (Magalhães, 1938; Del Pozo, 1968; Ismail _et al_., 1973; Stahnke, 1978).

The respiratory arrhythmias were explained by actions of the venoms on the central nervous system (Magalhães, 1938; Del Pozo 1968) or carotid bodies (Patterson and Wooley, 1972; Ismail _et al_., 1973). As the mechanism of the arrhythmias were not completely known, our group reinvestigated the subject using a purified toxin obtained from the venom of _Tityus serrulatus_ (Freire-Maia _et al_., 1970, 1973, 1976a).

We have shown that scorpion toxin, depending upon the dose, produced either stimulation or paralysis of the respiratory movements of rats. The gasping type of breathing produced by the toxin was not related to asphyxia and showed a fairly regular pattern. The respiratory movements between two gasps were irregular in rate and amplitude (ataxic breathing) or were absent (periodic breathing).Bilateral section of vagus nerves and denervation of carotid bodies prevented the gasping, ataxic and periodic respiration induced by the toxin. The apnea recorded in intact rats after toxin injection was of long duration in comparison with that observed in denervated animals. Moreover, bilateral vagotomy abolished periods of apnea observed between gasping respirations. These data seem to indicate that the respiratory arrhythmias produced by scorpion toxin in the rat are mainly due to stimulation of peripheral receptors,being therefore reflex in nature.

As the respiratory arrhythmias could be induced by stimulation of peripheral nerve endings by scorpion toxin (Freire-Maia _et al_., 1973)we decided to study the possible effects of the local anesthetic lidocaine on these arrhythmias. We showed that intravenous injection of lidocaine abolished transiently the respiratory arrhythmias (tachypnea, ataxic and gasping breathings). These experiments did not show, however, the site of action of lidocaine. Experiments were then conducted to observe the participation of the vagus nerves in the effects of the toxin. We have shown that the local anesthesia of the cervical vagus nerves with lidocaine abolished the apnea but did not change the bradycardiac effect, whereas the arterial pressure increased to values higher than the controls. Based on these data, and on the findings of Paintal (1973) who showed that stimulation of J receptors in lungs by phenyldiguanide produces apnea, bradycardia and hypotension, we presented the hypothesis that scorpion toxin acting on J receptors produces apnea and hypotension, of reflex nature (Freire-Maia _et al_., 1976a). Recently, we have shown that apnea induced by scorpion toxin, in rats, was accompanied by an increase in frequency and/ or amplitude of action potentials in cervical vagus nerves and abolition of the potentials in phrenic nerves. Bilateral vagotomy was followed by the return of both the action potentials in phrenic nerves and the respiratory movements. These data confirm the hypothesis that the apnea induced by scorpion toxin is due to reflex stimulation of vagal afferent fibers.

C. Effects on the neuromuscular system

Several investigators have described complex effects of scorpion venoms in laboratory animals (see References in Del Pozo and Anguiano, 1947 and Zlotkin and Shulov, 1969). The effects of Mexican scorpion venoms (_Centruroides suffusus suffusus_ and _Centruroides noxius_) were investigated by Del Pozo and Anguiano (1947) on cat striated muscle. According to these authors intravenous injection of venom induced fascicular contractions secondary to spinal activity.

Single maximal stimuli aplied to a poisoned muscle elicited contractions of greater amplitude and duration than in control experiments. Scorpion venom also presented competitive effects with curare.

Adam and Weiss (1959,1966) have shown that venoms of African scorpions(*Leiurus quinquestriatus*) added to denervated preparations of skeletal muscle induced a contracture of the muscle. A slow depolarization of the muscle membrane was observed, until the threshold level of the action potential was reached. This direct effect was similar to that induced by veratridine. On the other hand, Benoit and Mambrini (1967) have shown that when venom of the same species (*Leiurus quinquestriatus*) was applied at the frog neuromuscular junction it induced an increase in the duration of the presynaptic nerve action potential and an increase in the mean number of quanta released by a nerve impulse. These different results could be explained assuming that the venom exert both pre and postsynaptic effects.

Parnas and Russell (1967) have investigated the effects of venoms of North American scorpions on the innervated crayfish deep extensor muscle preparation. The first effect observed was excitatory, and characterized by spontaneous activity of the muscle; this was followed by complete block of electrical response to indirect stimulation of the nerve. Nerve conduction was not affected by scorpion venom, even when there was a complete block of the indirectly stimulated muscles. This indicates that the scorpion venom probably exerts its deleterious effects at the neuromuscular junction.

Katz and Edwards (1972) have studied the effects of venom of the Mexican scorpion *Centruroides suffusus suffusus* in the isolated frog sartorius nerve-muscle preparation. In the presence of the venom, single shocks applied to the nerve produced repetitive responses in both nerve and muscle, but reduction of the sodium concentration in the bathing fluid abolished the repetitive activity. According to the authors the site most accessible to the action of the venom is the exposed area of the axon near its termination. On the other hand, according to Yarom and Meiri (1972) the venom of the scorpion acts directly on the muscle membrane altering the calcium flux, but no ultrastructural lytic or disruptive lesions have been found in muscles exposed to the venom.

Vital Brazil *et al.*, (1973) have shown that the venom of the South American scorpion *Tityus serrulatus* induces the release of an acetylcholine-like substance from the innervated but not from the denervated rat diaphragm. The release of this substance could account for the twitches observed and also for the decurarizing activity of scorpion venom, first reported by Del Pozo and Anguiano (1947). A toxin purified from the venom of *Tityus serrulatus* did not induce pathological changes in diaphragm of mice, but alterations in the diaphragm nerve endings were reported (Böhm *et al.*, 1974). A presynaptic action was also reported to be responsible for spontaneous contractions induced by a purified toxin from the venom of *A. australis* (Lin *et al.*, 1975). On the other hand, crude venom of *Androctonus australis* scorpion induced a direct muscular effect on a paralysed locust-nerve-muscle preparation (Walther *et al.*, 1976).

Electrophysiological studies on the action of tityustoxin, purified from the venom of *Tityus serrulatus*, on rat phrenic nerve-diaphragm muscle preparation, have shown that the toxin transiently potentiated both the direct and indirect elicited muscle contractions and prolonged the half-relaxation time. The data indicated that the toxin had a presynaptic and postsynaptic action at the neuromuscular junction. An increase of sodium permeability evoked by toxin led to depolarization of pre and postsynaptic membranes. The initial alterations of the muscle twitch were due to a postsynaptic effect at the sarcolemmal membrane, where the toxin delayed sodium inactivation and prolonged the active phase of muscle contraction. On the other hand, the scorpion toxin had two sites of action presynaptically: it depolarized the nerve terminal, facilitating the spontaneous release of transmitter (acetylcholine) and acted at the membrane of the unmyelinated nerve terminal arborization, prolonging the sodium current. The repetitive response to single shocks aplied to the nerve was explained by the prolongation of the sodium currents (Warnick *et al.*, 1976).

The data summarized in this article indicate,therefore, that scorpion venoms of several species have pre and/or postsynaptic actions at the neuromuscular junction.

D. Effects on the gastrointestinal system

Clinical findings in scorpion poisoning include gastrointestinal symptoms, such as excessive salivation, nausea, vomiting and diarrhea (Zlotkin *et al.*, 1978; Campos *et al.*, 1980). We will try to explain in this section the mechanism of action of scorpion toxin on secretions induced by salivary glands, gastric mucosa and pancreas; moreover, the mechanism of action of the toxin on gastrointestinal motility will be also discussed.

1. Salivary secretion

A sialagogue effect was described in humans stung by scorpions (Waterman, 1938; Magalhães, 1946). An intense sialagogue effect, induced by *Tityus serrulatus* scorpion venom in mice, was abolished by atropine (Diniz and Valeri, 1959). On the other hand, the salivation induced by small doses of scorpion venom in dogs was due to excitatory action on the central and peripheral nervous system, while the effect induced by massive dose of the venom was explained by a nicotine-like action (Samaan and Ibrahim, 1959).

Our group studied the mechanism of salivary secretion induced by a purified toxin of *T. serrulatus* in rats (Catanzaro *et al*., 1978). We showed that the toxin increased not only the flow, but also the kallikrein and amylase secretions. Atropine abolished almost totally the flow, confirming previous data in mice. *In vivo* and *in vitro* experiments showed that the amylase secretion induced by toxin was blocked almost totally by reserpine, phenoxybenzamine or propranolol. These data suggest that catecholamines released by the toxin act on *alpha* and *beta* adrenergic receptors, increasing the amylase secretion. On the other hand, the release of kallikrein induced by toxin depended mostly on a cholinergic effect. Therefore, the increased salivary secretion (flow, amylase and kallikrein) induced by scorpion toxin in rats was due to cholinergic and adrenergic effects. Our group also showed that the actions of scorpion toxin on the kallikrein and amylase secretions, per minute, were more effective than those induced by pilocarpine and isoproterenol, respectively (Catanzaro *et al*., 1978). Scorpion toxin also stimulated the flow of saliva and increased the secretion of sodium, potassium and kallikrein, from both submandibular and parotid glands of rats. The mechanism of action involved stimulations of adrenergic and cholinergic receptors (Andrade *et al*., 1981).

2. Gastric secretion

Our group showed that an i.v. bolus injection of scorpion toxin (*T. serrulatus*) in urethane anesthetized rats induced a dramatic increase in volume, acid and pepsin output of gastric juice and a significant decrease in its pH. Hexamethonium did not prevent the gastric secretion elicited by toxin, whereas atropine or cimetidine abolished partially or totally the toxin effects. Acute bilateral cervical or abdominal vagotomy did not prevent the effects of toxin on gastric secretion. On the other hand, *in vitro* experiments showed that scorpion toxin increased the H^+ and pepsin output of the isolated frog mucosa. Lidocaine and atropine prevented these effects, whereas cimetidine prevented totally the effect on acid secretion. Based on the *in vivo* and *in vitro* experiments it was suggested that the changes in gastric secretion induced by scorpion toxin, in the rat, were due to the release of chemical mediators from postganglionic autonomic nerve fibers, which would act through muscarinic and H^2-receptors stimulation (Gonzaga *et al*., 1979; Cunha-Melo *et al*., 1983).

Venom from the scorpion *Buthus quinquestriatus* decreased the volume of gastric juice in rats, as compared with saline-injected control animals. However, the titratable acidity and pepsin concentration were increased (Mohamed *et al*., 1980). The authors suggest that there is a synergism between atropine and the scorpion venom regarding to gastric acid secretion. These results are different from those reported by our group with a toxin purified from *Tityus serrulatus* scorpion venom, since the gastric secretion evoked by the toxin was abolished in part by atropine (Gonzaga *et al*., 1979; Cunha-Melo *et al*., 1983). On the other hand, venom from *Leiurus quinquestriatus* increased the gastric secretion in rats, which was not completely abolished by bilateral vagotomy, atropine or cimetidine (Ghoneim *et al*., 1984).

Recently, we have shown that scorpion toxin (*Tityus serrulatus*) induces the release of acetylcholine and histamine from rat stomach (Cunha-Melo *et al*.,1987). Based on these findings and previous results with the blocking agents atropine and cimetidine, we think that scorpion toxin exerts its action upon the rat stomach by releasing acetylcholine directly from its nerve endings stores and by releasing histamine directly or indirectly from histaminocytes . Release of gastrin from pyloric antrum could also contribute to the overall response *in vivo* (Cunha-Melo, personal communication). From the medical point of view it would be necessary to observe carefully those suffering from peptic ulcers who are victims of scorpion stings (El--Asmar, 1984).

3. Pancreatic secretion

Acute pancreatitis was reported in humans stung by scorpion *Tityus trinitatis* (Waterman, 1938; Poon-King, 1963; Bartholomew, 1970). Acute pancreatitis was also induced in dogs injected with *T. serrulatus* scorpion venom (Machado and Silveira, 1974).The venom of *T. trinitatis* induced an increase in both volume and amylase secretion from the pancreas of anesthetized dogs (Bartholomew *et al*., 1975). This venom also evoked exocrine secretion in the isolated perfused canine pancreas (Bartholomew *et al*., 1976). Amylase was released from rat pancreatic slices by venom of the scorpion *T. trinitatis* (Sankaran *et al*., 1977). According to these authors, hexamethonium and tubocurarine had no effect on the venom-induced amylase release, ruling out the possibility of actions of the venom at the ganglia or "at the nerve-organ level". They suggested that the venom acted directly on muscarinic receptors. On the other hand,the *in vitro* amylase secretion induced by venom of scorpion *Tityus serrulatus* was explained by the release of acetylcholine from pancreatic nerves (Gallagher *et al*., 1981).

Our group studied the effects of a purified scorpion toxin,from *Tityus serrulatus*,on pancreatic secretion, in anesthetized rats. A bolus injection of scorpion toxin caused a striking increase in flow rate, protein content, kallikrein and amylase activities of the pancreatic juice. Sub-diaphragmatic bilateral vagotomy did not prevent the pancreatic secretion induced by toxin, but pre-treatment of the rats with atropine blocked the secretion evoked by toxin.It was suggested that the pancreatic secretion induced by scorpion toxin was due to actions of acetylcholine, released from postganglionic nerve fibers, on muscarinic receptors (Novaes *et al*., 1982). This hypothesis was supported by *in vitro* experiments (Gallagher *et al*., 1981).

As far as the pathogenesis of acute pancreatitis induced by scorpion toxin is concerned, it was suggested that it could be explained by a greatly increased exocrine output of the pancreas, associated with an outflow obstruction (Bartholomew *et al*., 1976). Kallikrein, released by scorpion toxin (Novaes *et al*., 1982), could also play a role in the pathogenesis of acute pancreatitis, after its activation by trypsin.

4. Intestinal motility

Scorpion venoms of several species contracted the smooth muscle of isolated intestine of guinea pig, dog, rabbit and rat (Diniz *et al*., 1978; Zlotkin *et al*., 1978). Experimental data showed that cocaine or atropine prevented the contraction of guinea pig ileum induced by *T.serrulatus* and *T. bahiensis* scorpion venoms (Diniz and Gonçalves, 1956). Moreover, incubation of segments of ileum with venom released an acetylcholine-like substance (Diniz and Torres, 1968). It was then concluded that the contraction of the guinea pig ileum evoked by the venom was indirect, through the release of an acetylcholine-like substance. A purified toxin from *Androctonus australis* venom induced contractions of the isolated guinea pig ileum which were explained by a postganglionic stimulation, with release of acetylcholine (Tazieffe-Depierre and Andrillon 1973; Tintipulver *et al*., 1976).

However, our group showed that atropine did not prevent totally the contraction evoked by *T. serrulatus* scorpion toxin either in rat or guinea pig ileum (Cunha-Melo *et al*., 1973; Freire-Maia *et al*., 1976c). But we also showed that physostigmine potentiated the contraction induced by scorpion toxin and that the toxin released acetylcholine from rat and guinea pig ilea through stimulation of sodium channels (Freire-Maia *et al.*, 1976b,c). We postulated , then, that the contraction of intestinal smooth muscle induced by scorpion toxin was due to the release of acetylcholine and another mediator. Based on indirect evidences we presented the hypothesis that this second mediator could be substance P (Cunha-Melo *et al*., 1973).

Scorpion toxin induced relaxation of isolated hen rectal caecum and also relaxation of the rat duodenum immersed in Tyrode solution containing atropine; the relaxations were prevented by tetrodotoxin and phentolamine plus propranolol (Freire-Maia *et al*., 1976 b,c). It was then concluded that the relaxations evoked by scorpion toxin were due to the release of catecholamines from nerve endings present in the intestine, with subsequent stimulation of alpha and beta adrenergic receptors.

Therefore, the contraction and/or relaxation of smooth muscle of the intestine induced by scorpion toxin are due to the release of chemical mediators, such as acetylcholine and catecholamines. Other mediators, such as substance P, could also be released.

Incubation of slices of rat ileum with scorpion toxin led to a decrease in the number of granular (dense) vesicles and a simultaneous increase in the number of agranular (clear) vesicles in the Auerbach plexus, as revealed by electron microscopy. It was suggested that the depletion of the granular vesicles could be related to the release of catecholamines or other active substances, such as substance P, from granular stores (Tafuri et al., 1974; Freire-Maia, 1983).

5. Effects of scorpion toxin on the release of acetylcholine

Incubation of slices of rat brain with a purified toxin extracted from Tityus serrulatus venom released acetylcholine, due to actions on sodium channels, since the release was prevented by tetrodotoxin (Gomez et al., 1973).

On the other hand, in vitro incubation of strips of guinea pig ileum with Tityus serrulatus scorpion venom released a substance not pharmacologically distinguishable from acetylcholine (Diniz and Torres, 1968). This release was prevented by tetrodotoxin (Tazieffe-Depierre and Andrillon, 1973; Diniz et al., 1974).

To study the effects of scorpion toxin on the ileum, our group performed experiments on isolated rat and guinea pig ileum. A purified toxin obtained from T. serrulatus venom was without effect when added to the organ bath with a piece of rat ileum immersed in Tyrode solution containing tetrodotoxin (TTX). However, after the Tyrode solution (plus TTX)was washed out and replaced by a solution without TTX, a strong contraction of the ileum was recorded . Addition of TTX to the bath brought the muscle back close to its original tone. A second wash with Tyrode solution without TTX was followed by contraction of the ileum, which was abolished, in part, by atropine. Moreover, Tyrode solution with TTX did not prevent the postsynaptic action of acetylcholine. These data indicated that the effect of scorpion toxin, blocked by TTX, was presynaptic. To study further this effect, slices of rat and guinea pig ilea were incubated with purified scorpion toxin. The data showed that the release of acetylcholine induced by toxin was prevented by TTX; however after washing the slices with the incubation fluid and reincubation (without further addition of scorpion toxin or TTX), a large increase in the amount of released acetylcholine was measured.

Our results seem to indicate that scorpion toxin binds to a site different from the TTX-binding site, but its physiological effect (e.g., release of acetylcholine) depends on an action on sodium-conducting pore of the channel (Freire-Maia et al., 1976c; Freire-Maia, 1983).

At about the same time Catterall (1975) reached a similar conclusion, that is, scorpion toxin and TTX bind to different sites in electrically excitable neuroblastoma cells.Moreover,scorpion toxin controls allosterically the activity of the site which transport sodium ions and is blocked by TTX (Catterall, 1980).

E. Effects on the spleen

We have shown,up to now,that scorpion toxin presents both cholinergic and adrenergic effects . As the spleen has an exclusively sympathetic inervation, we thought worthwhile to sudy the effects of scorpion toxin on the isolated rat spleen strips. We showed that the contraction induced by toxin was not affected by hexamethonium, but was prevented by tetrodotoxin , guanethidine, reserpine or phenoxybenzamine. It was then concluded that the contraction of spleen strips evoked by scorpion toxin was due to release of catecholamines from sympathetic nerve endings with subsequent activation of alpha adrenergic receptors (Freire-Maia et al., 1976b, c).

F. Effects on the blood

1. Blood-clotting

Poisoning by Buthus tamulus scorpion venom led to a "diffuse intravascular coagulation" or "defibrination syndrome" (Devy et al., 1970; Reddy et al., 1972). On the other hand,Hamilton et al. (1974) showed that the venom of Palamneus gravimanus had a procoagulant activity, through activation of factor X. But, at high concentrations P. gravimanus presented an anticoagulant activity, through a delay in the thrombin clotting time. The Leiurus quinquestriatus scorpion venom had only a marked anticoagulant activity. These data indicate that, depending on the scorpion species, it would be possible to observe intravascular thrombosis or hemorrhage . Centruroides sculpturatus scorpion venom caused a sustained platelet aggregation in dogs. The neurotoxic fractions extracted from the venom did not mimic this effect (Longenecker and Longenecker Jr. 1981). The authors suggested that epinephrine, released by the venom, could induce the platelet aggregation and this, in turn, could contribute to the defribrination syndrome described by other authors.

2. Converting enzyme

Tityus serrulatus scorpion venom potentiated the action of bradykinin on isolated smooth muscle preparations (Araujo and Gomez, 1976). Later, it was shown that high concentrations of *Centruroides sculpturatus* scorpion venom inhibited the angiotensin converting enzyme (Longenecker *et al*., 1980). However, none of the neurotoxins isolated from the venom were inhibitory. The presence in scorpion venoms of substances which inhibit the converting enzyme and potentiates the actions of bradykinin are of interest and need further investigation.

3. White blood cells

A striking neutrophil leukocytosis was found in all cases of severe scorpion poisoning in children (Campos *et al*., 1980). For this reason we thought worthwhile to study the possible effects of scorpion toxin on the leukocyte count in the rat.Intravenous injection of a scorpion toxin, obtained from *Tityus serrulatus* venom, into anesthetized and unanesthetized rats induced leukocytosis, due to a significant increase of total number of neutrophils (Beker and Freire--Maia, 1983; Beker *et al*., 1985). This effect was suggested to be mediated by catecholamines released by the toxin.

G. Effects on the kidney

As we have previously said (see chapter A1, Hypertension), venoms from scorpions *Centruroides sculpturatus* and *Leiurus quinquestriatus* release catecholamines, which in turn acting on beta adrenergic receptors in rat kidneys release renin (La Grange,1977). On the other hand,injection of *Buthus minax* scorpion venom into unanesthetized rats caused a significant decrease in urine volume possible due to the release of the antidiuretic hormone (Ismail *et al*., 1978). According to the authors, urinary sodium, potassium and calcium were also significantly decreased in the first day of venom injection.

Finally, *Tityus serrulatus* scorpion venom decreased renal plasma flow, urine and sodium excretion, in anesthetized dogs. These effects were assumed to be due to the release of catecholamines from renal nerve endings (Xavier *et al*., 1986).

H. Metabolic effects

The complex effects evoked by scorpion toxin, described in this review, may interfere with the metabolic processes of the organism (El-Asmar, 1984). We will describe some of the metabolic effects of scorpion toxin.

1. Hyperglycemia and glycogenolysis

Scorpion venoms of several species induced hyperglycemia (Magalhães, 1938; Anguiano *et al*., 1956; Freire-Maia and Ferreira, 1961; Mohamed *et al*., 1972; El Asmar *et al*., 1974).

The mechanism of hyperglycemia is complex. According to Mohamed *et al*., (1972) the hyperglycemia evoked by venom from scorpion *Buthus quinquestriatus* was due to excessive hepatic output of glucose elicited by serotonin present in the venom. But, venoms of other species do not have serotonin in their composition. According to Anguiano *et al* (1956) the hyperglycemic effect induced by *Centruroides suffusus* in the cat was due to stimulation of nuclei in the central nervous system, which in turn induced the release of catecholamines from adrenal medulla. But, Freire-Maia and Ferreira (1961) showed that adrenalectomy in dogs did not prevent the hyperglycemia evoked by *Tityus bahiensis* venom in dogs; moreover,ganglionic blockade did not prevent the hyperglycemic effect, suggesting a peripheral effect of the venom; finally, a sympatholytic drug (clorpromazine) prevented the appearance of hyperglycemia. On the other hand, El Asmar *et al*. (1974) showed that *Buthus minax* venom induced hyperglycemia in rats and that alpha adrenergic blockade with tolazoline prevented the effect. As we have said in this review, scorpion venoms of several species release catecholamines. It seems likely that the catecholamines, by stimulating alpha adrenergic receptors, could increase the hepatic glycogenolysis and/or inhibit the insulin release. Actually, inhibition of insulin release by scorpion venom was reported by Johnson et al. (1976). Finally, an increased glucagon secretion induced by scorpion venom could contribute to the hyperglycemic effect (Johnson and Ensinck, 1976).

It is concluded that scorpion venom releases catecholamines by a peripheral effect and that the amines increase the hepatic glycogenolisis, through alpha adrenergic stimulation, with a subsequent hyperglycemic effect. An increase in glucagon secretion and/or an inhibition of insulin secretion could contribute to the appearance of hyperglycemia following scorpion venom injection.

2. Minerals

An increase in potassium level and a decrease in sodium level in plasma were observed following injection of Buthus quinquestriatus venom (Mohamed et al., 1954; Tash et al., 1982). On the other hand, injection in rats of Buthus minax for 5 days caused an increase in K^+ but no change in Na^+ level (Ismail et al., 1978).

3. Acid-base balance

Injections of crude venom of Leiurus quinquestriatus in rats caused metabolic alkalosis, which was compensated by respiratory acidosis. These effects explain the lack of change of blood pH following the venom administration (Tash et al., 1982). According to El-Asmar (1984) the metabolic alkalosis could be explained by an increase in HCl secretion in the stomach (Gonzaga et al., 1979; Mohamed et al., 1980; Cunha-Melo et al., 1983; Ghoneim et al., 1984;Cunha-Melo et al., 1987), whereas the respiratory acidosis could be due, at least in part, to pulmonary edema (Freire-Maia et al., 1978).

Injection of Fraction 1, a lethal fraction separated from the venom of L. quinquestriatus, induced a metabolic acidosis, which was aggravated by respiratory acidosis. As a consequence, this fraction decreased the blood pH of the rat (Tash et al., 1982).

The investigators interested in other metabolic effects induced by scorpion venom could read the review by El-Asmar (1984).

I. Central nervous system

The pathophysiology of scorpion poisoning was associated for several years with effects of the venom on the central nervous system (Waterman, 1938; Magalhães, 1938,1946; Del Pozo,1968; Osman et al., 1973; Efrati, 1978).

Intracerebroventricular (ICV) injection of crude venoms of the scorpions Centruroides sculpturatus and Vejovis spinigerus in cats induced neurological and respiratory disturbances and death of the animals (Russell and Bohr, 1962). On the other hand, Osman et al. (1973) showed that ICV injection of crude venom of Leiurus quinquestriatus in rabbits induced hyperthermia, restlessness, struggling and sometimes convulsion, urination and defecation. The pupils were fully dilated and the ears were cold.

Our group studied the ICV effects of a toxin purified from the Tityus serrulatus scorpion venom, in unanesthetized rats. Immediately after the injection, the following signs were observed: impairment of righting reflexes, tremors, twitching, hyper-reactivity, convulsions, extensor rigidity, peddling, opisthotonus, respiratory arrhythmias, pulmonary edema and death (Lima et al., 1975). The pulmonary edema was prevented by a previous injection of guanethidine in adrenalectomized rats. It was then suggested that the pulmonary edema was due to the release of catecholamines from adrenal glands and postganglionic nerve endings,as a consequence of excitation of central autonomic structures by scorpion toxin (Almeida et al., 1976).

In urethane-anesthetized rats, the ICV injection of scorpion toxin did not induce pulmonary edema. The toxin caused dramatic cardiovascular and respiratory effects, consisting of hypotension, tachypnea, hyperpnea, ataxic and gasping breathing. Following these initial effects, the toxin induced arterial hypertension and hyperpnea. The early respiratory arrhythmias and hypotension were related to central muscarinic mechanisms(Lima and Freire-Maia, 1977). As incubation of rat brain slices with scorpion toxin released acetylcholine (Gomez et al., 1973) we assumed that this mediator, released by toxin,could induce the early respiratory arrhythmias and hypotension. On the other hand, the hypertensive effect induced by toxin was partially prevented by ICV phenoxybenzamine (Lima and Freire-Maia, 1977). As noradrenaline (NA) was released by scorpion toxin from synaptosomes prepared from rat brain (Moss et al.,1974), we assumed that ICV injection of scorpion toxin released NA from brain structures, with subsequent activation of central alpha adrenergic receptors,leading to a peripheral arterial hypertension.

We think that either the ICV injections of scorpion toxin (e.g., Lima and Freire-Maia, 1977) or the incubation of rat brain slices with the toxin (Gomez et al., 1973; Moss et al., 1974; Dolly et al., 1978) have an important academic interest. But, based on 20 years of research in the field we think that subcutaneous, intramuscular or intravenous injections of scorpion toxin produce their effects through peripheral actions (Freire-Maia and Diniz, 1970; Freire-Maia et al., 1973, 1974, 1976a; Freire-Maia, 1983). This assumption is corroborated by experiments which showed that following intramuscular or intraperitoneal injections of ^{125}I -labelled scorpion venom, the lowest radioactivity was found in the brain (Ismail et al., 1974).

J. Chemical composition and mechanism of action

Several polypeptide neurotoxins active on mammalian tissue have been isolated and purified from scorpion venoms of many species (see reviews in Rochat et al.,1979; Possani et al., 1984). On the other hand, scorpion venoms of several species(*Tityus serrulatus*, *Tityus bahiensis*, *Palamneus gravimanus*, *Hadrurus arizonaensis*, *Vejovis spinigerus*, *Paroroctnus mesaensis* and others) contain a high molecular weight protein with hyaluronidase activity (Diniz and Gonçalves, 1960; Wright et al., 1977; Possani et al., 1977). It seems likely that hyaluronidase may contribute to the toxicity of the crude venoms, by promoting the spread of the neurotoxins through the tissues (Wright et al., 1977). *Tityus serrulatus* venom does not present phospholipase, cholinesterase, phosphodiesterase, protease, amylase or fibrinolytic activities (Diniz and Gonçalves, 1960; Possani et al., 1977). But,scorpion venoms of other species present some of these enzymatic activities. So, cholinesterase was detected in *Vejovis spinigerus* scorpion venom (Russell,1967) and alkaline phosphatase was present in the venom of the scorpion *Palamneus gravimanus* (Wright et al., 1977). Finally, some scorpion venoms contain autacoides in their composition, such as serotonin in *Leiurus quinquestriatus* (Adam and Weiss, 1958) and histamine in *Palamneus gravimanus* (Ismail et al., 1975).

We think that it would be important to keep in mind the presence of enzymes or autacoides in scorpion venoms, when one try to explain the mechanism of action of some crude venoms.

K. Mechanism of action at molecular level

It is out of the purpose of this review on the pathophysiology of scorpion poisoning to study in details the mechanisms of action of scorpion toxins at the molecular levels. Many investigators have shown that mammalian scorpion toxins are low molecular weight proteins, of about 7000 daltons and composed of a single polypeptide chain cross-linked by four disulfide bridges (Rochat et al., 1979). Some crude scorpion venoms present also in their compositions toxins which are specific to insects or crustaceans (Zlotkin et al., 1978).

It seems likely that the majority of the effects of the mammalian toxins on the body are due to direct actions on sodium channels (Catterall, 1980; Couraud and Jover, 1984). According to Koppenhöfer and Schmidt (1968) and Narahashi et al. (1972) the effects of *Leiurus* and *Buthus* scorpion venoms were explained by a delay in the sodium inactivation, whereas Cahalan (1975) showed that *Centruroides* scorpion venom induced the appearance of a new sodium current. Based on these different data, Cahalan (1975) presented the hypothesis that venoms from scorpions of the Old World (e.g., *Buthus*) delay the sodium inactivation, while venoms from scorpions of the New World (e.g., *Centruroides*) induce the appearance of a new sodium current.

On the other hand, Catterall (1980) showed that there are three separate toxin receptor sites associated with sodium channel. Receptor site I binds tetrodotoxin and saxitoxin, which inhibit ion transport.Receptor site II binds the liposoluble toxins veratridine, batrachotoxin, aconitine and grayanotoxin. These toxins alter both activation and inactivation of sodium channels. Receptor site III binds scorpion toxin and sea anemone toxin. These toxins inhibit inactivation of sodium channel. Moreover, and according to Couraud et al. (1982), toxins purified from scorpions originating from Africa or Asia (e.g. *Androctonus australis*, *Leiurus quinquestriatus* and *Buthus occitanus*) are called α-scorpion toxins and bind to the receptor site III, whereas toxins purified from North Americans scorpions(e.g.*Centruroides sculpturatus*) are called β-scorpion toxins and bind to a different receptor site in the sodium channel (site IV). On the other hand, toxins purified from the South American scorpion *Tityus serrulatus* have different bindings on sodium channel. Then, tityustoxin or TsTX (Gomez and Diniz, 1966)binds to receptor site III, being therefore an α-scorpion toxin, whereas TsTX I (Toledo and Neves,1976), also called γ-toxin (Possani et al., 1977) and T_1 VIII (Sampaio et al., 1983), binds to the same receptor site as Centruroides, being therefore a β-scorpion toxin (Jover et al., 1980; Couraud et al., 1982; Barhanin et al., 1982).

It seems likely that the physio-pharmacological effects induced by scorpion toxins are due to actions on specific sites of sodium channels, with a subsequent depolarization of the membranes. The respiratory arrhythmias are due, at least in part, to depolarizations of visceral afferent fibers, induced by the toxin (Freire-Maia, 1983), whereas the other effects described in this review are mainly due to release from nerve endings of chemical mediators such as acetylcholine and catecholamines.

TREATMENT

Scorpion toxicity and human accidents

According to Bücherl (1978) the mean yield of venom obtained by electric extraction from *Tityus serrulatus* scorpions was 0,07 mg, whereas the LD50 value was 0,016 mg of venom, intravenously injected in 20 g mice (or 0,8 mg/kg). On the other hand, the *T. serrulatus* scorpion sting may cause the death of 3-5% of school children and 15-20% of babies and young children (Bücherl, 1978), indicating that the toxicity of this venom is much higher to humans than to laboratory animals, such as the mice.

Our clinical experience

From January 1972 to December 1987 (16 years period), 3.860 patients stung by scorpions were admitted at the Toxicological Center of the Hospital João XXIII, Belo Horizonte, Brazil. From these patients, 2.822 (73%) were adults and 1.038 (27%) were children from 0 to 14 years old. The scorpion were usually classified as *Tityus serrulatus* Lutz and Mello, 1922.

Clinical findings.

The symptomatology in adults consisted usually of pain at the site of sting. They were observed during 2 or 3 hours. When the pain was severe, the patients received an injection of an analgesic, e.g., dipirone.

From the 1.038 children attended at the Hospital, 168 (16,18%) presented a severe picture of scorpion poisoning. The most prominent clinical findings in these patients are shown in Table 1.

These clinical findings are similar to those induced by *Tityus trinitatis* (Poon-King, 1963), *Buthus tamulus* (Santhanakrishnan and Raju, 1974), *Centruroides sculpturatus* (Rimsza et al., 1980) and *Leiurus quinquestriatus* (Efrati, 1949; Hershkovich et al., 1985). Some differences are, however, remarkable among the findings of the latter authors and our data; then, pain was present in 100% of our patients, whereas Hershkovich et al.(1985) did not describe this symptom in their patients; on the other hand, priapism is present in 55% of their patients, whereas it was noted only in 1% of our patients. The reasons for such differences are not known.

Patients with high risk or main physiological system instability following a scorpion sting must be admitted to an Intensive Care Unit, for constant clinical evaluation and electrocardiographic monitoring (Campos et al., 1979, 1980; Freire-Maia and Campos, 1987). This type of treatment was also recommended by Rimsza et al. (1980) and Goyffon et al. (1982).

We have treated, in a 16 years period, 2.822 adults and 1.038 children stung by scorpions of the genus *Tityus* (usually *T. serrulatus*). The mild cases of intoxication were treated with symptomatic measures, whereas the severe cases were treated with symptomatic measures, support of vital functions and intravenous injection of antivenom. The following parameters were charted: pulse rate, arterial blood pressure, respiration rate and urine flow. The patients underwent continuous electrocardiografic monitoring to permit the early diagnosis and treatment of cardiac arrhythmias, and ventilatory support through oxygentherapy or positive pressure respiration. Pain was abolished by injection of dipirone (40-80 mg/kg/day). Vomiting, present in 86% cases, could induce electrolyte and acid-base imbalances, or even dehydration, and was treated by intravenous injection of metoclopramide (0.5 - 1.0 mg/kg), followed by oral administration of the same drug, 2-3 times a day. Hyperthermia was controlled with dipirone and/or tepid water sponging. In cases of cardiac failure and pulmonary edema the treatment consisted of support of vital functions, limb tourniquet to decrease the venous return and

Table 1. Clinical findings of severe scorpion poisoning by *Tityus serrulatus* in children (168 cases)

CLINICAL FINDINGS	No of CASES	%	CLINICAL FINDINGS	No of CASES	%
Pain at site of sting	168	100	Congestive heart failure	25	15
Vomiting	144	86	Acute pulmonary edema	20	12
Tachycardia	126	75	Hypothermia	19	11
Tachypnea	94	56	Bradycardia	17	10
Profuse sweting	79	47	Pallor	17	10
Restlessness	54	32	Tremors	14	08
Somnolence	42	25	Arterial hypertension	12	07
Abnormal breathing sounds	39	23	Decrease of capillary perfusion	10	06
Cardiac arrhythmias (other than			Mental confusion	10	06
tachycardia or bradycardia)	30	18	Cardiac arrest	08	05
Hyperthermia	29	17	Convulsion	08	05
Dehydration	29	17	Cyanosis	07	04
Dyspnea	26	16	Dizziness	07	04
Prostation	26	16	Shock	05	03

Other findings were found in less than 3% of the patients.

antivenom (Butantan Institute, São Paulo, Brazil), intravenously injected at a dose of 20-40ml. We have also injected digitalis and a diuretic agent (furosemide) in some patients presenting severe sinus tachycardia and clinical evidences of congestive heart failure and pulmonary edema.

We do not recommend atropine for our patients as a routine therapeutic measure, since experimental data had shown that it potentiated the hypertensive effect and increased the severity of the pulmonary edema induced by scorpion toxin in the rat (Freire-Maia *et al*., 1974, 1978). But, when scorpion venom produces a severe bradycardia (caused by sinus arrest or complete A-V block) then atropine (0.005-0.02 mg/kg) should be i.v. injected as an emergence measure.

We do not recommend also the routine use of propranolol for our patients, because experimental data have shown that although it prevents the appearance of sinus tachycardia, it does not prevent either A-V block in anesthetized rats (Freire-Maia *et al*., 1974) or pulmonary edema in unanesthetized rats (Freire-Maia *et al*., 1978).

As far as the use of alpha adrenergic blocking agents in scorpion poisoning, clinical investigations are needed to evaluate the efficacy of these agents in cases of severe arterial hypertension induced by scorpion venom in humans (Rimsza *et al*., 1980; Gueron and Ovsyshcher, 1987; Freire-Maia and Campos, 1987).

Some investigators recommend phenobarbital and/or diazepam in patients presenting restlessness (Stahnke, 1978; Rimsza *et al*.,1980). We do not prescribe these drugs to our children poisoned by scorpion venom because they could cause sedation in the patients or even precipitate a respiratory paralysis.

Cardiac arrhythmias other than sinus tachycardia and sinus bradycardia were present in 18% of the patients. The arrhythmias were the following: ventricular ectopic beats, complete A-V heart block, sinus arrest and wandering pacemakers. The ectopic beats or the wandering pacemakers disappeared from 12 to 48 hours after the sting, without prescription of antiarrhythmic drugs.

In some cases of circulatory shock we prescribed hydrocortisone to our patients. On the other hand some authors recommend the use of antihistamines to patients stung by scorpions. Our group do not recommend the routine use of an antihistamine to children stung by scorpions. As there is the possibility that histamine is involved in the genesis of pulmonary edema and increased gastric secretion induced by scorpion toxin (Freire-Maia et al., 1978; Cunha-Melo et al.,1987), we think that clinical investigations should be made to evaluate the efficacy of H_1 and H_2 histamine receptor blockers in the treatment of scorpion poisoning.

Antivenom. According to Gueron and Ovsyshcher (1984, 1987) there is no value of antivenom in the treatment or prevention of the cardiovascular manifestations of scorpion poisoning. We do not agree with this statement (Campos et al., 1979, 1980; Freire-Maia and Campos, 1987;and this paper).

We have demonstrated that i.v. injection of scorpion antivenom before scorpion toxin almost totally prevented the cardiovascular and respiratory effects induced by i.v. toxin in the rat (Freire-Maia et al., 1976a). These experiments clearly show that antivenom is an important therapeutic measure to neutralize the circulating venom. As the scorpions do not usually inoculate the venom directly into the blood but into interstitial tissue, we recommend i.v. injection of antivenom immediately after the admission of children, severely poisoned by scorpions, at the Emergency Hospital, in order to neutralize the circulating venom and the venom which is being absorbed from the site of the sting into the circulation (Campos et al ., 1980).

On the other hand, it seems likely that antivenom or immunoglubulins injected i.v. could act at the tissue level the following day (Ismail et al., 1983). Therefore,it would be very important to treat with symptomatic measures the patients in an Intensive Care Unit, besides the administration i.v. of antivenom. Moreover, the vital functions should be supported (artificial ventilation, correction of hydroelectrolytic disturbances,etc.).

Gueron and Ovsyshcher (1984), reporting the incidence of fatal cases of scorpion envenomation, have said that "Efrati in 1949 reported 27%, and in other comunications it ranged from 3.5 to 60%..." (Efrati, 1949). In Brazil Magalhães (1938) reported a mortality rate of 3.5% without antivenom and 1.8% in patients who received antivenom. With our method of treating benign cases with symptomatic measures and severe cases of poisoning with symptomatic measures, support of vital functions and antivenom in an Intensive Care Unit, this rate decreased to 0.26% (Campos et al.,1979,1980). The value of serotherapy can also be demonstraded in Israel, where the mortality rate is high when the treatment of scorpion poisoning does not include the antivenom (Gueron and Ovsyshcher, 1984, 1987) and low when the treatment includes the administration of antivenom (Herskovich et al.,1985). In Tunisia,the severe cases of poisoning by scorpions are caused by *Androctonus australis* and *Androctonus aeneas*; the serotherapy with a specific antivenom is considered the main element of the therapeutics (Goyffon et al.,1982).

Finally, we would like to stress, once more, that from 3.860 patients stung by scorpions in a 16 years period, and treated by our group, the mortality rate was very low, that is, 0.28%. It is important to stress, also, that all patients who died were children, admitted to the Emergency Hospital more than 3 hours following the sting.

Acknowledgements

This paper was supported by the Brazilian agencies FINEP and CNPq. One of the authors (LFM) is reciptient of a fellowship from CNPq. The authors thank Dr. A.D. Azevedo, Dr. J. R. Cunha-Melo and Dr. C.R. Diniz for their comments on a preliminary version of this review, and Mrs.Maria Celia Silva Costa, for typing the manuscript.

REFERENCES

Adam, K.R. and C. Weiss (1958). The occurence of 5-hydroxytriptamine in scorpion venom. J. exp. Biol., 35, 39-41.

Adam, K.R. and C.Weiss (1959). Action of scorpion venom on skeletal muscle. Br. J. Pharmac. 14, 334-339.

Adam, K.R. and C. Weiss (1966). Some aspects of the pharmacology of the venoms of african scorpions. Mem. Inst. Butantan, 33, 603-614.

Almeida, A.P., N.C. Alpoim and L. Freire-Maia (1982). Effects of a purified scorpion toxin (tityustoxin) on the isolated guinea pig heart. Toxicon, 20, 855-865.

Almeida, H.O., E.G. Lima and L. Freire-Maia (1976). Mechanism of acute pulmonary edema induced by intracerebroventricular injection of scorpion toxin (tityustoxin) in the unanesthetized rat. Toxicon, 14,435-440.

Andrade, S.P., R.A.S. Santos and W.T. Beraldo (1981). Comparative study of the action of purified scorpion toxin (tityustoxin) on the submandibular and parotid glands of the rat.

Toxicon, 19, 255-261.

Anguiano, G., C. Beyer and M. Alcárâz (1956). Mecanismo fisiológico de la hiperglicemia causada por el veneno de alacrán. Bol. Inst. Est. Med. Biol., 14, 93-101.

Araujo, R.L. and M.V. Gomez (1976). Potentiation of bradykinin action on smooth muscle by a scorpion venom extract. Gen. Pharmac.. 7, 123-126.

Azevedo, A.D., J.R. Cunha-Melo and L. Freire-Maia (1979). Arterial hypertension and pulmonary edema induced by catecholamines in unanesthetized rats. Pharmacol. Res. Comm., 11, 157-167.

Azevedo, A.D., A.B. Silva, J.R. Cunha-Melo and L. Freire-Maia (1983). Cardiovascular and respiratory effects induced by a purified scorpion toxin (tityustoxin) in unanesthetized rats. Toxicon, 21, 753-759.

Barhanin, J., J.R. Giglio, P. Leopold, A. Schmid, S.V. Sampaio and M. Lazdunski (1982). Tityus serrulatus venom contains two classes of toxins - Tityus γ toxin is a new tool with a very high affinity for studying the Na^+ channel. J. Biol. Chem., 257, 12553-12558.

Bartholomew, C. (1970). Acute scorpion pancreatitis in Trinidad. Br. med. J., 1, 668-670.

Bartholomew, C., J.J. Murphy, O. Fitzgerald and K.F. McGeeney (1975). Action of Tityus trinitatis venom on the canine pancreas. Toxicon, 13, 87.

Bartholomew, C., J.J. Murphy, O. Fitzgerald and K.F. McGeeney (1976). Experimental studies on the etiology of acute scorpion pancreatitis. Br. J. Surg. 63, 807-810.

Beavallet, M., J. Cheymol, F. Bourillet and M. Roch-Arveiller (1972). Contribution à l'etude d'action de venins de scorpions sur la sécrétion médullo-surrénale.J.Physiol. (Paris), 345A.

Beker, M.A.C.L. and L. Freire-Maia (1983). Neutrophil leukocytosis induced by injection of tityustoxin in the anesthetized rat. Brazilian J. Med. Biol. Res., 16, 478.

Beker, M.A.C.L., N.P. Silveira and L. Freire-Maia (1985). Effects of tityustoxin on the leukocyte count in unanesthetized rats. Brazilian J. Med. Biol. Res., 18, 772A.

Benoit, P.R. and J. Mambrini (1967). Action du venin de scorpion sur la jonction neuromusculaire de la grenouille. J. Physiol. (Paris), 59, 348.

Beraldo, W.T. and W. Dias da Silva (1966). Release of histamine by animal venoms and bacterial toxins. In O. Eichler and A. Farah (Ed.), Handbook of Experimental Pharmacology, Vol.XVIII/1, Springer-Verlag, Berlin, pp.334-366.

Böhm, G.M., S. Pompolo, C.R. Diniz, M.V. Gomez, A.F. Pimenta and J.C. Netto (1974). Ultrastructural alterations of mouse diaphragm nerve endings induced by purified scorpion venom (tityustoxin). Toxicon, 12, 509-511.

Braun, K., Stern, S., Werkson, S. and Yalon, S. (1970). Hemodynamic and electrocardiographic changes induced by scorpion venom: an experimental study. Toxicon, 8, 126.

Bücherl, W. (1978). Venoms of Titynae. A. Systematics, Distribution, Biology, Venomous Apparatus, etc. of Titynae; Venom Collection, Toxicity, Human Accidents and Treatment of Stings. In S. Bettini (Ed.), Arthropod Venoms, Springer-Verlag, Berlin, pp. 371-379.

Cahalan, M.D. (1975). Modification of sodium channel gating in frog myelinated nerve fibres by Centruroides sculpturatus scorpion venom. J. Physiol. (London), 244, 511-534.

Campos, J.A., O.A. Silva, M. Lopez and L. Freire-Maia (1979). Signs, symptoms and treatment of severe scorpion sting in children. Toxicon, 17 (suppl. 1), 19.

Campos, J.A., O.A. Silva, M. Lopez and L. Freire-Maia (1980). Signs, symptoms and treatment of severe scorpion poisoning in children. In D. Eaker and T. Wadström (Ed.), Natural Toxins, Pergamon, Oxford, pp. 61-68.

Catanzaro, O.L., R.A.S. Santos, O.M. Parra, R.M. Santos, L. Freire-Maia and W.T. Beraldo(1978). Effect of scorpion toxin (tityustoxin, TsTX) on the salivary gland of the rat, in vivo and in vitro. Agents Actions, 8, 119-124.

Catterall, W.A. (1975). Cooperative activation of action potential Na^+ ionophore by neurotoxins. Proc. Natl. Acad. Sci. USA, 72: 1782-1786.

Catterall, W.A. (1980). Neurotoxins that act on voltage-sensitive sodium channels in excitable membranes. Annu. Rev. Pharmacol. Toxicol. 20, 15-43.

Celeste Henriques, M., G. Gazzineli, C.R. Diniz, and M.V. Gomez (1968). Effect of the venom of the Tityus serrulatus on adrenal gland catecholamines. Toxicon, 5, 175-179.

Cheymol, J., F. Bourillet, M. Roch-Arveiller and J. Heckle (1974). Action cardiovasculaire de trois venins de scorpions Nord Africains (Androctonus australis, Leiurus quinquestriatus, Buthus occitanus) et de deux toxines extraites de l'un d'entre eux. Toxicon, 12, 241-248.

Corrado, A.P., A. Antonio and C.R. Diniz (1968). Brazilian scorpion venom (Tityus serrulatus), an unusual sympathetic postganglionic stimulant. J. Pharmac. Exp. Ther., 164, 253-258.

Corrado, A.P., F. Ricciopo Neto and A. Antonio (1974). The mechanism of the hypertensive effect of Brazilian scorpion venom (Tityus serrulatus, Lutz and Mello). Toxicon, 12, 145-150.

Couraud, F. and E. Jover (1984). Mechanism of action of scorpion toxins. In A. Tu (Ed.), Handbook of Natural Toxins, Vol. 2, Marcel Dekker, New York, pp. 659-678.

Couraud, F., E. Jover, J.M. Dubois and H. Rochat (1982). Two types of scorpion toxin receptor sites, one related to the activation the other to the inactivation of the action potential sodium channel. Toxicon, 20, 9-16.

Cunha-Melo, J.R., L. Freire-Maia, W.L. Tafuri and T.A. Maria (1973). Mechanism of action of purified scorpion toxin on the isolated rat intestine. Toxicon, 11, 81-84.

Cunha-Melo, J.R., H.M.S. Gonzaga, F. Alzamora and L. Freire-Maia (1983). Effects of purified scorpion toxin (tityustoxin) on gastric secretion in the rat. Toxicon, 21, 843-848.
Cunha-Melo, J.R., A.P. Almeida, H.M.S. Gonzaga, M.V. Gomez and L. Freire-Maia (1987). Effect of scorpion toxin on gastric histamine and acetylcholine content in the rat. Brazilian J. Med. Biol. Res. 20, 393-401.
Del Pozo, E.C. (1968). Farmacologia de los venenos de los Centruroides Mexicanos. Rev. Invest. Salud Publica (Mexico), 28, 51-66.
Del Pozo, E.C. and L.G. Anguiano (1947). Acciones del veneno de alacran sobre la actividad motora del musculo estriado. Rev. Inst. Salub. Enferm. Trop., 8, 231-263.
Devi, C.S., C.N. Reddy, S.L. Devi, Y.R. Subrahmanyam, H.V. Bhatt, G. Suvarnakumari, D.P. Murthy and C.R.R.M. Reddy (1970). Defibrination syndrome due to scorpion venom poisoning. Br. Med. J., 1, 345-347.
Diniz, C.R. (1978). Chemical and pharmacologic aspects of Tityinae venoms. In S. Bettini (Ed.), Arthopod Venoms, Springer-Verlag, Berlin, pp. 379-394.
Diniz, C.R. and J.M. Gonçalves (1956). Some chemical and pharmacological properties of Brazilian scorpion venoms. In E. Buckley and N. Porges (Ed.), Venoms, Am. Assoc. Adv. Sci., Washington, pp. 131-139.
Diniz, C.R. and V. Valeri (1959). Effects of a toxin present in a purified extract of telson from the scorpion Tityus serrulatus on smooth muscle preparations and in mice. Archs. int. Pharmacodyn. 71, 1-12.
Diniz, C.R. and J.M. Gonçalves (1960). Separation of biologically active components from scorpion venom by zone electrophoresis. Biochim. biophys. Acta, 41, 470-477.
Diniz, C.R. and J.M. Torres (1968). Release of an acetylcholine-like substance from guinea-pig ileum by scorpion venom. Toxicon, 5, 227-236.
Diniz, C.R., A.F. Pimenta, J. Coutinho Netto, S. Pompolo, M.V. Gomez and G.M. Böhm (1974). Effect of scorpion venom from Tityus serrulatus (tityustoxin) on the acetylcholine release and fine structure of the nerve terminals (1974). Experientia (Basel), 30, 1304-1305.
Dolly, O.J., C.K. Tse, J.W. Spokes and C.R. Diniz (1978). Effects of β-bungarotoxin and tityustoxin on uptake and release of neurotransmitters. Bioch. Soc. Trans., 6, 652-654.
Efrati, P. (1949). Poisoning by scorpion stings in Israel. Am. J. Trop. Med., 29, 249-257.
Efrati, P. (1978). Epidemiology, symptomatology and treatment of Buthinae stings. In S. Bettini (Ed.), Arthropod Venoms, Springer-Verlag, Berlin, pp. 312-317.
El-Asmar, M.F. (1984). Metabolic effect of scorpion venom. In A. Tu (Ed.), Handbook of Natural Toxins, Vol. 2, Marcel Dekker, New York, pp. 551-575.
El-Asmar, M.F., O.H. Osman and M. Ismail (1973). Fractionation and lethality of venom from the scorpion Buthus minax, (L.Koch). Toxicon, 11, 3-7.
El-Asmar, M.F., S.F. Soliman, M. Ismail and O.H. Osman (1974). Glycemic effect of venom from the scorpion Buthus minax (L. Koch). Toxicon, 12, 249-251.
Fayet, G., F. Couraud, F. Miranda, S. Lissitzky (1974). Electro-optical system for monitoring activity of heart cells in culture: application to the study of several drugs and scorpion toxins. Eur. J. Pharmac. 27, 165-174.
Freire-Maia, L. (1983). Neurotoxins as tools for physiological investigation. Physiologist, 26, 381-390.
Freire-Maia, L., and M.C. Ferreira (1961). Estudo do mecanismo da hiperglicemia e da hipertensão arterial, produzidas pelo veneno de escorpião, no cão (Abstract in English). Mem. Inst. Oswaldo Cruz, 59, 11-22.
Freire-Maia, L., and C.R. Diniz (1970). Pharmacological action of a purified scorpion toxin in the rat. Toxicon, 8, 132.
Freire-Maia, L., and J.A. Campos (1987). Response to the Letter to the Editor by Gueron and Ovsyshcher - On the treatment of the cardiovascular manifestations of scorpin envenomation. Toxicon, 25, 125-130.
Freire-Maia, L., R.M. Ribeiro, and W.T. Beraldo (1970). Effects of purified scorpion toxin on respiratory movements in the rat. Toxicon, 8, 307-310.
Freire-Maia, L., A.D. Azevedo, and V.P. Costa Val (1973). Respiratory arrhythmias produced by purified scorpion toxin. Toxicon, 11, 255-257.
Freire-Maia, L., G.I. Pinto, and I. Franco (1974). Mechanism of the cardiovascular effects produced by purified scorpion toxin in the rat. J. Pharmac. exp. Ther., 188, 207-213.
Freire-Maia, L., A.D. Azevedo, and E.G. Lima (1976a). Pharmacological blockade of the cardiovascular and respiratory effects produced by tityustoxin in the rat. In A. Ohsaka, K. Hayashi, and Y. Sawai (Ed.), Animal, Plant, and Microbial Toxins, Vol. 2, Plenum, New York, pp. 287-298.
Freire-Maia, L., J.R. Cunha-Melo, H.A. Futuro-Neto, A.D. Azevedo, and J. Weinberg (1976b). Cholinergic and adrenergic effects of tityustoxin. Gen. Pharmac., 7, 115-121.
Freire-Maia, L., J.R. Cunha-Melo, M.V. Gomez, W.L. Tafuri, T.A. Maria, S.L. Calixto, and H.A. Futuro-Neto (1976c). Studies on the mechanism of action of tityustoxin. In A. Ohsaka, K. Hayashi, and Y. Sawai (Ed.), Animal, Plant, and Microbial Toxins, Vol. 2, Plenum, New York, pp. 273-285.

Freire-Maia, L., H.O. Almeida, J.R. Cunha-Melo, A.D. Azevedo, and J. Barroso (1978). Mechanism of the pulmonary edema induced by intravenous injection of scorpion toxin in the rat. Agents Actions, 8, 113-118.
Gallagher, S., H. Sankaran and J.A. Williams (1981). Mechanism of scorpion toxin-induced enzyme secretion in rat pancreas. Gastroenterology, 80, 970.
Garcia Leme, J., A.F. Pimenta, M. Raulino-Filho and C.R. Diniz (1978). Sensory nerves and inflammation: evidence for the release of a neurogenic permeability factor by tityustoxin. J. Path., 124, 165-176.
Ghoneim, K., F.M. Tash, A.S. Eifiky and M.F. El-Asmar (1984). Effect of scorpion (Leiurus quinquestriatus H and E) venom on gastric secretion. Egyptian J. Biochem., 2, 73-87.
Gomez, M.V. and C.R. Diniz (1966). Separation of toxic components from the Brazilian scorpion-Tityus serrulatus - venom. Mem. Inst. Butantan, 33, 899-902.
Gomez, M.V., M.E.M. Dai and C.R. Diniz (1973). Effect of scorpion venom, tityustoxin, on the release of acetylcholine from incubated slices of rat brain. J. Neurochem., 20, 1051-1061.
Gonzaga, H.M.S., F. Alzamora, J.R. Cunha-Melo and L. Freire-Maia (1979). Gastric secretion induced by scorpion toxin. Toxicon, 17, 316-318.
Goyffon, M., M. Vachon and N. Broglio (1982). Epidemiological and clinical characteristics of the scorpion envenomation in Tunisia. Toxicon, 20, 337-344.
Gueron, M. and R. Yaron (1970). Cardiovascular manifestations of severe scorpion sting. Clinicopathologic correlations. Chest, 57, 156-162.
Gueron, M. and I. Ovsyshcher (1984). Cardiovascular effects of scorpion venoms. In A. Tu (Ed.) Handbook of Natural Toxins, Vol. 2, Marcel Dekker, New York, pp. 639-657.
Gueron, M. and I. Ovsyschcher (1987). Letter to the Editor - What is the treatment for the cardiovascular manifestations of scorpion envenomation? Toxicon, 25, 121-124.
Gueron, M., J. Stern and W. Cohen (1967). Severe myocardial damage and heart failure in scorpion sting. Am. J. Cardiol., 19, 719-726.
Gueron, M., R.J. Adolph, I.L. Grupp, M. Gabel, G. Grupp and N.O. Fowler (1980). Hemodynamic and myocardial consequences of scorpion venom. Am. J. Cardiol. 45, 979-986.
Grupp, G., I.L. Grupp, M. Gueron, F. Adolph and N.O. Fowler (1980). Direct myocardial effects of the yellow scorpion (Leiurus quinquestriatus) venom on contractile force of isolated guinea pig atria and papillary muscles. IRCS Med. Sci., 8, 666-667.
Habermehl, G.G. (1981). Venomous animals and their toxins. Springer-Verlag, Berlin, pp. 21-31.
Hamilton, P.J., D. Ogston and A.S. Douglas (1974). Coagulant activity of the scorpion venoms Palamneus gravimanus and Leiurus quinquestriatus. Toxicon, 12, 291-296.
Hassan, F. (1984). Production of scorpion antivenin. In A. Tu (Ed.), Handbook of Natural Toxins, vol. 2, Marcel Dekker, New York, pp. 577-605.
Hershkovich, Y., Y. Elitsur, C.Z. Margolis, N. Barak, S. Sofer and S.W. Moses (1985). Criteria map audit of scorpion envenomation in the Negev, Israel. Toxicon, 23, 845-851.
Ismail, M., O.H. Osman and M.F. El-Asmar (1973). Pharmacological studies of the venom from the scorpion Buthus minax (L. Koch). Toxicon, 11, 15-20.
Ismail, M., G. Kertesz, O.H. Osman and M.S. Sidra (1974). Distribution of ^{125}I labelled scorpion (Leiurus quinquestriatus H & E) venom in rat tissues. Toxicon, 12, 209-211.
Ismail, M., M.F. El-Asmar and O.H. Osman (1975). Pharmacological studies with scorpion (Palamneus gravimanus) venom: evidence for the presence of histamine. Toxicon, 13, 49-56.
Ismail, M., O.H. Osman and D. Petkovic (1976). Electrocardiographic studies with scorpion (Buthus minax, L. Koch) venom. Toxicon, 14, 79-83.
Ismail, M., K.A. Gumaa, O.H. Osman and M.F. El-Asmar (1978). Effect of Buthus minax (L.Koch) scorpion venom on plasma and urinary electrolyte levels. Toxicon, 16, 385-392.
Ismail, M., A.M. Shibl, A.M. Morad, and M.E. Abdullah (1983). Pharmacokinetics of ^{125}I-labelled antivenin to the venom from the scorpion Androctonus amoreuxi. Toxicon, 21, 47-56.
Johnson, D.G. and J.W. Ensinck (1976). Stimulation of glucagon secretion by scorpion toxin in the perfused rat pancreas. Diabetes, 25, 645-649.
Johnson, D.G., D.P. Henry, J. Moss and R.H. Williams (1976). Inhibition of insulin release by scorpion toxin in rat pancreatic islets. Diabetes, 25, 198-201.
Jover, E., F. Couraud and H. Rochat (1980). Two types of scorpion neurotoxins characterized by their binding to two separate receptor sites on rat brain synaptosomes. Biochem. Biophys. Res. Comm., 95, 1607-1614.
Katz, N.L. and C. Edwards (1972). The effect of scorpion venom on the neuromuscular junction of the frog. Toxicon, 10, 133-137.
Koppenhöfer, E. and H. Schmidt (1968). Incomplete sodium inactivation in nodes of Ranvier treated with scorpion venom. Experientia (Basel), 24, 41-42.
La Grange, R.G (1977). Elevation of blood pressure and plasma renin levels by venom from scorpions, Centruroides sculpturatus and Leiurus quinquestriatus. Toxicon, 15, 429-433.
Langer, S.Z., E. Adler-Graschinsky, A.P. Almeida and C.R. Diniz (1975). Prejunctional effect of a purified toxin from the scorpion Tityus serrulatus. Naunyn-Schmiedebergs Arch. Pharmac., 287,243-259.

Lima, E.G. and L. Freire-Maia (1977). Cardiovascular and respiratory effects induced by intracerebroventricular injection of scorpion toxin (tityustoxin) in the rat. Toxicon, 15, 225-234.

Lima, E.G., H.O. Almeida, M.V. Gomez and L. Freire-Maia (1975). Acute pulmonary edema induced by injection of tityustoxin into the lateral ventricles of rats. Toxicon, 13, 205-206.

Lin, S., W. Tseng and C.Y. Lee (1975). Pharmacology of scorpion toxin II in the skeletal muscle. Naunyn Schmiedebergs Arch. Pharmac., 289, 359-368.

Longenecker, G.L. and H.E. Longenecker Jr.(1981). Centruroides sculpturatus venom and platelet reactivity: Possible role in scorpion venom induced defibrination syndrome. Toxicon, 19, 153-157.

Longenecker, G.L., H.E. Longenecker Jr., D. Watt, C.G. Huggins and C.A. Peterson (1980). Inhibition of the angiotensin converting enzyme by venom of the scorpion Centruroides sculpturatus. Toxicon, 18, 667-670.

Machado, J.C. and J.F. Silveira Filho (1976/77). Indução de pancreatite hemorragica aguda no cão por veneno escorpiônico de T. serrulatus. Mem. Inst. Butantan, 40/41, 1-9.

Magalhães, O.C. (1938). Scorpionism. J. Trop. Med. Hyg., 41, 393-399.

Magalhães, O.C. (1946). Escorpionismo. IV Memória. Monografias Inst. Oswaldo Cruz, Imprensa Nacional, Rio de Janeiro, pp 1-220.

Mazzotti, L. and M.A. Bravo Becherelle (1961). Escorpionismo en la Republica Mexicana. Rev. Inst. Salubr. Enf. Trop. 21, 3-19.

Mohamed, A. H., H. Rohayem and O. Zaki (1954). The action of scorpion toxin on blood sodium and potassium. J. Trop. Med. Hyg. 57, 85-87.

Mohamed, A.H., M. Hani-Ayobe, M.A. Beskharoun and N.A. El-Damarawy (1972). Glycemic responses to scorpion venom. Toxicon, 10, 139-149.

Mohamed, A.H., S. Ahmed, M.S. El Fikey and M.K. Ibrahim (1980). Gastric secretion and ulceration induced in the rat by an extract from scorpion (B. quinquestriatus) telsons. Toxicon, 18, 619-624.

Moss, J., T. Kazic, D.P. Henry and I.J. Kopin (1973). Scorpion venom-induced discharge of catecholamines accompanied by hypertension. Brain Research, 54, 381-385.

Moss, J., N.B. Thoa and I.J. Kopin (1974). On the mechanism of scorpion toxin-induced release of norepirephrine from peripheral adrenergic neurons. J. Pharmac. exp. Ther., 190, 39-48.

Narahashi, T.B., I. Shapiro, T. Deguchi, M. Scuka and C.M. Wang (1972). Effects of scorpion venom on squid axon membranes. Am. J. Physiol., 222, 850-857.

Novaes, G., O.L. Catanzaro, W.T. Beraldo and L. Freire-Maia (1982). Effect of purified scorpion toxin (tityustoxin) on the pancreatic secretion of the rat. Toxicon, 20, 847-853.

Oliveira Antonio, M.P., F. Fernandes, J.A. Gonçalves Jr. and M. Rocha e Silva (1973). Pharmacological analysis of the mediators involved in the acute pulmonary edema produced in rats by adrenealine. Agents Actions, 3, 383.

Osman, O.H., M. Ismail and T. Wenger (1973). Hyperthermic response to intraventricular injection of scorpion venom: role of brain monoamines. Toxicon, 11, 361-368.

Paintal, A.S.(1973).Vagal sensory receptors and their reflex effects.Physiol.Rev.,53, 159-227.

Parnas, I. and F.E. Russell (1967). Effects of venoms on nerve, muscle and neuromuscular junction. In F.E. Russell and P.R. Saunders (Ed.), Animal Toxins, Pergamon, Oxford, pp. 401-415.

Patterson, R.A. and D. Wooley (1972). Effect of scorpion venom Centruroides sculpturatus on the carotid body and superior cervical ganglion of the cat. In A. de Vries and E. Kochva (Ed.), Toxins of Animal and Plant Origin, Gordon and Breach, New York, pp. 741-748.

Poon-King, T. (1963). Myocarditis from scorpion stings. Br. med. J., 1, 374-377.

Possani, L.D. (1984). Structure of scorpion toxins. In A. Tu (Ed.), Handbook of Natural Toxins, Vol. 2, Marcel Dekker, New York, pp 513-550.

Possani, L.D., A.C. Alagon, P.L. Fletcher Jr. and B. Erickson (1977). Purification and properties of mammalian toxins from the venom of the Brazilian scorpion Tityus serrulatus Lutz and Mello. Archs Biochem. Biophys., 180, 394-403.

Ramos, A.O. and A.P. Corrado (1954). Efeito hiperpiético do veneno de escorpião (Tityus serrulatus e Tityus bahiensis). An. Fac. Med. Univ. São Paulo, 28, 81-98.

Reddy, C.R.R.M., G. Suvarnakumari, C.S. Devi and C.N. Reddy (1972). Pathology of scorpion venom poisoning. J. Trop. Med. Hyg. 75: 98-100.

Rimsza, M.E., D.R. Zimmerman and P.S. Bergeson (1980). Scorpion envenomation. Pediatrics, 66, 298-302.

Rochat, H., P. Bernard, and F. Couraud (1979). Scorpion toxins: chemistry and mode of action. In B. Ceccarelli and F. Clementi (Ed.), Advances in Cytopharmacology, vol. 3, Raven, New York, pp. 325-334.

Rossi, M.A., A.L. Ferreira and S.M. Paiva (1974). Fine structures of pulmonary changes induced by Brazilian scorpion venom. Arch. Pathol., 97, 284-288.

Rothschild, A.M. and A. Castania (1976). Contribution of vasopressor and plasma kininogen changes towards acute adrenaline pulmonary edema in the rat. Naunyn-Schmiedeberg's Arch. Pharmac., 295, 177-181.

Russell, F.E.(1967). Comparative pharmacology of some animal toxins. Fed. Proc., 26, 1206-1224.
Russell, F.E. and V.C. Bohr (1962). Intraventricular injection of venom. Toxic. appl.Pharmac., 4, 165-173.
Samaan, A. and H.H. Ibrahim (1959). The effects of scorpion venom on salivary secretion. Archs int. Pharmacodyn., 72, 249-264.
Sampaio, S.V., C.J. Laure and J.R. Giglio (1983). Isolation and characterization of toxic proteins from the venom of the Brazilian scorpion Tityus serrulatus, Toxicon, 21, 265-277.
Sankaran, H., C. Bartholomew, O. Fitzgerald and K. F. McGeeney (1977). Secretory effect of the venom of the scorpion Tityus trinitatis on rat pancreatic slices. Toxicon, 15, 441-446.
Santhanakhishman, B.R. and V.B. Raju (1974). Management of scorpion sting in children. J. trop. Med. Hyg. 77, 133-135.
Savino, E.D. and O.L. Catanzaro (1979). The effects of tityus toxin on the isolated rat portal vein. lRCS: med. Sci., 7, 317.
Silva, T.L. (1950). Escorpionismo em Ribeirão Preto. Notas sobre epidemiologia e profilaxia. Arch. Hig. Saude Pública (São Paulo), 15, 79-90.
Stahnke, H.L. (1950). The Arizona scorpion problem. Ariz. Med., 7, 23-29.
Stahnke, H.L. (1978). The genus Centruroides (Buthidae) and its venom, In S. Bettini (Ed.), Arthropod Venoms, Springer-Verlag, Berlin, pp. 277-307.
Tafuri, W.L., T.A. Maria, L. Freire-Maia and J.R. Cunha-Melo (1974). Effect of the scorpion toxin on the granular vesicles in the Auerbach's plexus of the rat ileum. J. Neural Transm. 35, 233-240.
Tash, F., K. Ghoneim, N. Swelam, M.F. Bassiony and M.F. El-Asmar (1982). Effect of a scorpion (Leiurus quinquestriatus H and E) venom on blood gases and acid-base balance in rat. Toxicon, 20, 802-805.
Tazieff-Depierre, F. (1971). Action de la tetrodotoxine sur la cardiotoxicité des venins de scorpion (Androctonus australis). C.R. Acad. Sci.(Paris), 273, 915-918.
Tazieff-Depierre, F. and P. Andrillon (1973). Sécrétion d'acetylcholine provoquée par le venin de scorpion dan l'iléon de cobaye et sa suppresion par la tétrodotoxin. C.R. Acad. Sci. (Paris), 276, 1631-1633.
Tintpulver, M., T. Zerachia and E. Zlotkin (1976). The action of different toxins derived from scorpion venom on the ileal smooth muscle preparation. Toxicon, 14, 371-377.
Toledo, D. and A.G. A. Neves (1976). Purification and partial characterization of a second toxin from the scorpion Tityus serrulatus. Comp. Biochem. Physiol., 55B, 249-253.
Vital Brazil, O., A.C. Neder and A.P. Corrado (1973). Effects and mechanism of action of Tityus serrulatus venom on skeletal muscle. Pharmacol. Res. Comm., 5, 137-150.
Walter, Ch., E. Zlotkin and W. Rathmeyer (1976). Action of different toxins from the scorpion Androctonus australis on a locust nerve-muscle preparation. J. Insect Physiol., 22,1187-1194.
Warnick, J.E., E.X. Albuquerque and C.R. Diniz (1976). Electrophysiological observations on the action of purified scorpion venom, tityustoxin, on nerve and skeletal muscle of the rat. J. Pharmac. Exp. Ther., 198, 155-167.
Waterman, J.A. (1938). Some notes on scorpion poisoning in Trinidad. Trans. Roy. Soc. Trop.Med. Hyg., 31, 607-624.
Waterman, J.A. (1957). Some notes on scorpion poisoning in Trinidad. Caribean med. J., 19, 113-128.
Wright, R.P., T.K. Chan, L. Honetschlager, D.E. Howell and G.V. Odell (1977). Enzymes and toxins of the scorpion venom Palamneus gravimanus. Toxicon, 15, 197-205.
Xavier, M.S., J.F. Cardini, R.P. Machado and F. Alzamora (1986). Effect of phentolamine on the renal action of norepinephrine and scorpion venom. Brazilian J. Med. Biol. Res. 19, 536A.
Yarom, R. and K. Braun (1970). Cardiovascular effects of scorpion venom, morphological changes in the myocardium. Toxicon, 8, 41-46.
Yarom, R. and U. Meiri (1972). Effect of scorpion venom on ultrastructure of frog sartorius muscle. Toxicon, 10, 291-294.
Yarom, R., S. Yallon, F. Notowitz and K. Braun (1974). Reversible myocardial damage by scorpion venom in perfused rat hearts. Toxicon, 12, 347-351.
Zlotkin, E. and A.S. Shulov (1969). Recent studies on the mode of action of scorpion neurotoxins. A review. Toxicon, 7, 217-221.
Zlotkin, E., F. Miranda and H. Rochat (1978). Chemistry and pharmacology of Buthinae scorpion venoms. In S. Bettini (Ed.) Arthropod Venoms, Springer-Verlag, Berlin, pp. 317-369.

TREATMENT OF VENOMOUS JELLYFISH STINGS

Joseph W. Burnett, M. D.

Division of Dermatology, Department of Medicine, University of Maryland School of Medicine, Baltimore, Maryland 21201 U.S.A.

ABSTRACT

Jellyfish venoms are mixtures of toxic and/or antigenic pathogenic polypeptides and enzymes. As newer therapeutic agents become available to treat the various reactions to stings by these animals, an accurate diagnosis of the type of syndrome and the offending species will be necessary. First aid therapy to inactivate nematocysts within tentacles still adhering to the victim's skin appears to be species-specific. Verapamil is an effective drug for jellyfish cardiotoxins. Hyperbaric oxygen may be a promising treatment to counteract the lethal or vasospastic effect of the venoms. Sting-induced cutaneous pain is difficult to treat because of its rapid onset and the fact that it results from intracutaneous injection of venom which requires a time delay before effective drug-induced analgesia can be achieved.

KEYWORDS

Jellyfish; Chironex; Pelagia; Physalia; Chrysaora; envenomation; lethality; dermonecrosis; vasopermeability; vasospasm.

Multiple envenomation syndromes caused by jellyfish stings can occur (Burnett and Calton, 1987a). The lesions may be localized or systemic and can vary widely in clinical severity. These disorders result from toxic or immunological reactions to various polypeptides and enzymes present in coelenterate venoms (Burnett and Calton, 1977; 1987b). These pathogenic mixtures are injected into the skin of man by means of the forceable projection of a venom-coated nematocyst thread into the dermis. As newer therapeutic agents become available to treat the various reactions to stings by these animals, an accurate diagnosis of the type of syndrome and the offending species will be necessary. First aid therapy to inactivate nematocysts within tentacles still adhering to the victim's skin appears to be species-specific.

Cutaneous Sting

The initial treatment of a cutaneous sting is to reassure the patient and immobilize the envenomated area of the body. These maneuvers stabilize cardiac output and reduce the pump action exerted by the skeletal muscles. It is essential to keep the venom localized in the skin and prevent rapid uptake of the toxic fractions into the systemic circulation.

The use of local heat is contraindicated since it increases the permeability of the venom. In one instance, visible erythematous lymphangitic spread could be seen on the extremity of an adult male who had immersed his arm in a 31°C water bath for 15 minutes following a *Physalia* sting. Cold compresses have not been effective against the pain. Pain is reduced as long as cold is applied to the sting site but returns once the extremity is rewarmed.

The neutralization of the nematocysts on the tentacles still adherent to the victim's skin is the next procedure. The use of vinegar for *Chironex* or *Physalia* stings, baking soda slurry in the case of *Chrysaora* stings and calcium salts for *Pelagia* stings (Hartwick *et al.*, 1980; Turner and Sullivan, 1980; Burnett *et al.*, 1983b; Salleo *et al.*, 1984) is recommended. It is essential that the first aid physician test the viability of the tentacle fragments after treatment with these first aid solutions before they are removed from the body. This testing can be done by elevating a small specimen and gently rubbing it against the rescuer's dorsal fingertips. Once the nematocysts have been disarmed, then manual removal of the remaining fragments can be attempted. Salicylates, non-steroidal analgesics or opiates should be administered systemically as necessary for pain. Parenteral *Chironex* anti-venom can be given early if the patient has been significantly stung by the box jellyfish. Topical or systemic corticosteroids or antihistamines and topical analgesics or anesthetics are ineffective against the cutaneous sting because the painful stimulus is too deep in the dermis to be quickly counteracted by a percutaneously administered drug (Burnett et al., 1975).

Recurrent Cutaneous Eruptions

Recurrent cutaneous eruptions are short lived lasting one to seven days (Burnett et al., 1983a; Burnett and Calton, 1987a, b). These lesions may occur from 5-30 days after the original sting and may occur up to four times (Burnett and Calton, 1987a). Topical or systemic corticosteroids or antihistamines are all ineffective. Presently, systemic administration of non-steroidal analgesics appears to be marginally effective and is being evaluated.

Vasospasm

Patients who develop vasospasm after jellyfish envenomation should be treated with adequate oxygenation and hydration (Williamson et al., 1988). Should the envenomation be due to box jellyfish, specific anti-venom should be administered. The patient should then be evaluated for anticoagulation or systemic vasodilators. Anti-platelet aggregators or sympathetic blockade should be considered. The progress of the peripheral pulses and the temperature of the affected part should be carefully monitored. In cases where the patient does not respond to prompt therapy consideration for surgical decompression and/or hyperbaric oxygen therapy should be given.

Systemic Symptoms

Patients who develop extracutaneous symptoms after jellyfish envenomation should be promptly placed on respiratory and cardiovascular support with adequate oxygenation (Williamson et al., 1984; Burnett and Calton, 1987a, b). Those victims stung by Chironex should receive intravenous anti-venom. At this point it is clinically difficult to differentiate anaphylaxis from the rapidly progressing cardiotoxic or respiratory action of the venom. The history of the patient's reaction to various envenomations should be sought and if anaphylaxis is suspected, epinephrine should be instantly administered (Togias et al., 1985). Most of these patients, however, will have a cardiotoxic reaction to the jellyfish venom. Cardiac monitoring should be undertaken and intravenous verapamil given at the first sign of any arrhythmia (Burnett and Calton, 1983; Burnett et al., 1985).

The "Irukandji" Syndrome

Presently the best treatment for "Irukandji" syndrome includes systemic analgesics and phentolamine. The use of Chironex anti-venom is contraindicated (Fenner et al., 1986a). Administration of opiates and diazepam provide symptomatic relief (Fenner et al., 1986b).

Hyperpigmentation, fat atrophy, neuritis and keloid

Cutaneous hyperpigmentation should be treated with frequent application of topical 2-3% alcoholic hydroquinone solutions. Keloids are difficult to resolve, but attempts may be made with intralesional corticosteroids and plastic surgical excision. There is no good therapy for fat atrophy, and peripheral neuritis should be managed with corticosteroids and physical therapy.

TREATMENT OF EXPERIMENTALLY INDUCED SYNDROMES

Several models simulating the clinical envenomations syndromes have been developed in animals. The results of numerous studies utilizing these models have been reported. Three common experimental systems include vasopermeability assays, measurement of dermonecrosis, and determination of in vivo lethality. Studies of the positive and negative effects of various pharmacological agents on the venom's ability to induce these syndromes have provided clues useful to the clinician. Because of this fact, a discussion of the results of drug-venom interaction in these experimental systems is warranted.

Vasopermeability

Non-steroidal analgesics and methysergide have given positive results against vasopermeability in animals

(Burnett and Calton, 1986). The species specificity of these drugs against the various venoms was striking. Methysergide was effective against *Chironex* and *Physalia* venom but not against that of *Chrysaora*. Indomethacin was effective against *Chironex* venom but not those of *Chrysaora* or *Physalia*, and piripost (6,9-deepoxy-6,9-(phenylimino)- 6,8 prostaglandin II (U-60,257) was found to be effective as a prophylactic agent against the vasopermeability activity of *Chironex*, *Physalia* and *Chrysaora* venoms. Piripost, a leukotriene inhibitor, was only transiently effective if given within three to seven minutes after venom challenge. Several drugs have been found to be ineffective against coelenterate venoms in the vasopermeability assay. Interleukin 2 administered at doses between 15,000 and 300,000 units daily for five days did not prevent the vasopermeability activity of *Chrysaora* venom. Corticosteroids administered prior to or post venom challenge did not affect the size of the Evans blue dye extravasation. Additionally, prior treatment with vinblastin or with an anti-serotonin agent LY53857 6-methyl-1-(1-methylethyl)-ergoline-8-carboxcylic acid, 2 hydroxy-1-methylpropol ester (Z)-2-butinedioate (1:1) was also ineffective in this assay system.

Dermonecrosis

Acetylsalicylic acid, H1 and H2 antihistamines, nitrogen mustards, and cromoglycate were not effective against the dermonecrotic activity of *Chrysaora*, *Physalia* or *Chironex* venoms. Captopril (50 mg/kg twice daily for five days i.p.) (Mazzocchio *et al.*, 1985) was ineffective in preventing the dermonecrotic activity of *Chironex*, *Chrysaora* and *Physalia* venoms. No prophylactic effect also was found with the use of cyclosporin 30 mg/kg p.o. for three days. Modified bradykinin molecules given in 10 mM concentrations at the time of venom challange or 10 minutes prior to injection did not prevent the dermonecrotic activity of the three jellyfish venoms listed above. The bradykinin analogs assayed were des-Arg-bradykinin, The 5,8 D-Phe^{7}-bradykinin, B-6769-des-Arg-9 Leu^{8} bradykinin. Phenindione or NDGA (nordihydroguiaretic acid), known leukotriene receptor blockers, did not prevent the dermonecrosis when administered in 100 uM amounts 30 minutes prior to challenge.

Lethality

The adenyl cyclase activator, forskolon, did not prevent the lethal action of intravenous *Chrysaora* venom when administered at the dosage of 0.05 ml of a 12 mM solution. Systemic calcium ions, adrenalin, papaverine, procaine, atropine, tolazoline and hydrocortisone do not affect the lethal activity of *Chironex* venom (Keen, 1970). Intravenous verapamil was found to be effective as a prophylactic or counteractant agent against *Physalia*, *Chrysaora* or *Chironex* venom challenges in mice or rats (Burnett and Calton, 1983; Burnett *et al.*, 1985). Preliminary data suggests that immediate hyperbaric oxygen therapy may also counteract the lethal effect of the venom. Perhaps the definitive therapy against the lethal effect of jellyfish venoms is verapamil plus hyperbaric oxygen (Myers, R.A.M., Marzella, L. and Burnett, J.W., unpublished data).

PREVENTION OF ENVENOMATION

Three techniques to prevent jellyfish envenomation have been investigated. Protective clothing or "Stinger suits" consisting of nylon thick meshed cloth completely covering the body except for a small area about the face are somewhat effective. However, these suits are cumbersome and not widely accepted. The application of petrolatum can diminish the cutaneous pain of tentacle contact when applied thickly (Burnett *et al.*, 1968). The thickness of the ointment may be decreased with the addition of polysorbate or a base, but these products are not satisfactory since the former washes off and the latter will produce desquamation. Silicone stop-cock greases, if applied at similar thicknesses, are also effective but these topical agents are difficult to use since they are gritty and thick.

Numerous studies on nets and enclosures have also been performed (Schultz and Cargo, 1969). Nets are ineffective because jellyfish fragments and small animals can penetrate the mesh. Enclosures whose perimeter is demarcated with air jets can be designed to keep jellyfish from designated swim areas. These air jet barriers are more effective than water jet fences because the latter are fouled more easily.

Twenty years ago an article on the subject of jellyfish envenomation therapy would have been brief and without much scientific fact. We were all standing by helplessly observing patients with these syndromes. If the next decade advances at a similar pace, excellent therapeutic procedures should be available.

TABLE 1. Treatment of Venomous Jellyfish Stings

	Effective	Ineffective
Prevention		
	stinger suits	nets
	air jets	water jets
	petrolatum - add silicone, polysorbate or base	
Cutaneous sting		
	immobilize stung area	heat or cold
	neutralize nematocysts on adherent tentacles	topical analgesics
	& test neutralized nematocysts before removal	topical or systemic
	systemic analgesics	corticosteroids or
	Chironex antivenom - if Chironex sting	antihistamines
Systemic symptoms		
	respiratory and cardiovascular support	
	oxygen	
	verapamil for cardiotoxicity	
	Chironex antivenom for Chironex stings	
	epinephrine for anaphylaxis	
Vasopermeability		
	piripost	Interleukin 2
	nonsteroidal analgesics	corticosteroids
	methysergide	other antiserotonin agents
Dermonecrosis		
		nitrogen mustard
		synthetic bradykinin
		acetylsalicylic acid
		antihistamines H1 and H2
		nordihydroguiaretic acid (NDGA)
		cromoglycate, vinblastin
		phenindione, captopril
		cyclosporin
Irukandji		
	phentolamine	*Chironex* antivenom
	systemic analgesics	
Lethality		
	verapamil	forskolin
	hyperbaric oxygen	
Recurrent cutaneous eruptions		
	? nonsteroidal analgesics	topical or systemic corticosteroids
	antihistamines	
Vasospasm		
	hydration	
	oxygenation	
	specific antivenom administration if due to box-jellyfish	
	systemic vasodilators	
	antiplatelet aggregators	
	sympathetic blockade	
	? surgery; ? hyperbaric oxygen	

Burnett, J.W. and G.J. Calton (1977) The chemistry and toxicology of some venomous pelagic coelenterates. Toxicon 15, 177-196.

Burnett, J.W. and G.J. Calton (1983) Response of the box-jellyfish (Chironex fleckeri) cardiotoxin to intravenous administration of verapamil. Med. J. Aust. 2, 192-194.

Burnett, J.W. and G.J. Calton (1986) Pharmacological effects of various venoms on cutaneous capillary leakage. Toxicon 24, 614-617.

Burnett J.W. and G.J. Calton (1987a) Jellyfish envenomation syndromes updated. Ann. Emerg. Med. 16, 1000-1005.

Burnett, J.W. and G.J. Calton (1987b) Venomous pelagic coelenterates: chemistry, toxicology, immunology and treatment of their stings. Toxicon 25, 581-602.

Burnett, J.W., G.J. Calton, H. Meier and A.P. Kaplan (1975) Mediators present in the nematocyst venoms of the sea nettle, sea wasp and Portuguese man-o'war. Comp. Bio. & Physiol. 51C, 153-156.

Burnett, J.W., C.S. Cobbs, S.N. Kelman and G.J. Calton (1983a) Studies on the serologic response to jellyfish envenomation. J. Amer. Acad. Dermatol. 9, 229-231.

Burnett, J.W., H. Rubinstein and G.J. Calton (1983b) First aid for jellyfish envenomation. So. Med. J. 76, 870-872.

Burnett, J.W., C.J. Gean, G.J. Calton and J.F. Warnick (1985) The effect of verapamil on the cardiotoxic activity of Portuguese man-o'war (Physalia physalis) and sea nettle (Chrysaora quinquecirrha) venoms. Toxicon 23, 681-689.

Burnett, J.W., L.H. Pierce Jr., U. Nawachinda and J.H. Stone (1968) Studies on sea nettle stings. Arch. Dermatol. 98, 587-589.

Fenner, P., D. Rodgers and J. Williamson (1986a) Box jellyfish antivenom and "Irukandji" stings. Med. J. Aust. 144, 665.

Fenner, P.J., J.A. Williamson, V.I. Callanan and I. Audley (1986b) Further understanding of, and a new treatment for, "Irukandji" (Carukia barnesi) stings. Med. J. Aust. 145, 569-574.

Hartwick, R., V.I. Callanan and J.A. Williamson (1980) Disarming the box-jellyfish. Nematocyst inhibition in Chironex fleckeri. Med. J. Aust. 1, 15-20.

Keen, T.E.B. (1970) Recent investigations of sea wasp stings in Australia. Med. J. Aust. 1, 266-270.

Mazzocchio, G., C. Robba, P. Rebuffat, G. Gottardo and G.G. Nussdorfer (1985) Effect of somatostatin on the zona glomerulosa of rats treated with angiotensin II or captopril, stereology and plasma hormone concentrations. J. Ster. Biochem. 23, 353-356.

Salleo, A., G. La Spada, G. Falzea and N.G. Denaro (1984) Discharging effects of anions and inhibitory effect of divalent cations on isolated nematocysts of Pelagia noctiluca. Molec. Physiol. 5, 25-34.

Schultz, L.P. and D.G. Cargo (1969) Sea nettle barriers for bathing beaches in upper Chesapeake Bay. Chesapeake Biological Laboratory, Solomons, Maryland, Ref. #69-69.

Togias, A.G., J.W. Burnett, A. Kagey-Sobotka and L.M. Lichtenstein (1985) Anaphylaxis after contact with a jellyfish. J. Aller. Clin. Immunol. 75, 672-675.

Turner, B. and J. Sullivan (1980) Disarming the blue bottle - Treatment of Physalia envenomation. Med. J. Aust. 2, 394.

Williamson, JA, J.W. Burnett, P.J. Fenner, V. Hach-Wunderle, L.Y. Hoe, and K.M. Adiga (1988) Acute regional vascular insufficiency following jellyfish envenomation. Med. J. Aust. (in press)

Williamson, J.A., L.E. La Ray, M. Wohlfart and P.J. Fenner (1984) Acute management of serious envenomation by box-jellyfish (Chironex fleckeri). Med. J. Aust. 141, 851-853.

DEVELOPMENT OF DRUG THERAPIES FOR SNAKE VENOM INTOXICATION

Richard D. Crosland

Pathology Division, U.S. Army Medical Research Institute of Infectious Diseases, Frederick, Maryland 21701-5011

ABSTRACT

I determined the efficacy of chloroquine, chlorpromazine, dexamethasone, and piracetam with respect to reducing the toxicity in mice of *Bungarus caeruleus* venom, *Bungarus multicinctus* venom and its neurotoxic components α-bungarotoxin and β-bungarotoxin, *Crotalus durissus terrificus* venom and its neurotoxic component crotoxin, and *Oxyuranus scutellatus* venom and its neurotoxic component taipoxin. Venom or toxin was administered i.p., followed immediately by an i.p. injection of the drug of interest. The effect of the drug on lethality caused by the venom or toxin was recorded 24 hr later. Chloroquine and chlorpromazine proved to be effective antagonists of the toxicity of *B. caeruleus* venom, *B. multicinctus* venom, and β-bungarotoxin without themselves being overtly toxic. Dexamethasone was similarly effective against the lethality of *O. scutellatus* venom and taipoxin. Piracetam was without effect on the lethality of any of the venoms or toxins. Protection from lethality was maximal when the drugs were administered immediately after the injection of venom or toxin.

KEYWORDS

snake venom; neurotoxin; chloroquine; chlorpromazine; dexamethasone; piracetam; therapy

INTRODUCTION

Antivenoms are the pharmacological agents currently used for treatment of intoxication due to snake venoms. Several factors, however, limit their usefulness. A given antivenom is effective against the venom from only a small number of species of snakes. In addition, some people are hypersensitive to antivenoms. Finally, antivenoms require refrigeration and are expensive --- two factors that limit their availability. Treatment of snake venom intoxication would be greatly enhanced if drugs could be found which would overcome these deficiencies of antivenoms.

Several potent snake venoms contain neurotoxins that constitute the most lethal components of the venom. The best studied of these venoms is that of the Formosan krait *Bungarus multicinctus*, which is the most poisonous snake in Taiwan, and whose bites have resulted in a 23% mortality rate (Kuo and Wu, 1972). The venom of *B. multicinctus* contains two neurotoxins that contribute to its toxicity. α-Bungarotoxin is a postsynaptic neurotoxin which binds to the nicotinic acetylcholine receptor at the neuromuscular junction and blocks muscle contraction stimulated by acetylcholine. β-Bungarotoxin is a presynaptic neurotoxin which inhibits the release of acetylcholine from neurons, also blocking muscle contraction (Chang, 1985). The two toxins work in concert to cause respiratory failure, which is the ultimate cause of death due to the venom of *B. multicinctus*. β-Bungarotoxin is the most toxic component of B. multicinctus venom and the most investigated of the snake presynaptic neurotoxins, making it useful to study in conjunction with the venom. Other snakes such as Bungarus caeruleus (Indian krait), Crotalus durissus terrificus (South American rattlesnake), and Oxyuranus scutellatus (taipan) have venoms with presynaptic neurotoxins that have an effect at the neuromuscular junction similar to that of β-bungarotoxin (Chang, 1985).

Although the biochemical mechanism of action of the presynaptic neurotoxins of snake venoms is unknown, it is possible that they act through a phosphatidate 2-acylhydrolase (EC 3.1.1.4) (trivial name: phospholipase A_2) activity (Chang, 1985). Chloroquine, chlorpromazine, dexamethasone, and piracetam have been shown to be effective inhibitors of non-neurotoxic phospholipase A_2 activities (Jain et al., 1984; Kato, et al., 1985; Nikolov and Koburova, 1984) and may therefore be effective antagonists of the toxicity of snake presynaptic neurotoxins and of the venoms of which they are a part.

MATERIALS AND METHODS

Materials

Bungarus caeruleus, B. multicinctus, C. durissus terrificus, and O. scutellatus venoms and α-bungarotoxin, β-bungarotoxin, and crotoxin were purchased from Miami Serpentarium Laboratories, Salt Lake City, UT. Taipoxin was the gift of Dr. John Middlebrook of this Institute. Lyophilized venoms and toxins (except crotoxin) were dissolved (1 mg/ml) in deionized water. Lyophilized crotoxin was dissolved (1 mg/ml) in 10 mM sodium phosphate, 10 mM ammonium acetate, pH 4.0; centrifuged at 3000 x g for 5 min; and the pellet discarded. Aliquots of venom and toxin solutions were stored at -20°C and were not refrozen after thawing. Further dilution of all venoms and toxins was performed using gel-phosphate buffer (0.2% gelatin, 0.4% sodium phosphate, pH 6.2). Chloroquine diphosphate and chlorpromazine hydrochloride were purchased from Sigma Chemical Co., St. Louis, MO. Dexamethasone sodium phosphate was purchased from LyphoMed, Inc., Rosemont, IL. Piracetam was the gift of Dr. Harvey Altman, Lafayette Clinic, Detroit, MI. All references to chloroquine, chlorpromazine, and dexamethasone imply their salt forms. All drugs were dissolved and/or diluted in 150 mM sodium chloride, 6 mM sodium phosphate (pH 7.2) (PBS).

Methods

Female ICR mice (20-30 g; Harlan Sprague-Dawley, Inc., Frederick, MD) were housed five per cage, maintained on a 12 hr light-dark (1800 - 0600) cycle, and allowed free access to food and water. The mice were injected i.p. with the venom or toxin of interest in gel-phosphate buffer, followed by an i.p. injection of either PBS (control) or drug in PBS. All doses, expressed per kg mouse, were adjusted for the weight of the animal, and were administered in a volume of 10 ml/kg. Almost all of the animals that survived 24 hr after the injection of venom or toxin recovered fully, and the number of animals that died within 24 hr was used as the measure of toxicity. Each experiment was repeated at least once (sometimes with different, but overlapping doses), and the data from the repeated experiments were combined. Each data point represents at least five mice. A p value associated with a change in LD_{50} due to drug treatment refers to the significance of the drug effect on the dose-response curve as calculated by logit analysis and not to the significance of the difference between LD_{50}s. Other tests of significance (two-tailed) were calculated by contingency analysis (overall and adjusted multiple post hoc comparisons). Statistical tests were considered significant when $p < .05$. Any comparisons not shown were not significant.

I determined dose-effects of drugs by injecting mice with venoms or toxins at dose levels that were targeted to be the minimal 100% lethal dose (usually about two times the respective LD_{50}). The injection of venom or toxin was immediately followed by a separate injection of drug. The resulting dose-response curve had to have a basically montonically increasing phase followed by a basically monotonically decreasing phase and demonstrate protection of at least 70% of the mice at at least one dose before further investigation of a particular drug-venom (toxin) combination was pursued. The ED_{50} of each effective drug was calculated by using data from the rising phase of its dose-response curve while its LD_{50} was similarly calculated using the declining phase.

The effect of a drug on the dose-response of venoms and toxins was determined by injecting mice with various doses of venom or toxin immediately followed by administration of drug. In most experiments no control mice survived 24 hr (data not shown on graphs).

I investigated the effect of injecting drugs at different time intervals both before and after the injection of amounts of venom or toxin targeted to be minimal 100% lethal doses. In most experiments no mice that received a 45-min preinjection or a 45-min postinjection of PBS alone survived 24 hr (data not shown on graphs).

RESULTS

Chloroquine

Dose-effect of chloroquine. The protective effect of various doses of chloroquine toward the toxicity of B. caeruleus venom, B. multicinctus venom, and β-bungarotoxin was similar, increasing with increasing amounts of chloroquine up to 20 mg/kg in the case of B. caeruleus venom and β-bungarotoxin and 40 mg/kg in the case of B. multicinctus venom (Fig. 1a). Higher doses of chloroquine resulted in a decline in effectiveness in all cases. The ED_{50} of chloroquine was 3.2, 6.3, and 5.4 mg/kg in the presence of B. caeruleus venom, B. multicinctus venom, and β-bungarotoxin, respectively. The LD_{50} of chloroquine was 80 mg/kg in the presence of B. caeruleus venom, 89 mg/kg in the presence of B. multicinctus venom, and 37 mg/kg in the presence of β-bungarotoxin. The therapeutic indices of chloroquine were 25, 14, and 7 in the presence of B. caeruleus venom, B. multicinctus venom, and β-bungarotoxin, respectively. Chloroquine provided little protection from C. durissus terrificus venom, crotoxin, O. scutellatus venom, or taipoxin (Fig. 1b).

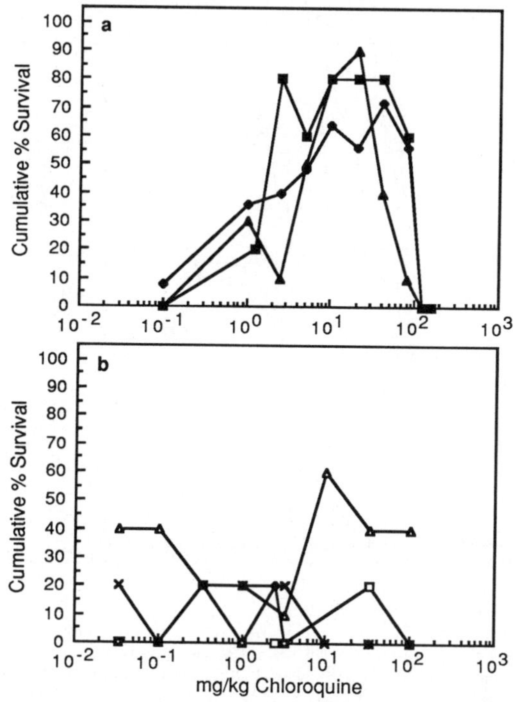

Fig. 1. Dose-response effect of chloroquine. (**a**) Mice were injected with 150 μg/kg of B. caeruleus venom (■), 75 μg/kg of B. multicinctus venom (◆), or 150 μg/kg of β-bungarotoxin (▲), followed immediately by a separate injection of various doses of chloroquine. Tests of significance: B. caeruleus venom; p (overall) = .0001, p (2.5, 10, 20, or 40 mg/kg vs. control) = .0030, p (5 or 80 mg/kg vs. control) = .034. B. multicinctus venom; p (overall) = .0001, p (1 mg/kg vs. control) = .0081, p (2.5 mg/kg vs. control) = .0036, p (5, 10, 20, or 40 mg/kg vs. control) = .0009. β-Bungarotoxin; p (overall) = .0001, p (10 mg/kg vs. control) = .0021, p (20 mg/kg vs. control) = .0007. (**b**) Mice were injected with 200 μg/kg of C. durissus terrificus venom (□), 100 μg/kg of crotoxin (Δ), 20 μg/kg of O. scutellatus venom (◇), or 2 μg/kg of taipoxin (✕), followed immediately by a separate injection of various doses of chloroquine.

Effect of chloroquine on dose-response of venoms and toxins. Chloroquine increased the LD_{50} of B. caeruleus venom 15 fold from 26 μg/kg to 400 μg/kg ($p < .0005$) (Fig. 2a). In fact, chloroquine protected 98% of the mice which received over four times a minimal 100% lethal dose of B. caeruleus venom. Chloroquine increased the LD_{50} of B. multicinctus venom 5.0 fold from 19 μg/kg to 95 μg/kg ($p < .0005$). Since chloroquine substantially increased the LD_{50} of B. multicinctus venom, I examined the effect of chloroquine on the neurotoxic components of the venom. Chloroquine had no effect on the LD_{50} of α-bungarotoxin (170 μg/kg to 240 μg/kg) ($p = .10$), but it increased the LD_{50} of β-bungarotoxin 17-fold from 7.8 μg/kg to 134 μg/kg ($p < .0005$) (Fig. 2b). In fact, chloroquine completely protected mice against the minimal dose of β-bungarotoxin (30 μg/kg) that killed 100% of the mice which received a saline postinjection. The effect of chloroquine on the LD_{50} of a mixture of α-bungarotoxin and β-bungarotoxin which approximated their relative proportions in B. multicinctus venom was the same as the effect of chloroquine on the LD_{50} of the native venom (Fig. 2a). Chloroquine increased the LD_{50} of the mixture 4.8 fold from 16 μg/kg to 77 μg/kg ($p = .001$). An injection of gel-phosphate buffer followed immediately by an injection of 17 mg/kg of chloroquine had no overt effect on mice when observed for 72 hr (N = 20).

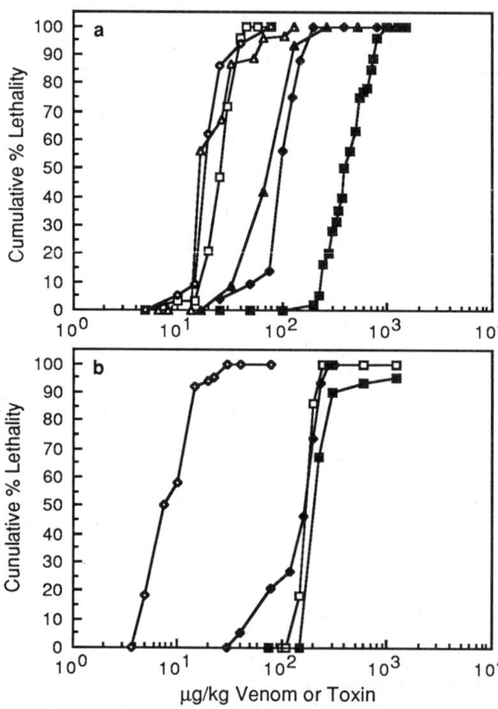

Fig. 2. Effect of chloroquine on the LD_{50} of venoms and toxins. Mice were injected with various amounts of venoms or toxins, followed immediately by a separate injection of either PBS (empty symbols) or 17 mg/kg chloroquine (filled symbols). (a) B. caeruleus venom (□,■); B. multicinctus venom (◇,◆); total weight of α-bungarotoxin:β-bungarotoxin::5:3 (by weight) (△,▲). (b) α-Bungarotoxin (□,■); β-bungarotoxin (◇,◆).

Effect of relative time of injection of chloroquine. Chloroquine provided maximal protection for mice from the effects of B. caeruleus venom, B. multicinctus venom, and β-bungarotoxin when it was administered immediately after (0 min) intoxication (Fig. 3). Good protection was also afforded when chloroquine was given 15 min before intoxication. Protection declined with increasing delay of administration of chloroquine after intoxication, but was still significant at 30 min. At 60 min postintoxication, chloroquine was ineffective.

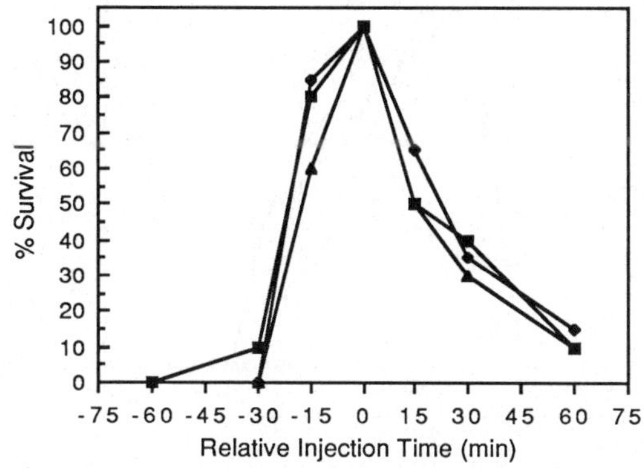

Fig. 3. Effect of relative time of injection of chloroquine. Mice were injected with 50 µg/kg of B. caeruleus venom (■), 75 µg/kg of B. multicinctus venom (◆), or 30 µg/kg of β-bungarotoxin (▲), each preceeded (negative times) or followed (0 and positive times) by an injection of 17 mg/kg of chloroquine. Tests of significance: B. caeruleus venom; p (overall) = .0001, p (-15 or 0 min vs. control) = .0007, p (15 min vs. control) = .0035, p (30 min vs. control) = .017. B. multicinctus venom; p (overall) = .0001, p (-15, 0, 15, or 30 min vs. control) = .0008. β-bungarotoxin; p (overall) = .0001, p (-15, 0, or 15 min vs. control) = .0007, p (30 min vs. control) = .0098.

Chlorpromazine

Dose-effect of chlorpromazine. Chlorpromazine protected mice from the toxicity of B. caeruleus venom, B. multicinctus venom, and β-bungarotoxin (Fig. 4a) while providing little protection from C. durissus terrificus venom, crotoxin, O. scutellatus venom, or taipoxin (Fig. 4b). When chlorpromazine did enhance survival, protection increased with increasing amounts of chlorpromazine up to 0.5 mg/kg in the case of β-bungarotoxin and 1 mg/kg in the cases of B. caeruleus venom and B. multicinctus venom. Higher doses of chlorpromazine resulted in a decline in protection. The ED_{50}s of chlorpromazine were 0.28, 0.10, and 0.27 mg/kg with respect to B. caeruleus venom, B. multicinctus venom, and β-bungarotoxin. Combining these values with LD_{50}s of 13, 7.2, and 13 mg/kg resulted in therapeutic indices of 46, 72, and 48 for B. caeruleus venom, B. multicinctus venom, and β-bungarotoxin, respectively.

Effect of chlorpromazine on dose-response of venoms and toxins. Chlorpromazine increased the LD_{50} of B. caeruleus venom 8.6-fold from 32 µg/kg to 275 µg/kg ($p < .0005$), of B. multicinctus venom 2.6-fold from 47 µg/kg to 120 µg/kg ($p = .012$), and of β-bungarotoxin 3.7-fold from 11 µg/kg to 41 µg/kg ($p = .004$) (Fig. 5). In the case of β-bungarotoxin, chlorpromazine completely protected mice from approximately twice a minimal 100% lethal dose of the toxin. In contrast, chlorpromazine had no effect on the LD_{50} of α-bungarotoxin, decreasing it from 240 µg/kg to 210 µg/kg ($p = .38$) (data not shown). An injection of gel-phosphate buffer followed immediately by an injection of 1 mg/kg of chlorpromazine had no overt effect on 20 mice when observed for 48 hr.

Effect of relative time of injection of chlorpromazine. Chlorpromazine provided maximal protection when it was injected immediately following (0 min) the injection of venom or toxin (Fig. 6). Only in the case of B. caeruleus venom, however, did chlorpromazine offer significant protection at other than 0 min. With this venom, chlorpromazine afforded a 70% survival rate when it was administered 15 min after intoxication. At 30 min its protection fell to a statistically non-significant 30%.

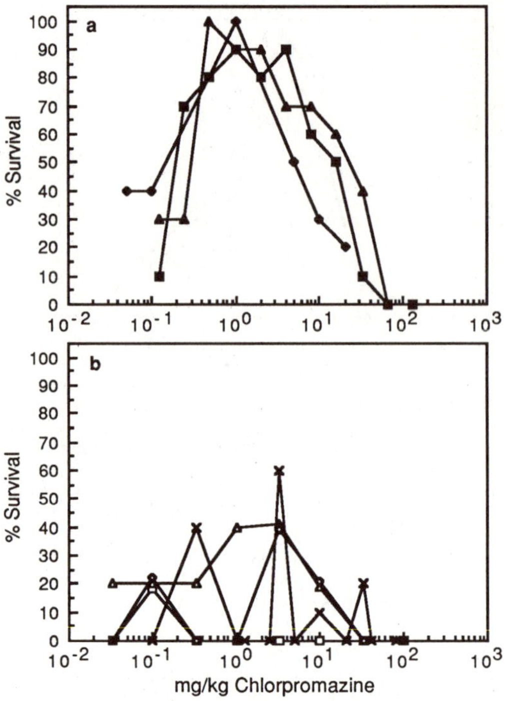

Fig. 4. Dose-response of chlorpromazine. (**a**) Mice were injected with 80 µg/kg of <u>B. caeruleus</u> venom (■), 75 µg/kg of <u>B. multicinctus</u> venom (◆), or 25 µg/kg of β-bungarotoxin (▲), followed immediately by a separate injection of various doses of chlorpromazine. Significance tests: <u>B. caeruleus</u> venom; p (overall) = .0001, p (0.25, 1, or 4 mg/kg vs. control) = .0011, p (0.5 or 2 mg/kg vs. control) = .0033, p (8 mg/kg vs. control) = .037. <u>B. multicinctus</u> venom, p (overall) = .0056, p (1 mg/kg vs. control) = .024; β-bungarotoxin, p (overall) = .0001, p (0.5, 1, or 2 mg/kg vs. control) = .0011, p (4 or 8 mg/kg vs. control) = .011), p (16 mg/kg vs. control) = .037. (**b**) Mice were injected with 200 µg/kg of <u>C. durissus terrificus</u> venom (□), 100 µg/kg of crotoxin (△), 20 µg/kg of <u>O. scutellatus</u> venom (◇), or 2 µg/kg of taipoxin (✕), followed immediately by a separate injection of various doses of chlorpromazine.

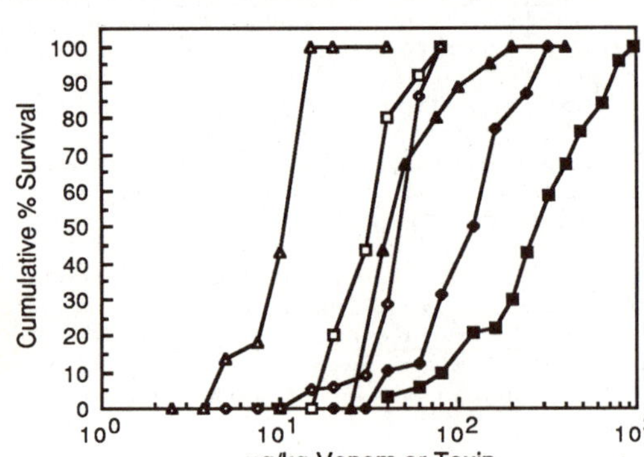

Fig. 5. Effect of chlorpromazine on the LD_{50} of venoms and toxin. Mice were injected with various amounts of venoms or toxin, followed immediately by a separate injection of either PBS (empty symbols) or 1 mg/kg chlorpromazine (filled symbols). <u>B. caeruleus</u> venom (□,■); <u>B. multicinctus</u> venom (◇,◆); β-bungarotoxin (△,▲).

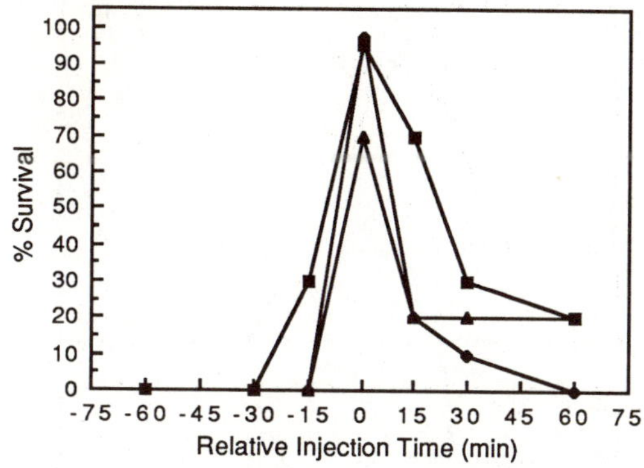

Fig. 6. Effect of time of injection of chlorpromazine relative to time of injection of venom or toxin. Mice were injected with 50 µg/kg of B. caeruleus venom (■), 80 µg/kg of B. multicinctus venom (◆), or 25 µg/kg of β-bungarotoxin (▲), each preceeded (negative times) or followed (0 and positive times) by an injection of 1 mg/kg of chlorpromazine. Tests of significance: B. caeruleus venom; p (overall) = .0001, p (0 or 15 min vs. control) = .0007. B. multicinctus venom; p (overall) = .0001, p (0 min vs. control) = .0007. β-bungarotoxin; p (overall) = .0001, p (0 min vs. control) = .0007.

Dexamethasone

Dose-effect of dexamethasone. Dexamethasone effectively protected mice from the toxicity of O. scutellatus venom and taipoxin (Fig. 7a). The ED_{50}s were 27 and 12 mg/kg, respectively. There was no declining phase to either dose-response curve, so no LD_{50}s or therapeutic indices could be calculated. With some reservation I deemed dexamethasone to be an ineffective antagonist of the toxicity of the other venoms and toxins (Fig. 7b). Dexamethasone presented a "sawtooth" dose-response curve over a wide range of concentrations with some of the venoms or toxins (e.g., B. multicinctus venom, crotoxin). I interpreted this phenomenon as an inconsistent or marginal protective effect which did not merit further immediate investigation. This conclusion was supported by dexamethasone's effect on the LD_{50} of B. multicinctus venom (see below).

Effect of dexamethasone on the dose-response of venoms and toxin. Dexamethasone increased the LD_{50} of O. scutellatus venom 3.5-fold from 22 µg/kg to 76 µg/kg ($p < .0005$) (Fig. 8). It completely protected mice from an 86% lethal dose of venom. Dexamethasone also increased the LD_{50} of taipoxin 4.0-fold from 2.5 µg/kg to 10 µg/kg ($p = .001$), completely protecting mice from a minimal 100% lethal dose of the toxin. Dexamethasone had no significant effect, however, on the LD_{50} of B. multicinctus venom, increasing it from 70 µg/kg to 120 µg/kg ($p = .10$) (data not shown). An injection of gel-phosphate buffer followed immediately by an injection of 48 mg/kg of dexamethasone in 20 mice made them lethargic and sleepy for several hr. After 24 hr all the mice had recovered, appeared normal, and remained so throughout the remainder of the observation period (24 more hr).

Effect of relative time of injection of dexamethasone. As with chloroquine and chlorpromazine, dexamethasone exhibited maximal protective action when it was administered immediately following intoxication with O. scutellatus venom or taipoxin (0 min, Fig. 9). In the case of O. scutellatus venom, moreover, protection was evident as long as 30 min after intoxication, whereas no such postintoxication protection was observed with taipoxin.

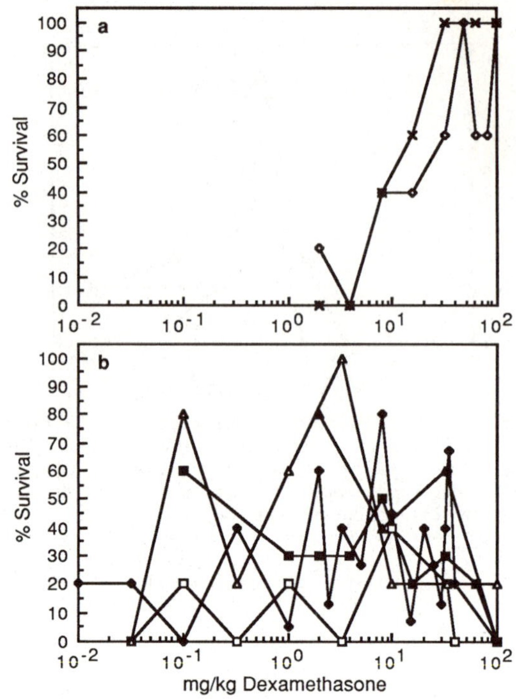

Fig. 7. Dose-effect of dexamethasone on venoms and toxins. (**a**) Mice were injected with 50 μg/kg of O. scutellatus venom (◇) or 5 μg/kg of taipoxin (✕), followed immediately by a separate injection of various doses of dexamethasone. Tests of significance: O. scutellatus venom; p (overall) = .0011, p (32 mg/kg vs. control) = .030, p (48 or 100 mg/kg vs. control) = .0009. taipoxin; p (overall) = .0001, p (32, 64, or 100 mg/kg vs. control) = .0056. (**b**) Mice were injected with 50 μg/kg of B. caeruleus venom (■), 80 μg/kg of B. multicinctus venom (◆), 25 μg/kg of β-bungarotoxin (▲), 200 μg/kg of C. durissus terrificus venom (□), or 100 μg/kg of crotoxin (△), followed immediately by a separate injection of various doses of dexamethasone.

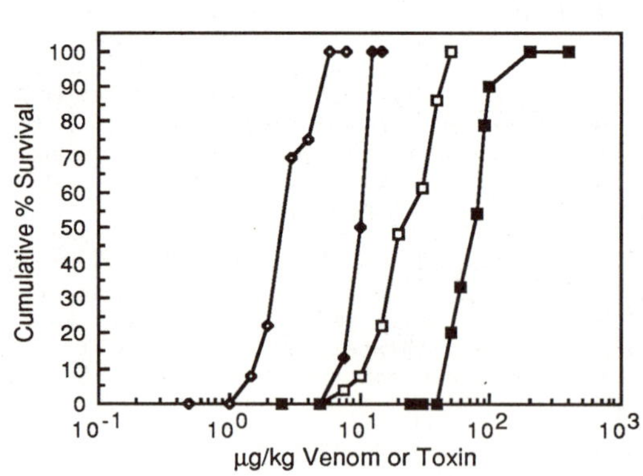

Fig. 8. Effect of dexamethsasone on the LD_{50} of O. scutellatus venom and taipoxin. Mice were injected with various amounts of O. scutellatus venom (□,■) or taipoxin (◇,◆), followed immediately by a separate injection of either PBS (empty symbols) or 48 mg/kg dexamethasone (filled symbols).

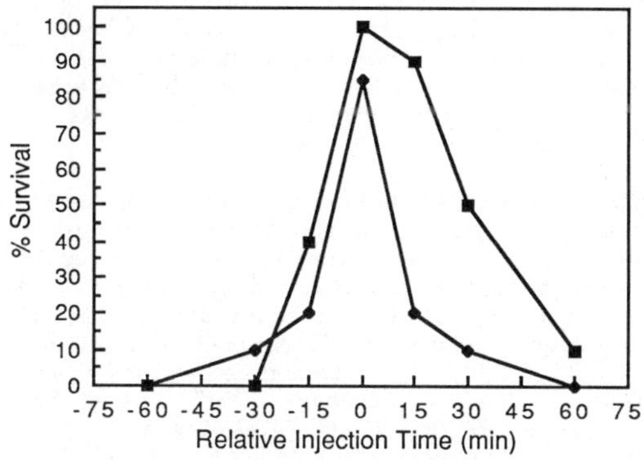

Fig. 9. Effect of time of injection of dexamethasone relative to time of injection of venom or toxin. Mice were injected with 20 µg/kg of O. scutellatus venom (■) or 4 µg/kg of taipoxin (◆), each preceeded (negative times) or followed (0 and positive times) by an injection of 48 mg/kg of dexamethasone. Tests of significance: O. scutellatus venom; p (overall) = .0001, p (0 or 15 min vs. control) = .0007, p (30 min vs. control) = .026. taipoxin; p (overall) = .0001, p (0 min vs. control) = .0007.

Dose-effect of piracetam. Piracetam did not effectively protect mice from the toxicity of any of the venoms or toxins tested (Fig. 10). Similarly to dexamethasone, piracetam produced a "sawtooth" dose-effect curve with crotoxin, but I deemed the effect not significant. No further investigation of the protective qualities of piracetam against the toxicity of any of the venoms or toxins was undertaken.

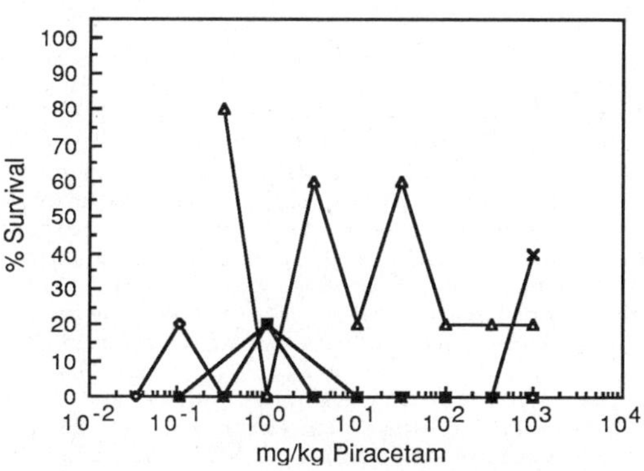

Fig. 10. Dose-effect of piracetam. Mice were injected with 40 µg/kg of B. caeruleus venom (■), 75 µg/kg of B. multicinctus venom, 50 µg/kg of β-bungarotoxin (▲), 200 µg/kg of C. durissus terrificus venom, 100 µg/kg of crotoxin (△), 20 µg/kg of O. scutellatus venom (◇), or 2 µg/kg of taipoxin (✕), followed immediately by a separate injection of various doses of chlorpromazine. Piracetam did not protect any mice that had been injected with B. multicinctus venom or C. durissus terrificus venom (data not shown).

DISCUSSION

I have shown that some drugs in clinical use in humans for other purposes can be effective antagonists in mice of the toxicity of some snake venoms and their presynaptic neurotoxins. Chloroquine and chlorpromazine antagonized the toxicity of B. caeruleus venom, B. multicinctus venom, and β-bungarotoxin, while dexamethasone antagonized the toxicity of O. scutellatuus venom and taipoxin. None of the drugs tested, however, had any marked effect on the toxicity of C. durissus terrificus venom or crotoxin, while piracetam had no effect on the toxicity of any of the venoms or toxins tested.

Chloroquine and chlorpromazine were optimally effective at mg/kg doses (20 and 1 mg/kg, respectively) which were slightly higher than the highest doses recommended for use in humans (Barnhart, 1987). This fact suggests that these drugs protected mice from venoms and toxin through mechanisms similar to those through which they produce their therapeutic effects in humans. This suggestion is buttressed by the observation that the optimal dose of these drugs alone caused no overt effect in mice. The optimal dose of dexamethasone (48 mg/kg), on the other hand, was approximately 50 times greater on a mg/kg basis than the maximal dose recommended for administration to humans (Barnhart, 1987). Additionally, the optimal dose of dexamethasone alone caused marked lethargy and sleepiness in mice. Both of these facts suggest that dexamethasone protected mice from the toxicity of O. scutellatuus venom and taipoxin through a mechanism other than that operative in human therapy.

Chloroquine increased the LD_{50} of B. caeruleus venom 15-fold, that of B. multicinctus venom 5-fold, and the LD_{50} of β-bungarotoxin 17-fold. Chloroquine had little effect on the LD_{50} of α-bungarotoxin. With a combination of α-bungarotoxin and β-bungarotoxin that approximated their relative proportions in B. multicinctus venom, however, chloroquine increased the LD_{50} the same amount (4.8-fold) that it increased the LD_{50} of the venom itself. This suggests that α-bungarotoxin and β-bungarotoxin account for the behavior of the venom with respect to chloroquine. It also suggests that α-bungarotoxin acted to decrease the potency of chloroquine with respect to β-bungarotoxin (reducing it 3-fold), even though chloroquine had little effect on α-bungarotoxin alone. Chlorpromazine increased the LD_{50} of B. caeruleus venom 8.7-fold, the LD_{50} of B. multicinctus venom 2.6-fold, and the LD_{50} of β-bungarotoxin 3.8-fold. Unlike chloroquine, the effect of chlorpromazine on the LD_{50}s of B. multicinctus venom and β-bungarotoxin was similar. Like chloroquine, chlorpromazine had no effect on the LD_{50} of α-bungarotoxin. Dexamethasone was effective against the toxicity of only O. scutellatuus venom and taipoxin, increasing their LD_{50}s by similar amounts, 3.5- and 4.0-fold, respectively.

Chloroquine, chlorpromazine, and dexamethasone were maximally effective against the toxicity of venoms and toxins when the drugs were administered immediately after intoxication. In general, only the first stage of intoxication (rapid respiration) was observed, and the mice remained normally active. At other times of administration of drug relative to intoxication, however, the drugs' effectiveness varied considerably. Chloroquine, for example, was the only drug to afford significant protection (60-85%) from toxicity when administered 15 min prior to intoxication. None of the drugs was effective when administered 30 or 60 min prior to intoxication. When administered 15 min after intoxication, chloroquine was also the only drug to provide significant protection (50-65%) from the toxicity of all the venoms and toxins against which it was effective at 0 min. Chlorpromazine was effective against only B. caeruleus venom, while dexamethasone was effective against only O. scutellatuus venom. At 30 min postintoxication, chloroquine was still the only drug to provide significant protection (30-40%) from the toxicity of all the venoms and toxin against which it was effective at 0 min. Chlorpromazine was not effective at all, while dexamethasone was effective against only O. scutellatuus venom. None of the drugs was effective when administered 60 min after intoxication.

My data provide support for the hypothesis that the presynaptic neurotoxic components of the venoms are the major cause of the toxicity of the venoms. Qualitatively, whenever a drug effectively antagonized the toxicity of a venom, it also antagonized the toxicity of that venom's presynaptic neurotoxin (when available for testing). Conversely, whenever a drug did not antagonize the toxicity of a venom, it did not antagonize the toxicity of that venom's presynaptic neurotoxin. Quantitatively, (with the exception of B. multicinctus venom and β-bungarotoxin), an effective drug increased the LD_{50} of a venom and its presynaptic neurotoxin by similar degrees.

Phospholipase A_2 activity is a common feature of presynaptic neurotoxins in snake venoms and may be the primary cause of their toxicity (Chang, 1985). Although not necessarily an indication of the drugs' effects on the phospholipase A_2 activity of the presynaptic neurotoxins I investigated, chloroquine, chlorpromazine, and dexamethasone have been found to be inhibitors of non-neurotoxic phospholipase A_2 activities (Jain et al., 1984; Kato, et al., 1985; Nikolov and Koburova, 1984). It is possible, therefore, that the drugs are acting through their anti-phospholipase A_2 activity to antagonize the toxicity of β-bungarotoxin and taipoxin and thus the toxicity of the venom from *B. multicinctus* and *O. scutellatuus*, respectively. This mode of action could also account for the the protective effect of chloroquine and chlorpromazine toward *B. caeruleus* venom because this venom has components with β-bungarotoxin-like activity (Lee et al., 1976). Chloroquine and chlorpromazine could be antagonizing the toxicity of these components in a manner similar to its action on β-bungarotoxin, thus providing protection from the venom.

β-Bungarotoxin, crotoxin, and taipoxin have similar effects on neuromuscular transmission, have phospholipase A_2 activity, and are thought to act through similar mechanisms (Chang, 1985). With respect to the effects of the drugs I investigated, however, the toxins are quite distinct. For example, in contrast to their effects on the venoms from the two snakes of the genus *Bungarus*, chloroquine and chlorpromazine did not protect mice from *C. durissus terrificus* venom or its presynaptic neurotoxin crotoxin, or *O. scutellatus* venom or its presynaptic neurotoxin taipoxin. Dexamethasone, on the other hand, protected mice from the toxicity of *O. scutellatus* venom and taipoxin, but was ineffective against the toxicity of the remainder of the venoms and toxins. Based on this admittedly few data, the three toxins appear to fall into three categories: β-bungarotoxin (and the β-bungarotoxin-like activity in *B. caeruleus* venom), antagonized by chloroquine and chlorpromazine only; crotoxin, antagonized by none of the drugs tested; and taipoxin, antagonized by dexamethasone only. In support of this categorization is evidence that β-bungarotoxin, crotoxin, and taipoxin bind at different sites on the presynaptic membrane (Chang and Su, 1980). The drugs may act to inhibit the binding of the toxins differentially, thus providing differential protection from their respective venoms. Alternatively, the drugs may have differential effects against the postbinding (phospholipase A_2?) activity of the three toxins, resulting in differential protection from their respective venoms. In any event, the differential effect of the drugs on the toxicity of the three toxins shows that characteristics elucidated about one toxin cannot be automatically ascribed to the other two.

ACKNOWLEDGEMENT

I thank Mr. Percival Cueto for his excellent technical assistance.

REFERENCES

Barnhart, E. R. (1987) *Physician's Desk Reference*, 41st Edition. Medical Economics Co., Oradell, NJ.

Chang, C. C. (1985) Neurotoxins with phospholipase A_2 activity in snake venoms. *Proc. Natl. Sci. Counc. B. ROC*, *9*, 126-142.

Chang, C. C. and M. J. Su (1980) Mutual potentiation at nerve terminals between toxins from snake venoms which contain phospholipase A activity: β-bungarotoxin, crotoxin, taipoxin. *Toxicon*, *18*, 641-648.

Jain, M. K., M. Streb, J. Rogers, and G. H. DeHaas (1984) Action of phospholipase A2 on bilayers containing lysophosphatidylcholine analogs and the effect of inhibitors. *Biochem. Pharmacol.*, *33*, 2541-2551.

Kato, N., K. M. Halprin, S. Matsuo, and J. R. Taylor (1985) Dexamethasone directly inhibits snake venom phospholipase A. *Biochem. Biophys. Res. Comm.*, *130*, 761-767.

Kuo, T. P. and C. S. Wu (1972) Clinico-pathological studies on snake bites in Taiwan. *J. Formosan Med. Assoc.*, *71*, 447.

Lee, C. Y., Y. M. Chen, and Mebs, D. (1976) Chromatographic separation of the venom of *Bungarus caeruleus* and pharmacological characterization of its components. *Toxicon*, *14*, 451-457.

Nikolov, R. and K. Koburova (1984) Inhibition of phospholipase A_2 *in vitro* by some anti-hypoxic drugs. *Meth. Find. Expt. Clin. Pharmacol.*, *6*, 429-431.

SUBJECT INDEX

(see Taxonomic Index pp.200)

A

B

F

G

H

N

P

R

T

Taxonomic Index

(See also Subject Index, p.177)

A

D

E

F

G

H

L

M

V